Leadership for
EVIDENCE-BASED
INNOVATION in
Nursing and Health Professions

Edited by

Sandra Davidson, PhD, MSN, RN
Assistant Professor, Faculty of Nursing
University of Alberta
Edmonton, Alberta, Canada

Daniel Weberg, PhD, MHI, BSN, RN
Director, Nursing Innovation
Kaiser Permanente
Oakland, California
Auxiliary Faculty
College of Nursing
Ohio State University
Columbus, Ohio

Tim Porter-O'Grady, DM, EdD, ScD, APRN, FAAN
Senior Partner, Tim Porter-O'Grady Associates, Inc.
Atlanta, Georgia
Associate Professor, Leadership Scholar
College of Nursing and Health Innovation
Arizona State University
Phoenix, Arizona

Kathy Malloch, PhD, MBA, RN, FAAN
President, KMLS, LLC
Glendale, Arizona
Professor of Practice
College of Nursing and Health Innovation
Arizona State University
Phoenix, Arizona
Clinical Professor
College of Nursing
Ohio State University
Columbus, Ohio

D0031805

JONES & BARTLETT
LEARNING

World Headquarters
Jones & Bartlett Learning
5 Wall Street
Burlington, MA 01803
978-443-5000
info@jblearning.com
www.jblearning.com

Jones & Bartlett Learning books and products are available through most bookstores and online booksellers. To contact Jones & Bartlett Learning directly, call 800-832-0034, fax 978-443-8000, or visit our website, www.jblearning.com.

The content, statements, views, and opinions herein are the sole expression of the respective authors and not that of Jones & Bartlett Learning, LLC. Reference herein to any specific commercial product, process, or service by trade name, trademark, manufacturer, or otherwise does not constitute or imply its endorsement or recommendation by Jones & Bartlett Learning, LLC and such reference shall not be used for advertising or product endorsement purposes. All trademarks displayed are the trademarks of the parties noted herein. *Leadership for Evidence-Based Innovation in Nursing and Health Professions* is an independent publication and has not been authorized, sponsored, or otherwise approved by the owners of the trademarks or service marks referenced in this product.

There may be images in this book that feature models; these models do not necessarily endorse, represent, or participate in the activities represented in the images. Any screenshots in this product are for educational and instructive purposes only. Any individuals and scenarios featured in the case studies throughout this product may be real or fictitious, but are used for instructional purposes only.

The authors, editor, and publisher have made every effort to provide accurate information. However, they are not responsible for errors, omissions, or for any outcomes related to the use of the contents of this book and take no responsibility for the use of the products and procedures described. Treatments and side effects described in this book may not be applicable to all people; likewise, some people may require a dose or experience a side effect that is not described herein. Drugs and medical devices are discussed that may have limited availability controlled by the Food and Drug Administration (FDA) for use only in a research study or clinical trial. Research, clinical practice, and government regulations often change the accepted standard in this field. When consideration is being given to use of any drug in the clinical setting, the health care provider or reader is responsible for determining FDA status of the drug, reading the package insert, and reviewing prescribing information for the most up-to-date recommendations on dose, precautions, and contraindications, and determining the appropriate usage for the product. This is especially important in the case of drugs that are new or seldom used.

Production Credits
VP, Executive Publisher: David D. Cella
Executive Editor: Amanda Martin
Associate Acquisitions Editor: Rebecca Myrick
Editorial Assistant: Danielle Bessette
Production Manager: Carolyn Rogers Pershouse
Associate Production Editor: Juna Abrams
Senior Marketing Manager: Jennifer Scherzay
VP, Manufacturing and Inventory Control: Therese Connell
Composition: S4Carlisle Publishing Services
Cover Design: Scott Moden
Rights & Media Specialist: Wes DeShano
Media Development Editor: Troy Liston
Cover Image: © solarseven/Shutterstock
Printing and Binding: Edwards Brothers Malloy
Cover Printing: Edwards Brothers Malloy

Library of Congress Cataloging-in-Publication Data
Names: Davidson, Sandra, 1973- , author. | Weberg, Daniel Robert, author. |
  Porter-O'Grady, Timothy, author. | Malloch, Kathy, author.
Title: Leadership for evidence-based innovation in nursing and health
  professions / Sandra Davidson, Daniel Robert Weberg, Tim Porter-O'Grady, Kathy Malloch.
Description: Burlington, Massachusetts : Jones & Bartlett Learning, [2017] |
  Includes bibliographical references.
Identifiers: LCCN 2015042802 | ISBN 9781284099416
Subjects: | MESH: Evidence-Based Nursing. | Nurse
  Administrators—organization & administration. | Organizational Innovation.
Classification: LCC RT89 | NLM WY 105 | DDC 610.73068—dc23 LC record available at http://lccn.loc.gov/2015042802

6048

Printed in the United States of America
20 19 18 17 16   10 9 8 7 6 5 4 3 2 1

Table of Contents

Contributors

Kevin Clouthier, MSc, MBA
Executive Director
Open Doors for Lanark Children and
Youth
Ontario, Canada

Gregory L. Crow, EdD, MSN, BSN, RN
Adjunct Faculty and Director of the
Vietnam Nurse Project
School of Nursing and Health
Professions, University of San Francisco
San Francisco, California
Consultant
Tim Porter-O'Grady Associates
Atlanta, Georgia

Gregory A. DeBourgh, EdD, RN, ANEF
Professor
School of Nursing and Health
Professions, University of San Francisco
San Francisco, California

Denise Duncan, RN
Executive Vice President
United Nurses Association
Union Health Care Professionals
San Dimas, California

Robert C. Geibert, EdD, EdM, BSN, BS, RN
Senior Staff Nurse II
Kaiser Permanente
San Rafael, California

Diane Heliker, PhD, RN
Professor
St. Xavier University
Chicago, Illinois

Cheryl Hoying, PhD, RN, NEA-BC, FACHE, FAAN
Senior Vice-President
Cincinnati Children's Hospital Medical
Center
Cincinnati, Ohio

Cathy Lalley, PhD, RN, MHI
Interim Director of Health Care
Innovation Programs
Arizona State University
Phoenix, Arizona

Joshua Rutkoff, BS
Associate Program Director
Coalition of Kaiser Permenente Unions
Pasadena, California

Dolora Sanares-Carreon, MPA, BSN, RN, NE-BC
Program Manager (Evidence-Based Practice)
University of Texas Medical Branch
Galveston, Texas

Jerry E. Spicer, DNP, RN, NEA-BC, FACHE
Vice President, Patient Care Services
Kaiser Permanent Foundation Hospitals, Southern California Region
Pasadena, California

Rayne Soriano, PhD, RN
Manager, Clinical Informatics
Care Delivery Information Technology
Kaiser Permanente
Oakland, California

Foreword

"And" is the new "Or."

The need for effective leadership in health care has never waned, but what it takes to be an effective leader, especially an effective nurse leader in today's healthcare environment, is changing rapidly. The challenges facing leaders and caregivers today are both daunting and exciting. As populations in all countries age, and as the burden of disease grows, we are seeing increasing demands on the care system. The pace of technological innovation and development has never been so fast. And never before have leaders had to manage four distinct generations within the same workforce. Rightfully, patients and staff are changing their expectations of how they should engage the healthcare system.

Amid all of these shifting circumstances and changing expectations, I am seeing some leaders focus down on the challenges immediately in front of them, relying only on their accumulated experience and wisdom and looking only as far as the walls of their facility. Yet I am seeing other leaders looking up and out—searching, with an open mind and a boundless curiosity, for new ideas on how to thrive in this new era and get to the Triple Aim (better care, better health, lower costs). These leaders understand that any health system extends far beyond the walls of any building, into the community, and into people's homes. They understand that they need to reject the this *or* that thinking that promotes antiquated notions of what healthcare providers should do and what effective health care is.

At the Institute for Healthcare Improvement (IHI), we see the path forward in the notion that *and* is the new *or*, and this book provides wonderful examples of this: how to integrate evidence *and* innovation; how to foster teamwork *and* professionalism; how to hear the voice of the patient *and* ensure the best standards of care.

In 2014, IHI launched the Leadership Alliance and supported the beginning of the 100 Million Healthier Lives initiative. Together these work to improve both health care (Leadership Alliance) *and* health (100M Healthier Lives). Success in both initiatives will rest on understanding how to link innovative models of care with the best science available, and this text can serve as a guide for exactly that.

The Leadership Alliance's credo is "care better than we've ever seen, health better than we've ever known, at a cost we can all afford." This simple but ambitious agenda needs *and* thinking. The challenges, for all of us, are how to spread evidence-based practice *and* how to create a culture of innovation and how to leverage both to improve care delivery and overall health and well-being.

The authors in this text offer tools, cases, and methods to help achieve best practice everywhere. And crucially, these tools, cases, and methods can be used in a way that protects and preserves two of the most precious resources we have in health care: nurses *and* the joy all nurses should, and deserve to, experience in their daily work.

My friends Tom Bodenheimer and Christine Sinsky published an article recently that argued that effective care for patients requires effective care of providers. This fourth aim (on top of the Triple Aim) is essential to securing and protecting the contributions to health that nurses make each and every day. The crisis of burnout among nurses (and all clinicians) is a clear and present danger to the health and well-being of our communities. The tools, cases, and methods described in this text have the potential to restore the joy that should rightfully be among the rewards for the hard, diligent work that nurses do. But we cannot do this, and will not do this, unless we choose *and* instead of *or.*

MAUREEN BISOGNANO
President and CEO
Institute for Healthcare Improvement
October 2015

Preface

EVIDENCE AND INNOVATION: THE EVOLUTION OF LEADERSHIP IN HEALTH CARE

There are rare occasions in the evolution of an industry when the foundations of practice are solid, the knowledge to advance the industry exists, and the tools for leaders to enact catalytic transformation are accessible. Now is one of those moments. The foundations of evidence-based practice, the research and practice of innovation and the evolving practice of leadership in health care, are poised to transform health care. This text emerged as a result of conversations among the editors and authors who jointly recognized the need for a different kind of resource in order to support healthcare transformation.

This text combines and reimagines two core concepts in the leadership of healthcare organizations: evidence-based practice and innovation. Evidence-based practice forms the foundation from which healthcare leaders can build a case for change, while the practice of innovation provides for the exploration of emerging and novel approaches to care delivery. The exponential growth of available research, advancing health care and information technology, and the pressing need to prepare current and future leaders to navigate the complex and dynamic contexts of health care were key drivers in the development of this text.

This book combines the two seemingly opposing concepts of innovation and evidence and provides examples and insights that allow leaders to build capacity for transformation. Until now, there has not been a comprehensive leadership text with an explicit focus on combining innovation and evidence onto one dynamic reference and guide for the leading evidence-based innovation.

This new text includes chapters that focus on understanding the landscape for evidence-based innovation, provides insight into the sources of evidence-grounded innovation, supports leaders in measuring innovation, and provides tools for spreading evidence-based innovation throughout organizations and the healthcare system as a whole.

Introduction

Healthcare organizations require both innovation and evidence-based practice to build systems that will support the future of care. Historically, evidence-based practice and healthcare innovation have been utilized separately and often perceived to be at odds with each other. This text seeks to illuminate the perspective that evidence-based practice and innovation practices are synergistic and symbiotic. This perspective requires the development of a foundational understanding of the knowledge, skills, and behaviors that are required of leaders to engage in the evidentiary dynamic of healthcare innovation. This text has been intentionally laid out to create sections that will build from one to the next in a way that will facilitate the development of these new leadership capacities.

SECTION 1: USING THE KNOWN TO LEAD THE UNKNOWN

The foundations of evidence-based practice and innovation are complex and interconnected. Section 1 will introduce the synergy of the two concepts and how they build the foundational floor of leadership and change. Leaders embarking on the journey of change need to first have a foundational understanding of the innovation and evidence-based framework (Chapter 1). Then they must build an understanding of the leadership behaviors and team dynamics that can influence change across the organization and system (Chapter 2). As leaders reflect on the impact of their behaviors on the team, they can begin to build a vision for a culture that embraces the evidentiary dynamic as an essential component of leadership, innovation, and organizational change (Chapter 3). Finally, the foundational understanding of innovation, evidence, leadership, and culture must align to a greater purpose, patient-centered care (Chapter 4). These first four chapters enable leaders to build a solid base from which to lead change in health care using the evidentiary dynamic and innovation processes.

SECTION 2: SUPPORTING INNOVATION THROUGH EVIDENCE

Evidence is generated by connecting data, experience, technology, and systems together in complex ways. Data to support evidence-based practices has traditionally come from publications and research studies. However, with the advances in technology and big data, new sources of evidence are emerging. Leaders must be aware of these new sources and how they can influence how we think about evidence, change, and outcomes in health care (Chapter 5). In complex healthcare organizations we cannot rely on passive diffusion of evidence to create systems change. Rather, leaders must work to create the culture and conditions that inculcate evidence-based practice and innovation. Chapter 6 will provide examples, tools, and resources for how leaders can build a business case for innovation through evidence. As new sources of evidence emerge and leaders build business cases for disrupting the status quo, leaders must develop new ways to view organizational activities and influence. Chapter 7 describes how leaders can leverage the complexity principles of emergence and disruption to shift toward a culture of evidence-based innovation amid highly complex and relational organizational structures. As healthcare organizations become more interdependent and complex, caregivers and leaders must rely less on memorization and standard practices and more on access to information at the right time and used in the right way for a particular context of care. Chapter 8 describes how access to just-in-time information can facilitate the implementation of innovation and evidence in real time.

SECTION 3: MEASURING INNOVATION

Measuring the outcomes of evidence-based practice and innovation is a core skill for leaders. This measurement can inform future strategy, provide insights into opportunities, and demonstrate that change is working (or failing). To measure innovation, leaders must understand how innovation and evidence emerge in an organizational culture (Chapter 9). As innovation emerges, measuring it using traditional methods, such as return on investment, research metrics, and prescribed projects outcomes, do not always work. Leaders must also look for patterns of change in team behavior, patient interactions, and organizational structures in addition to traditional metrics. Chapter 10 provides a new view into measuring change through the recognition of patterns of change across constellations of healthcare contexts. Listening to the conversational life of an organization can provide leaders with ongoing formative feedback to inform innovation work. Leaders embarking on building the capacity for change must also recognize that failure is always an option. Failure informs the dynamic and complex work of evidence-based innovation, and leaders should learn to seek out failure and embrace the learning that results. Chapter 11 provides a lens through which to view failure as a rich source of evidence, innovation metrics, and a source of dynamic and positive change.

SECTION 4: INNOVATION AND EVIDENCE AS AN INTEGRATED AND ITERATIVE PROCESS

The leadership journey is informed by evidence and experience. Section 4 provides leaders with real examples of innovation and evidence in action while providing insights and solutions to common barriers that might be faced in the implementation of evidence-based innovation leadership. New ways of working and evidence require an evolving workforce. Chapter 12 provides leaders with examples and content to begin to build the workforce of the future in health care. Chapter 13 provides leaders with strategies and ideas to overcome resistance to change within teams, organizations, and the healthcare system as a whole. Chapter 14 describes emerging educational paradigms, challenges, and opportunities for consideration as leaders seek to create educational programs that will prepare the next generation of healthcare providers. Chapter 15 describes how individuals and teams with differing viewpoints can collaborate to build dynamic and innovative partnerships for profound change. Finally, Chapter 16 reinforces the concepts developed throughout the text to create a new framework for the leadership of evidence-based innovation that is both integrative and emergent.

Evidence and Innovation: Using the Known to Lead into the Unknown

Evidence-Based Practice and the Innovation Paradigm: A Model for the Continuum of Practice Excellence

Tim Porter-O'Grady and Kathy Malloch

The secret of change is to focus not on fighting the old but on building the new (p. 113).[1]

CHAPTER OBJECTIVES

Upon completion of this chapter, the reader will be able to:

1. Define and outline the key components of a cybernetic dynamic model of evidence-based practice and innovation.
2. Outline the critical interdependencies between evidence and innovation that are indispensable to creating appropriate action and achieving sustainable outcomes.
3. Identify the essential processes associated with linking evidence and innovation that are vital to advancing positive change.

INTRODUCTION

One of the most challenging issues related to intersecting evidence and innovation is the perception that they are fundamentally different. In fact, evidence and innovation are critical partners in a continuum of relationships, and their interaction is essential to accurate and sustainable outcomes (Melnyck & Overholt, 2014).

It is easy to differentiate evidence-based practice (EBP) and innovation by definition. EBP represents a more solid and factual foundation that is the product of deep

---

[1] Spoken by the character Socrates in Millman, D. (1984). *Way of the peaceful warrior: A book that changes lives.* Tiburon, CA: HJ Kramer.

study or research incorporating all related elements derived from multiple sources, from disciplined research to experiential applications (Spencer, Detrich, & Slocum, 2012). Innovation, on the other hand, demonstrates a more generative but just as rigorous process that leads to something new and changes our circumstances and lives (Morrar, 2014). Clearly, both are dynamic processes with clear structures, stages, and disciplines that lead definitively to an impact or a product. Each relates to the other insofar as one (evidence) serves as the foundation for the other (innovation) (Hofbaur, Murawski, Karlsson, & Freddie, 2013).

This notion of evidence and innovation as a dynamic is critical to understanding the multidimensional nature of both. Dynamics suggests that there is an element of both interaction and impact (Rook, 2013). Also implied is the continuous nature of this interaction as indicated by a cybernetic (closed loop) process that ultimately changes the environment, the system, and people (Pickering, 2014). The assumption here reflects the level of complex interactions between elements and components of a process in a way that influences what those processes do, how they work, and the future change the action of this relationship creates on processes and products (**Figure 1-1**).

Figure 1-1 Evidence and innovation dynamic

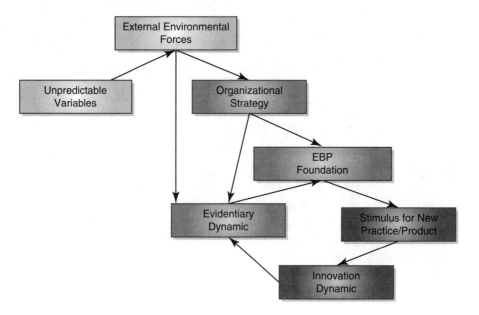

Discussion

How does EBP serve as the foundation for innovation? What is the relationship between the two? Do you think that evidence is always the foundation upon which innovation is built? On the other hand, can innovation emerge instantaneously, free from a relationship or interaction with any other environmental or organizational forces?

WHY EVIDENCE AND INNOVATION?

Much transformation and essential change is occurring in the healthcare delivery system. Indeed, the very foundation of the delivery of health care is shifting from a volume foundation to value drivers (Shaw, Asomugha, Conway, & Rain, 2014). Elements of a new concept associated with Triple Aim objectives are now forming the premise cornerstone of the future delivery of health care. These Triple Aim objectives reflect the shifting change in the broader landscape of technology and clinical science and are radically altering the context and framework for health service delivery (Costich, Scutchfield, & Ingram, 2015). These products of the digital age now create the possibility for generating and managing big data in a way that provides a high level of usefulness and applicability never seen in the history of human experience, especially in the healthcare system (Simpao, Ahumada, Galvaz, & Rehman, 2014). In fact, one of the major objectives of the Patient Protection and Affordable Care Act of 2010 (PPACA) and the Centers for Medicare and Medicaid Services (CMS) in healthcare transformation can be identified as the Triple Aim (service satisfaction, quality metrics, and affordability). It requires the aggregation, generation, and utilization of large pools of data, which clearly enumerate scientific and practice evidence, for the provision of clearly enumerate scientific and practice evidence the provision of clinical services (**Figure 1-2**).

One of the most dramatic impacts of this digital reality is the ability to aggregate, integrate, and coordinate huge composites of data and to sort through it in meaningful ways to obtain significant information that provides value in defining, interpreting, and evaluating the vast variety of healthcare activities in an unlimited array of arrangements. In fact, the larger the data pool becomes, the more difficult it is to manage, yet the more vital it is to systematically organize it and accelerate its usefulness in making decisions, taking action, and evaluating the impact. Management of these huge pools of data now becomes a significant, indeed vital, challenge in the appropriate provision of health care and the evaluation of its effectiveness (Wills, 2013).

It is out of these foundations that evidentiary dynamics have emerged. EBP is a formal process associated with this notion of evidentiary dynamics, which serves as the

Figure 1-2   Triple-aim objectives

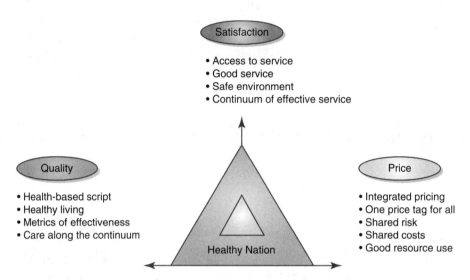

complex driver of the fluidity necessary to understand the interactions and relationships embedded deep within the evidentiary process. Evidentiary dynamics is merely a term that alludes to the complex array of individual elements (agents) that must operate in concert to produce a value that is both meaningful and useful in making decisions and taking action. In evidentiary dynamics, it is the confluence of the full range of facts, factors, elements, and influences that, when converged, deliver a message that has meaning and value for the receiver (Malloch & Porter-O'Grady, 2010).

WHAT IS EVIDENCE?

Evidence is simply the accumulation of facts and factors that provide conclusive insight into the legitimacy, accuracy, and viability supporting a particular process or action. Because of the veracity of the evidence and its generalizability, it serves as a foundation or the floor of an action that establishes a rational and justifiable basis upon which to undertake the action and to utilize it as a standard for performance. An EBP serves as the foundation of our actions in health care for patients by ensuring that the minimum standards of viability, appropriateness, and safety have been established and can be replicated with a high level of assurance such that consistent impacts and outcomes can be achieved. Until such evidence is eclipsed by newer and more relevant data to suggest a change in practice and behavior, the current evidence in practice serves as the standard (C. Brown, 2014).

However, since evidence is dynamic, a static or permanent foundation for practice is never created in an evidence-based environment. Evidentiary dynamics suggests the continuous exploration, discernment, and, ultimately, creation of new information, insights, and practices. These processes imply an ongoing currency—a continual production of data that suggests an aggregation of existing practices and the generation of new knowledge that emerges from those practices. This knowledge-based practice evolves into new research outcomes and changes that are suggested by enhancements and best practices drawn from both experience and new interpretations of data (Porter-O'Grady & Malloch, 2014).

In evidence-based processes and practices, a mosaic of actions and interactions become necessary to assure both relevance and viability in a way that positively influences clinical practice. Structures of EBP are grounded in effective data systems that demonstrate a high degree of interoperability, fluidity, flexibility, and portability. All these elements or characteristics are associated with the capacity to make just-in-time decisions and undertake dynamic and continuously modified clinical practice. To do so, both the information system and the practitioner must find that the components of the information and the characteristics of clinical practice have the capacity to change quickly in ways suggested by emerging evidence. Two dynamics must occur in concert to make these practices real. First, the evidence-driven data systems must yield accurate, immediate, and relevant data related to particular practices in a relatively short period of time and in a useful manner. Second, the users' approach to practice must be fluid and flexible enough so practice processes can be immediately adjusted and changed in a way that incorporates these changes into the normative delivery of specific patient care. Of course, both of these objectives are highly problematic if the information systems are not sufficiently responsive to the data or if people tend to perpetuate ritual and routine instead of embrace relevant and immediate recommended changes to practice. Our clinical history is grounded in volume that is certified and sanctified by an endless array of mechanisms founded in ritualistic protocols, procedures, and practices that almost prevent individuals from being available to recommended improvements in practices without a great deal of personal and organizational drama and trauma (McNelis, Ironside, Zvonar, & Ebright, 2014).

EVIDENCE AS A REQUIREMENT FOR PRACTICE

EBP implies a generalized availability and practitioner readiness to incorporate sometimes substantive adjustments into practice in relatively short periods of time as an ordinary operational mechanism for undertaking clinical work (Lubejko, 2014). This is precisely the reason that evidence-based processes must be incorporated into the structural components of operating clinical practices so they become the prevailing format for clinical work activities and the normative way of doing clinical business.

Case Example: Designing and implementing EBP

Sally Brown, RN, MSN, has just become the new director of medical–surgical services in her hospital. An initial assessment of the clinical structure supporting care indicated that much of practice in a medical–surgical setting was grounded on policy and procedure, historic practice routines, and individual nursing experience. Recently the organization had committed to lean strategies to minimize practice variability and errors in clinical practice. The staff members had not robustly engaged these efforts and seemed lost in bridging their own nursing approaches in a more formal process that set new parameters for their practice.

Sally believed that EBP was essential to build solid practice foundations that would lead to more data-based practices, reduce variability, strengthen professional and patient care relationships, and advance quality nursing practice on all medical–surgical units. She knew she would have to initiate an effective plan in a series of steps to structure EBP and to gain staff engagement in its implementation.

Prior to a process of implementation, Sally knew that a structured approach to EBP would be required to formalize EBP as a part of nursing clinical work. The first steps of implementation were grounded on the plan function beginning with three steps—ask, acquire, and appraise, to include the following:

- Raise key questions with staff regarding the safe care of individual patients, episodes, populations, and communities.
- Define and search legitimate sources of data regarding these questions of care.
- Select care priorities and processes that are most important to particular patient care activities or interventions.
- Clarify specific and definable goals with regard to care and intervention and the intended impact and outcome the related activities would produce.
- Clarify and study existing evidence related to effective EBP programs elsewhere, as well as interventions and standards specifically related to aligned patient care events, episodes, or interventions in other settings.

As Sally and her design and implementation team pursued building a framework for EBP, the following key questions related to effective implementation needed to be specifically addressed by the clinical leaders:

- How are the insights, views, and experiences of providers and patients included in the EBP considerations?
- How was the implementation design specifically tailored to the unique characteristics of units and care groups, including consideration of role, competencies, unit culture, patient characteristics, and past practices?

- How were successful models from other organizations and institutions accessed and analyzed to determine their relevance and viability in informing the development of EBP at Sally's institution?
- How was the design and implementation team educated, supported, and resourced, and how was their work communicated to all stakeholders?
- Were metrics established to measure progress and challenges ahead of understanding, commitment, and application of strategies for EBP implementation?
- When adjustments were made in the implementation plan, were they noted and evaluated for effectiveness and impact?
- Is evaluation continuous, does the produced data inform and influence subsequent action and provide an opportunity for necessary change, and does it include staff engagement?

Sally recognized that these are simply initial essential steps and stages in designing and creating the beginning structures for a dynamic evidence-based process for each unit. Guided by a consistent and systematic approach for the medical–surgical services as a whole, each unit of service and clinical teams is able to adapt the processes and questions to their unique culture in specific patient populations. Continuous evaluation of the framework helps Sally make sure the EBP plan is appropriate and effective and the implementation achieves the intended impact.

As organizations become more amenable to value drivers and responsive to the Triple Aim of service excellence, metrics of high-level quality, and affordability, they will have to increasingly embed deeply within their cultures an operating milieu that requires an accelerating level of responsiveness to just-in-time practice changes, that demonstrate their availability to evidence that points to an immediate change.

Also of immediate interest in relationship to particular significance of evidentiary dynamics in the clinical workplace is the increasingly necessary and growing emergence of transdisciplinary care models in patient-centered delivery systems (Nandan & Scott, 2014). Each discipline brings its own clinical culture, practices, and applications to patient service in a way that is clearly and uniquely valuable in meeting patient needs. However, it is becoming increasingly evident that value is influenced and moderated by the degree of integration and goodness of fit between the activities of any one discipline and the actions of all disciplines involved in patient care (Pilon, 2015). Current research suggests that the interface of clinical activity of each discipline with the work of other disciplines is fragmented, often not aligned, and may even represent divergent goals for care (Starck & Rooney, 2015). Past mechanisms for communication among disciplines have been highly compartmentalized, vertically oriented, and structured in ways that often make it cumbersome and difficult. Research has shown that these mechanisms significantly reduce the ability of practitioners and organizations to change practices or create innovative solutions to improve care (Weberg, 2013).

From the patient's perspective, individual increments of care and service operate at a low level of comprehension. The only interest is that all clinical activities of essential stakeholders converge in a way that positively affects the patient experience, improves the patient's condition, and advances the patient's healthcare experience. What individual practitioners provide for the patient, from the patient's perspective, is often amorphous and indeterminate. The patient hopes that all the practices of key stakeholders demonstrate a high level of synthesis that, when coalesced, results in improvement and moves the patient to a higher likelihood of health. It may be a good thing that the patient is not aware of how limited communication is among providers and how difficult it is to coalesce clinical goals, interactions, and communications in a way that assures a concerted, tightly woven clinical alignment rather than a patchwork quilt of somewhat isolated clinical events.

One of the significant challenges of EBP is the centrality of communication and integration of clinical stakeholders around an interfaced clinical plan of action. This plan should be clearly enumerated—to provide significant opportunity for demonstrating how well-grounded in evidence the individual and collective clinical action is, and to demonstrate how mutually supportive both the evidentiary data and clinical action is in practice. Lack of coordination is certainly becoming less acceptable as evidentiary principles now more broadly drive practice planning and decision making. Yet improving tool sets and mechanisms must be refined in the practice environment in a way that reflects a strong foundation in team-based clinical practices that are subjected to well-defined models of care delivery and ongoing mechanisms for evaluating impacts and effectiveness (Sheikh, George, & Gilson, 2014).

Sustainable EBP will increasingly be dependent on the capacity of team-based practice to ground itself in collective efforts to link and integrate discipline-specific practices in a community of practice for the convergence of effort that yields direct patient-centered benefits and impacts. Evidence of the degree of interface and goodness of fit of clinical effort will be as critical a part of the dynamics of evidence-grounded processes as will the clinical activities themselves. Transdisciplinary evidence-based mechanisms and processes are quickly becoming the foundation for future practice and the tool set for viable value-based practices.

A good part of establishing EBP as a foundation for future practice is eliminating rituals and routines that reflect the linear and procedural orientation to practice and moving to value-based practice that demonstrates clinical impact, care outcomes, and sustainable health (**Figure 1-3**). Evidence suggests the capacity for meaningful change. The meaningfulness of change requires the ability to understand the foundations for decisions and actions, comprehend the shifts that are occurring in real time, and translate those shifts into relevant response and action. The commitment to past practice

Figure 1-3 From volume to value to practice

Yesterday:	*Tomorrow:*
• Procedural	• Evidence
• Positional	• Mobile
• Subordinated	• Partnered
• Task/ritual/routine	• Impact/making a difference
• Volume of work	• Value of practice
• Hospital-based	• Continuum-focused
• Treatment/intervention	• Health, patient-centered

and well-established activities and routines simply because they have been proven effective is a direct impediment to using those same processes as a reference point for improving practice. If emerging evidence coming out of improvements or revelations in the science—or the failure or success of current practices, or even emerging innovations that elevate practices and outcomes—fail to change past practice, it then ceases to be relevant and viable (Belar, 2014).

Many practitioners hold to the values of what they were taught or believe that if it was good enough for them to learn, it is still good enough today, along with similar beliefs that suggest a sort of dictatorship of history. This notion that good practices are fixed and finite results in a rather strident connection to functionalism. At the institutional level, the same behaviors are represented by the infrastructure of policy, procedure, protocol, standardization, and so forth. From either the personal or institutional perspective, these patterns of behavior represent practice as a series of tasks and checklist items that, if completed properly, can assure safe patient care activity and positive outcomes. They assume that basing the plans and processes of care on metrics that suggest value and positive impact is a stronger and more sustainable approach to obtaining and advancing health. The issue here is not one of value for these tasks and practices; instead, it is an issue of perspective.

STANDARDIZATION AND EVIDENCE

Certainly, the use of safe practices, routines, and protocols provide significant value to good and safe patient processes and positive impacts. However, such standards need to be seen as foundations for practice in a way that establishes the foundation of practice upon which all practitioners firmly stand. These protocols suggest an agreement of basic practices and processes that reflect minimum expectations for relevance and safety that simply cannot be transgressed or violated. These foundations suggest to the practitioner that good practice is grounded in solid principles and that as those principles remain valid, the foundation simply represents the ground of practice upon which all professionals stand for their individual and collective professional work.

It must be posited, however, that establishing the base of the foundations of practice does not itself assure practice excellence. Safety, for example, is a minimum right of expectation of every patient. Maintaining a safe environment for patient care should not be considered a measure of excellence. A safe environment is a basic expectation and right of patients in their interactions and experiences with the health system. A high level of safety is a low level of measure for patient care because it is a basic expectation that every practitioner should demonstrate at all times in all actions. Regardless of the principle or the foundation promulgated, patient care providers must clearly recognize that upholding those principles and foundations with a high level of consistency does not imply excellence; instead, it simply reflects both understanding and compliance with basic practice principles.

This same insight holds true for the process of standardization. Standardization reflects a basic set of principles or protocols that are proven effective and adhered to consistently in a way that demonstrates a good measure of value and positive impact for the patient (Merry & Hamblin, 2012). Recognizing that, no one should suggest that organizations or individuals can standardize their way to excellence. While standardization represents the consistent application of the foundation of our practice, excellence represents a reach toward the ceiling of our practice. Standardization represents the ground we stand on, and excellence represents a reach to different higher levels of service and care delivery that, once achieved, become the new foundation of our practice—a new foundation upon which to reach anew toward a ceiling (excellence) that raises our practice and enhances the patient experience.

EVIDENCE AS MOVEMENT

As stated at the beginning of this chapter, EBP is a dynamic. As such, it suggests constant activity and movement. Such practices indicate that when foundations are laid and principles are established, the work of practitioners is to use those foundations as a premise for setting out on a journey that ultimately challenges them in a way that will result in advancements, improvements, and enhancements of patient care practices and clinical outcomes. While evidence is predominantly about establishing principles and foundations through dynamic activity, it creates the drive—the urge, if you will—to grow, improve, and advance action and impact. Therefore, deeply implied in evidentiary dynamics is the suggestion for creativity and innovation, which are forces that are essential to improvement and advancement.

The leader in EBP environments is challenged to create a context where evidence-based processes serve as the dynamic impetus for mindfully reflecting and analyzing professional practices and clinical behavior as an ongoing requisite for data-driven patient care. The evidence-grounded leader recognizes that an environment essential to evidence is energized by rigorous and methodological, yet creative and imaginative, relationships and processes that move beyond existing evidence as professional staff reach for improvement, enhancements, and innovative opportunities for advancing practice (Aarons, Ehrhart, Farahnak, & Hurlburt, 2015). This notion of movement is fundamental to the understanding of EBP. Movement, in a complexity framework, suggests that nothing remains static or the same. The universe is in constant motion, both continuously constructing and deconstructing energy and matter everywhere. Therefore, nothing in existence can remain static or unchanged. The forces of this positive and negative energy are constantly operating to both create and deconstruct. The same can be said for human dynamics, including clinical practice. If practice is not always changing and improving, it is not simply doing nothing (remaining static). Because practice is itself a dynamic, if it is not improving, it is regressing. This regression is ultimately seen in accelerating levels of risk, diminishing rates of improvement, and continuing challenges to patient safety, care relevance, and positive outcomes. There is ample evidence to suggest that the slavish addiction to permanent ritual and routine, policies and procedures, tasks and processes, ultimately results in diminishing performance and decelerating metrics of value and patient impact (Grimmer, Dizon, Milanese, King, & Beaton, 2014).

Discussion

How do we understand this notion of movement in light of clinical practice? Is movement always either negative or positive? What do we mean by the statement that there is nothing static in the universe? How do we keep EBP from becoming negative (ritual, routine, nonrelevant, etc.)? How does EBP lead to the potential for creativity and innovation?

INNOVATION AND EVIDENCE

Evidence and innovation are dynamic partners within the same continuum. The innovative practice leader is always grounded in the evidence and uses that evidence as the footing from which creative energies are generated to advance and change the care experience. At the same time, the evidence-grounded innovator values and respects both the discipline and the rigor of the scientific process for its use and the translation of its products into practice. This attachment to the exactitudes of analysis guide the evidence-based innovator in validating good processes, disciplining the translation of innovation in ways that represent a high level of relevance that result in a strong demonstration of positive impacts (Porter-O'Grady & Malloch, 2014).

The relationship between evidence and innovation can be described as cybernetic. The definition of *cybernetic* is the science of communication and control that looks at the controlled yet interactive and continuous relationship of elements within a system and their dynamic influence on each other. Cybernetic systems are usually closed-system mechanisms that loop continuously, determined by how processes move within them and the relationships among elements in the system. Cybernetic systems are generally cyclical, dynamic, and highly interactive. Each component or part of the system is interdependent, with other parts representing a continuous flow that begins at one place, loops through other elements of the process, and ends up where the process began. It is this cybernetic relationship between evidence and innovation that is described subsequently in this chapter and forms the foundation for the interdependent interaction between evidence and innovation (Porter-O'Grady & Malloch, 2016).

The evidence-based innovator understands the relationship among the firm foundation of principles, protocols, and standards supported by the evidence. At the same time he or she recognizes that this foundation represents only half the work of good practice. The other half of the work of good practice is represented by faithful commitment to the movement from firm principles and foundations toward new, emerging, and innovative practices that produce new technologies, models of care, and clinical activities that advance both the experience and the health of the patient. Furthermore, the evidence-based innovator acknowledges the overriding need for the commitment and engagement of the practice community and represent in their own attitudes and practices a constant mobilization toward the creative, the innovative, and the new as they grapple with the improvement and advancement of practice.

The innovative milieu grounded in evidentiary dynamics provides the kind of context that frees practitioners to discern, debate, and delineate new insights, practices, collaborations, technologies, and configurations for patient care. Rather than being constrained by evidence-based structures and processes, the evidence-grounded innovator represents both the commitment to the rigors of evidence and of the freedom to embrace the generativity embedded in exploring opportunities for enhancement, enrichment, change, and invention. For example, EBP with regard to patient falls, establishes a set of principles and processes that best demonstrate safe foundations for limiting the dangers and risks of patient falls in particular circumstances. These safety protocols establish a consistent floor for the practice of all professionals and generate a standard that influences everybody's action and serves as the foundation of their relationship with high-risk patients. Assuming this standard is in place, the emergence of a new digital device or software that helps practitioners remotely monitor and follow these patients and alerts providers of the potential risks of falls or compromises in safety, changes the landscape of practice. This innovation, therefore, calls into question existing standards and protocols related to falls and patient safety and asks practitioners to create a new framework or foundation that now includes the application and utility of the new technology in establishing future safe fall-prevention practices. Here, existing EBP standards served as the floor (some would say impetus) for good practice, and the emerging innovation created the challenge for the stretch away from existing practices that caused the need to reexamine and recalibrate evidence-based foundations to reflect the application of the emerging technology. While evidence provided the floor of good practice, innovation created the opportunity to stretch toward a new ceiling for good practice.

Where evidence demands grounding in the rigors of scientific process and analysis, innovation requires an environment that is open, responsive, reflective, challenging, and enabling (Bleich, 2014). The innovative practice leader needs to reflect upon his or her skill set regarding the capacity to be responsive, discursive, flexible, and challenging. Both the discipline of evidence and the requisites of innovation require the leader to create an environment in which practitioners can fully experience their autonomy and represent it in patterns of practice that are themselves open, discerning, discursive, responsive, and collaborative, representing a sustainable culture of innovation and creativity. Indeed, the environment must be truly professional, representing a full engagement of the professional practice community in both defining the foundations of its practice (evidence) and exploring the rich possibilities of the future of practice (innovation). More often than not, organizations that have embraced shared governance and the Magnet Recognition Program have demonstrated the best partnership between organization and profession. The mutual commitment between healthcare organizations and healthcare professionals to affirm the foundations of good practice (evidence) and advance the interests of excellence and creativity (innovation) serves as the best frame for sustainable positive impact on the patient healthcare experience.

None of these dynamics or practices can be sustained, however, without an appropriate context and infrastructure that provides the medium for assuring fluid and meaningful movement along the evidence–innovation continuum. Just as shared governance assures autonomy in professional practice and creates a structure that advances the ownership of each professional in his or her own practice and in the obligations of the profession, the evidence and innovation relationship needs good structure to support it (A. Brown, 2014). As in all human activity, there is an overarching need for a strong interface between structures that create the vessel supporting action and a process discipline that provides a rigorous yet progressive vehicle for advancing practice, adapting to change, and creating the new and different. This model further provides the essential interface between evidence and innovation that accurately enumerates the action of each in the contribution of both to advancing good practice and to improving the nation's health care.

THE CYBERNETIC MODEL FOR EVIDENCE AND INNOVATION

A model that is cybernetic demonstrates an approach to systems analysis that describes its elements, characteristics, and relationships within a closed loop structure that continually feeds back upon itself (Paul, Muller, Preiser, Neto, & Marwala, 2014). These cybernetic structures are dynamic and in continuous movement, where in the relationship among each and all of its constituents is continuously interacting. This dance of interaction describes the life of the system and shows how that system functions and interacts in a way that creates meaningful emerging and growing change. This same cybernetic infrastructure operates in the relationship between evidence and innovation, demonstrating their inherent interface and the part each plays individually, and with and upon the other in a way that advances and changes practice.

Discussion

The PPACA created a catalyst for fundamental changes in healthcare transformations. The convergence of sociopolitical, technological, and economic forces evidencing the need for change in the American healthcare system created the conditions that make existing models of care decreasingly relevant or useful. As a result, healthcare leadership was stimulated (some would say required) by the demands for deconstructing a volume-based system and creating a value-based system. Embedded inside the demand for change was the need for the inclusion of new healthcare infrastructure, technologies, delivery models, metrics, and person-centered clinical approaches. All these emerging demands and opportunities have forever and radically shifted the foundations for building the future of health care.

In these circumstances, how did the PPACA act as a catalyst for shifting your own organizational and clinical foundations toward new service structures and clinical practices? How did the architecture of your health system change to meet the demands of the more person-centered and mobility-based care delivery system? What personal impact has the catalyst of the PPACA created in your own practice and service delivery?

Gather a team of four to seven colleagues and explore the following questions:

- What are the short-term and immediate shifts in clinical practice that must occur now as the foundations for future service changes?
- What kind of clinical partnerships will need to emerge in order to address a more integrated and bundled model of clinical service for episodes of care, populations, and the continuum of care?
- How do you communicate the demands for changes in clinical practice and the need for innovating approaches to health service delivery to colleagues and clinical partners in a way that helps them engage necessary changes?

Context describes the frame within which all action and change occurs in a cybernetic process. Although the process is a closed-loop dynamic, it occurs within a larger environment in which the forces that create the conditions for change are in constant flux. This vortex of continuous, cyclical, and dynamic interaction at the environmental level creates the landscape within which organizational and individual action unfold. In human dynamics, there is a constant interface between sociopolitical, technological, and economic forces that are interchangeably congruent and discordant and create the conditions within which the agents of change operate (Porter-O'Grady & Malloch, 2010). At times in this complex environment, these sociopolitical, technological, and economic forces converge to create conditions that require a concerted response and force communities and individuals to address their impact and give substance to their actions. This is no less true in the relationship between evidentiary dynamics and innovation. Here, as at any point of convergence in response to the environment, the aggregation of the evidence provides a critical demand for change and transformation in the structures, processes, and impact of human activity. In health care this means that the complex dance among health system, provider, and user (including individuals, populations, communities, and society as a whole) requires a constant awareness of the impact of these broad environmental forces that are particular and specific in order to grow, improve, and advance change—in short, to innovate (Schartinger, Miles, Saritas, Amanatidou, & Giesecke, 2015).

THE CYBERNETIC PROCESS AND RISK AS FUEL FOR EVIDENCE AND INNOVATION

Much of the energy fueling EBP comes out of the significant knowledge deficit and wide variability in clinical practices in nursing and other healthcare professions. This wide variability creates a high degree of risk. Further, variability implies a wide latitude of permissible behavior that fails to reflect and demonstrate already well-defined parameters for safe and appropriate practice in a wide variety of clinical settings. This variability is perhaps one of the most concerning in dangerous aspects of nondefinitive care practices that result in high patient risk every year.

These gaps in professional practice create not only a high degree of risk, but also questions with regard to exactly what practices are appropriate, meaningful, and viable. The assumption is that we know little about which particular foundations produce or influence specific outcomes. The truth is, however, that we know much more about these relationships than is often evidenced in the wide variety of practice settings across the nation. This lack of a uniform, disciplined, and aligned set of foundations for practice that are clearly and specifically enumerated across institutions and environments is not only a great threat to effective health care but also provides a great opportunity for healthcare leaders (Kaplan, Witkowski, Abbot, Guzman, & Higgins, 2014).

The development of an organized and systematic approach to managing knowledge is a critical effort to actually successfully handling it. Knowledge regeneration and application approaches require a comprehensive framework that can be used regularly and stands the test of time. Not only that, the model or approach must be able to adapt to the continuing influences that unfold in the environmental, developmental, strategic, tactical, and priority setting activities of systems and people today, especially in this digital, value-driven age. There is a fundamental demand to assure that there is a strong cause-and-effect relationship between action and consequences. The value equation requires that there be a meaningful relationship between the actions undertaken and the impact desired. This critical relationship defines the constant focus and activity of clinical leadership as they begin to unfold, first, foundations that ensure a set of solid principles that ground clinical action and, second, the capacity to change practice as quickly as the evidence indicates a need for change.

Because of the activities that must be centered at the point of service, organizational support structures and activities that enable this point-of-service locus of control must be designed in a way that assures that practice is nimble, fluid, and flexible. Ownership of the obligations of practice must be deeply embedded in the practitioners. This ownership must be evidenced by their capacity to make decisions, take action, evaluate impact, and change actions quickly to accommodate the need for accuracy and relevance. The further away from the point of service the decisions related to these activities are made, the slower the response time, the greater the opportunity for error, and the less likely that the response will be accurate and appropriate (Cristofoli, Markovic, & Meneguzzo, 2014).

In addition to the need for point-of-service driven responses is the requirement for increasing the accuracy and veracity of clinical action and data. The more specific and detailed information is with regard to the appropriateness and viability of clinical activity, the more useful it is. The ability to assess metrics specifically and clearly is critical to determining their veracity and impact on the patient experience. Also, the clarity of specific actions help define in a uniform and precise way how those actions perform. Furthermore, as we become clear about the performance of specific clinical actions, we can also get a stronger sense of the interface of those individual actions with other related actions in a way that helps us assess the comprehensive impact of these interfaced and related actions. Keep in mind that from the patient's perspective, that interest is in impacts and outcomes on the patient experience. The patient is generally unaware of the particular and unique activities of any one discipline or provider. The patient is aware, however, of the impact of the collective action of all providers on his or her clinical experience. Therefore, it becomes critical that clear and specific clinical behavior enumerated by any one discipline be strongly correlated, linked, and integrated with activities of other providers in a way that demonstrates the comprehensive impact of the collateral and collective contribution of all providers. This is a fundamental characteristic of the cybernetic process. It is also a central element of good EBP management and demonstrates the essence of seamless patient-centered care (Davis, Mahanna, Joly, Zelek, & Riley, 2014).

In addition, any cybernetic evidence–innovation model requires that the intersections and relationships among components demonstrate a flow of effort that is progressive, reflects the value of each component in subsequent steps, and ultimately demonstrates the seamless interface between each component. This must occur in a way that creates a systematic approach to addressing knowledge creation, generation, application, evaluation, and adaptation. Furthermore, it is essential that the innovation process be applicable at any stage of the cybernetic process so that whatever variables or variances that require particular responses can be addressed in those places where action is necessary. Here again, the more specific and particular the application is in each phase, the more utility it demonstrates in addressing the particular issue at a given point in the cybernetic process. Such a cybernetic model must also have embedded in it the flexibility necessary to adjust and adapt timing, intervention, dramatic environmental shifts, or the products of evaluation in a way that moves to quick resolution and sustainable solutions. The cybernetic process must also be understood and have high utility at the point of service where practitioners of all kinds can use it, understand its application to their own practice, and tease out its mechanisms and use them as a vehicle for assessing and adjusting their own practices (Yolles, 2010). In short, the model must make sense and have a high degree of utility in the practice environment. At the same time, it must be relevant to the organization at large and useful at the senior levels of the organization where environment and system meet, providing an opportunity for the system to make the same kind of adjustments that are expected to be seen in practice decisions at the point of service.

CYBERNETIC EVIDENCE AND INNOVATION MODEL

Models serve as a composition of integrated and interacting concepts and elements. The use of models helps both capture and encapsulate whole notions that are comprised of particular elements, components, and phases. A cybernetic model demonstrates the action of the integration and interface among elements and components of the model, how they relate and interact, and how they feed back upon themselves to contribute to the dynamic (cybernetic) nature of the model. This modeling lends itself well to the evidence–innovation continuum insofar as it enumerates their essential relationship, the characteristics that lend utility to processes and applications of EBP, and the innovation enterprise.

In the case of the evidence–innovation cybernetic model, the forces driving human activity—enterprise, social, political, and economic—create the contextual framework for all the activities influenced by and responsive to those environmental forces. These forces can be seen as a series of continuous winds that blow out of the broad contextual environment that influences human action and creates forces that require a specific response in a particular way, as evidenced in human action and continuous change. The degree of effectiveness of the action and change is directly related to the goodness of fit between the character of the forces (our so-called winds) and the impact of the action. This impact is visualized positively by resulting enhancement, improvement, change, or innovation. Because these winds are constantly blowing and carrying with them the seeds of change and adjustment that is generated out of immediate past and current creative thinking, ideation, formation, or production, they constantly influence knowledge creation and generation, which then initiates the cybernetic cascade through a system. In the case of evidence and innovation, cybernetic cascade begins with knowledge creation, research, and generation, and influences and informs practice, and advances particular expertise. This movement then forms and deepens clinical insights and values, which drives the creation of a strong culture. In the case of health care, it influences service and care, and provides the framework for clinical action, which ultimately creates an impact, outcome, or particular change.

Because this process is cybernetic all along the way, incomplete and unformed notions and actions demonstrate gaps in knowledge creation, generation, and application and require a response if negative results are to be minimized or avoided. Each of these gaps provide the engine for innovation out of which comes new ideas, processes, applications, and products that, when created, enhance, advance, or transform both process and product. And because this dynamic is cybernetic, it continues to feed back upon itself, unceasingly informing and advancing both knowledge and action (**Figure 1-4**) (Porter-O'Grady & Malloch, 2014).

KNOWLEDGE CREATION AND RESEARCH

Structure

Healthcare organizations, to be relevant, are in the knowledge management business. In patient care, it is critical that the most relevant and often most recent technologies, models, and mechanisms for delivering patient services be utilized to compete and thrive in the healthcare arena. Knowledge is, therefore, one of the central critical tools that is essential to the organization's work. The many types of professionals that work in concert related to any particular patient process depend both on their own capacity to generate and use contemporary clinical knowledge and the commitment of other disciplines to do the same. This mutual expectation with regard to knowledge currency, appropriateness, and viability is a critical assumption upon which the disciplines

Figure 1-4   Cybernetic interface of innovation and evidence

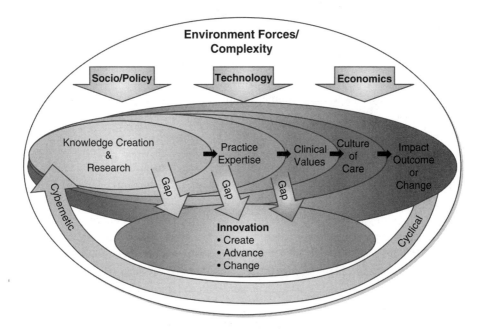

depend to successfully do their own work. Physicians assume that nurses are utilizing the most recent and relevant skills in caring for their patients in a way that facilitates clinical outcomes and positive impact. Nurses, on the other hand, expect that physicians, social workers, physical therapists, and other professionals are utilizing their own contemporary best practices in their roles to advance patient interests and ensure positive outcomes (De Bruijne, 2010).

The truth, however, lies somewhere short of the assumptions made by each discipline regarding its own practice and the practice of others. The precision associated with a tight fit between evidence-grounded best practices and the actual practices of professions does not necessarily demonstrate a strong cause–effect relationship between knowledge and practice. Questions are raised with regard to whether a large segment of practices are based essentially on assumptions, rituals, routines, or protocols that have simply stood the test of time but have never been rigorously validated through close examination that addresses viability and impact. The foundations of EBP over the past decade has raised the specter of how well structured this cause-and-effect relationship is embedded in the healthcare organization's expectations and in the normative practices of each of the disciplines.

Organizations and professions that are committed to relevance and viability recognize that embedded in the structure of the organization and its relationship to the professions must be a framework that makes knowledge creation and management a normative part of the relevant work of the organization. Creative design around laying the foundations of managing the generation, utility, and application of viable knowledge calls the organization to engage its professional members in a way that requires each to commit to a formal process related to the evidence-grounded management of knowledge. Creativity and innovation are embedded in the design of such structures; evidence-based insights and practices are the products of the work undertaken in such a structure.

Increasingly, collaboration among the disciplines in a way that reflects value-based principles and commitment to the Triple Aims of meaningful service, health impact, and price effectiveness are vital in today's environment (Hansen, 2013). Increasingly, the focus of each discipline will be evidenced in the character of the relationship with partner disciplines, the clarity of their interdependence, the specificity of their clinical partnership, and the collaborative and coalescing impact on the high reliability, high viability related to patient outcomes. The historic compartmentalized, segmented, and vertically siloed insulation of the disciplines from each other is not a sustainable premise upon which a viable knowledge management system can be built.

Embedded inside the knowledge management system is the information infrastructure that allows the organization to use just-in-time and highly mobile mechanisms to change and adapt practices in a way that reflects emerging clinical research and new knowledge generation. Many of the associated issues with the management of new and emergent knowledge and its generation and utility, such as big data, electronic medical records, supportive shared governance structures, innovation and failure, and so forth, are related to knowledge that is generated from the innovation process. The relationship between the emergence of knowledge affecting relevant practice and the capacity of practitioners to access and translate that knowledge in a relatively short period of time demonstrates the organization's capacity to innovate. The ability of the practitioners to utilize and apply that knowledge in their own practices demonstrates their commitment to be continuously relevant, current, and evidence-based (Dalkir, 2013). Here again, evidence and innovation are both points of reference along the same continuum. The organization's innovation in this scenario is reflected by well-defined and systematic knowledge management structure and also by functional flexibility and adaptability that stimulate practice change in the face of new evidence. Practice change in the ideal infrastructure can be made easily and fluidly when the emerging evidence suggests that change is appropriate. Gone from that structure should be the long-term, ineffective, and pedantic policy and procedure process. In its place should be an effective, linked, interoperative, and continuous information management infrastructure that informs clinical team members at the point of service about the products of evidence and research generated by continuous small testing, comparative practices, and intersystem measures of comparative effectiveness. Adapting these mechanisms as a way of doing business creates an effective and useful operating infrastructure that is responsive to innovation, grounded in evidence, and dynamic in application.

These emerging evidence-grounded innovations will require a new compact within and among health professions. The often rote addiction to past practices, rituals, and routines often found in the disciplines must give way to a more reflexive and adaptive model of clinical practice that reflects a basic understanding that change is a fundamental attribute of the work of these professions and that, when validated as viable and appropriate, is evident in the processes and applications associated with that work.

The role of innovation in the evidence–innovation continuum is evidenced by a continuously systematic flexibility and personal adaptability that is apparent when the evidence indicates that there is a need for a change in practice. The trajectory of innovation is always an improvement in practice, a relevant new practice, and the continuous and growing positive impact on individual and population health. While evidence-based methodology is the means to improve and advance practice, innovation is the driver that requires the organization to develop mechanisms and focused testing of evidence-grounded approaches, draw comparisons, build practices based on best practices, and participate in a comprehensive, systematic, multisite undertaking of comparative effectiveness analysis in order to establish strong population-associated best practices (Grant, Guthrie, Entwistle, & Williams, 2014).

Institutional structures and methodologies linking innovation and EBP demonstrate their commitment to effective knowledge management through strong information-based systems that support ongoing research and clinical data management (Quinn, Huckel-Schneider, Campbell, Seale, & Milat, 2014). Fluid and flexible mechanisms, that make information availability and utility a systems characteristic for those delivering healthcare services, are critical components of effective patient care. Here again, evidentiary dynamics and methodologies are the means for assuring best practices, and innovation is the medium that provides the enabling dynamic and impetus for continuously pushing the walls of currency in the organizations and the professions that continuously reach for practice excellence. The innovation framework in the organization stimulates the search for gaps between current practices and the potential for excellence. These gaps create the urge to analyze and examine current practices, products, and behaviors in the interests of refining, improving, or changing practice in the interest of advancing service excellence and health (**Figure 1-5**). It is out of these gaps that true innovation emerges, the results of which are to actually change or create new culture, practices, products, and behaviors.

Figure 1-5   Environment forces/complexity

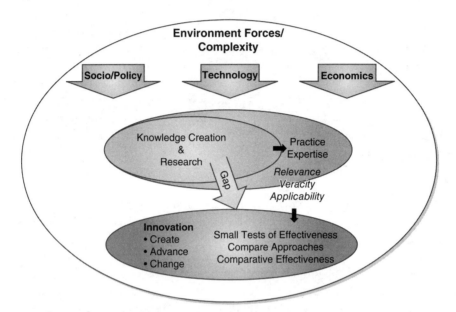

PRACTICE EXPERTISE: TRANSLATION TO IMPACT

Evidence of viability and effectiveness is the constant driver for practice excellence. This continuous and dynamic journey is essentially a disciplined process that represents an intentional yet continuous march toward improvement, enhancement, and change (innovation). As previously indicated, practice change reflects the rigors of good knowledge management, research, and comparative effectiveness processes. At the same time, evidence-based dynamics also reflect the more relational interactional and experiential elements and characteristics embedded in the acts and interactions of practice. While the consistencies and rigors of the science of evidence are the essential platform upon which providers stand to make judgments regarding their practices, the relationships and interactions embedded in the dynamic of practice also provide relevant insights and information that positively or negatively affect the healthcare experience. Issues associated with the more subjective and relational aspects of health service driven by political, social, cultural, ethnic, regional, familial, and personal variables and vagaries strongly influence the viability and sustainability of health. Failure to incorporate these more collateral characteristics influencing the health service experience, quality metrics, and the social, emotional, and financial price of health care can clearly affect its positive viability and sustainability.

Case Example: Innovation as the culture of care

Ben Jones, RN, DNP, is a health system chief nursing officer (CNO). He recognized that with all the changes that are unfolding in the health system while moving toward value-based care and accountable care models, many changes would have to occur in the structures and processes of nursing. He knew that many of the adaptations and changes in practice would have to be driven by clinical and management leadership very close to the point of service. His problem was that the organization has historically been very hierarchical and vertical, with a strong management-driven work environment. This clearly needed to change.

Ben realized that the significance of the change means that a shift in the culture would have to emanate from every place in the health system. He believed that nurses were positioned to provide leadership in making this cultural change because nursing is one of the central activities of the health system. He began to plan for systematically implementing a culture change that would support an environment of innovation throughout the nursing service.

Ben's first issues were as follows:

- Who do I need to include in the initial deliberation and design process to best strategize how we might affect the nursing culture?
- How would the nursing vision and mission need to change in order to give purpose and direction to the shift in the nursing culture of care?
- In a value-driven care model, patients and partners need to be at the table. How do we form this process so discussions and decisions are informed and competent?
- How do we avoid creating a department/office/center of innovation that is isolated and independent from the ownership of innovation at the point of service and engage the stakeholders?

The necessary elements for a structure of innovation are as follows:

- Ben realized, after detailed study, that some essential principles were needed to guide the leadership in their work of creating a culture that supports innovation. These principles include the following:
  - Wherever innovation occurs in a system, it must align with the systems environmental requirements and strategic priorities that guide and direct the innovation choices and actions anywhere in the system.
  - Successful innovation is never driven from the top of the system. Innovation is always generated from the work of the system and best engages stakeholders that are closest to the system's point of service.

- Formal structures must be developed for framing, informing, guiding, and rewarding innovation in a way that makes innovation a normative part of everyone's work and continually engages them.
  - Innovation is a discipline/process. Its various mechanics, stages, and phases can be defined and learned. A dynamic, available, and ongoing innovation learning process must be incorporated into the development activities of the organization so that every stakeholder can access and understand the elements and applications of innovation.
  - Recognition and reward are part of the lifeblood of innovation and must be structured into the dynamics of innovation. This critical element is utilized liberally to sustain energy, motivation, and commitment to innovation.
  - Regular assessment and evaluation of the supported innovation mechanisms and processes in the organization helps determine the viability of the innovation program, the effectiveness of innovation activities, the impact of innovation, and the required needs for adjustment or accommodation to accelerate the effectiveness of innovation.

Ben recognized that if the health systems innovation program is to be successful, particular themes must guide leadership to assure that innovation is viable, effective, and sustainable:

- Innovation is tied to mission.
- Innovation must advance the success of the organization and the individual.
- Innovation is best directed from the point of service.
- Innovation requires recognition.
- Innovation is a team activity. No innovation is successful if unilaterally controlled.
- Innovation is a disciplined process and must be structured into the organization's way of doing business.
- Failure is a fundamental element of all innovation; it must be accepted, accommodated, and even celebrated.
- Innovation leaders must become comfortable with risk takers, brokers, contrarians, out-of-the-box thinkers, actors, and creative noise.
- A system of just-in-time communication, decision making, and movement accompanies the innovation process and requires an immediate response and quick turnaround from leaders and stakeholders.

Within the context of this practice framework, evidence-based dynamics support, indeed require, the inclusion of the collateral and collaborative mechanisms that generate insights, algorithms, and service approaches, experiences, and data that reflect evidence emanating from sociocultural contexts, population/group history and experience, collective wisdom, tradition, and regional practices (Sarkadi, Sampaio, Kelly, & Feldman, 2014). Keep in mind that the patient brings a set of beliefs and notions about health care, about him- or herself, and about his or her relationship to the world. This informs the patient's interaction with the healthcare system, health professionals, and family. All these elements combine to create a contextual framework for the patient that informs and guides his or her thinking and conversation with regard to personal health and his or her role and relationship with the healthcare system. Much of the concepts associated with this patient-centered dynamic creates the frame for the relationship and interaction among the individual, the family, and health professionals. In addition, the patient brings past experiences related to personal health, his or her health journey, and the healthcare system. All these combine to create the conditions in which the patient and provider meet and operate under the rubric of the healthcare system. This complex array of interactions creates the frame within which all healthcare activities will unfold and guides the thinking, communication, and interaction among all these players (Damie, 2014).

For the care of professionals, evidence for practice expertise generates out of their own history, experiences, gained insights, shared wisdom, policies, and standards. Reliance on these factors is served as the backdrop to much of practice and has created a cultural overlay that values particular traditions, approaches, and practices that define the role of the provider. As the social, political, and technological landscape change and produce a paradigm shift in a way that transforms these experiences within a new set of conditions, many of the traditions and established practices are challenged with regard to their relevance and viability. Still, they have stood the test of time, and dependence upon them have provided some of the impetus and information that has ultimately generated new insights and emerging practices. This historical context creates another frame within which practice is defined, challenged, and changed and therefore must be valued. As it is valued, practice expertise and experience must be incorporated into the evidentiary dynamic as a part of lending insight, context, and wisdom to the host of other evidentiary factors driven by analysis, research, and data synthesis.

Experience too comes with its contribution to the gap between what we have done traditionally and what emerges out of the processes of knowledge management in EBP. Often the connection between practice experience and knowledge management creates the landscape for innovation. Additionally, the convergence or divergence between practice experience and knowledge management creates the catalyst for generating either validation or contest out of which will spawn emerging shifts in understanding and practice. The tension between what is known, what is experienced, and what is anticipated ensures that the evidentiary dynamic continually moves within the individual practitioner resulting in the identification of gaps requiring the need for innovation. The elements of the patient's experience and insights, the provider's clinical practice experience, and the science associated with knowledge management each contribute

Figure 1-6 Cybernetic application of practice expertise

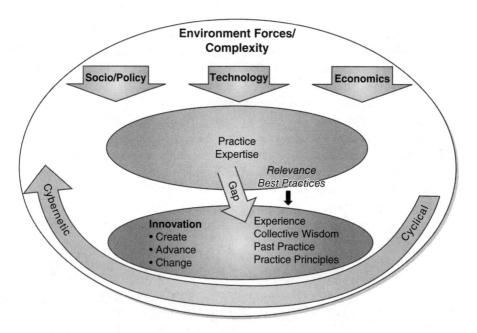

to the other and collectively provide information that, when coalesced, leads to an understanding that enhances the patient experience, improves the quality of care, and effects the economics of service delivery (**Figure 1-6**).

INDIVIDUAL, PERSONAL, AND CULTURAL VALUES AND PRACTICES

Health care is not provided in a sterile, scientific, evidentiary cocoon. Because health service is a human dynamic, it comes with individual, family, community, tribal, cultural, and societal beliefs, practices, and behaviors that have an equally significant impact on the healthcare dynamic, as do the clinical and scientific variables. These traditions are deeply embedded in faith, families, and cultures in a manner that often defines the fundamental characteristics of people in a way that influences who they are and what they do. Along with these characteristics come the personal attributes, tools, and processes they use for meeting the challenges, accommodations, and circumstances of their lives. All these devices are incorporated into health practices and influence personal and collective choices that ultimately influence individual and community health.

Many cultural beliefs and practices demonstrate some level of evidence about the impact on quality of life and health, but some do not. Yet all practices have some relevance to EBP when they are incorporated into the full range of understanding regarding persons and populations. Aggregating this information with more objective and data-driven sources of clinical evidence creates a composite frame of reference for the healthcare community that guides their partnership with the patient in a way that better informs both patient and provider about what is potentially viable and sustainable in relation to health.

Except for practices that are clearly dangerous or debilitating, evidence-based providers must accommodate in their data integration these personal and communal beliefs and cultural characteristics that more fully inform the caregiving community of all the circumstances that inform healthcare choice making in person-centered best practices. Insightful and culturally competent providers are aware of the synergy between culture and care and find ways to use tactical choices from both arenas in planning and executing the best care approaches. Out of this evidence-based foundation in the partnership among culture and care, personal practices, faith and belief, and healing processes emerge new and innovative paradigms. These new connections or insights, when added to the evidentiary foundations for care, may positively influence the creation of more effective models or approaches to advance health. Indeed, many of these culturally specific health practices may serve as the vehicle for gaining engagement and ownership for science-based, evidence-grounded clinical practices that may have otherwise been rejected if approached solely on their own merits (Napier, Ancarno, Butler, Calbrese, & Charter, 2014).

Discussion

Many cultures provide alternative models or service supports as a part of their caring culture (e.g., doula, promatora, medicine man, shaman, curandera, etc.). As health care moves to more person-centered models and approaches, community, family, and culturally based healing and health support systems will become increasingly important. Partnerships among these various family and community health supports and formally trained health professionals will be critical to build a culture of health and healing.

What kind of different thinking will help professionals bring to the interdisciplinary table other partners and health service delivery mechanisms? In what way is person-centered care different from patient-centered care, and what does it mean to providers? What is your organization doing to expand the inclusiveness of care partners, family, and community and what is it doing to plan for continuum of care services?

In these circumstances the partnership between evidence and innovation becomes more definitive. Care providers and practitioners from the involved traditions now must meet on common ground to delineate and negotiate the most effective evidence-based choices that can be made within the vagaries and variables of a particular culture. The innovation arises out of this communion between the individual or community and the provider in ways that suggest unique negotiated approaches that both meet the cultural health norms of the user and incorporate the data-driven practices of the provider. This communication and interaction between person and provider demonstrates the best in both evidence and innovation. Evidence demands that both bring to the table a clear delineation of the impact of both culture and data and determine how each serves as a medium for the other in making effective health choices. Innovation, on the other hand, requires that the stakeholders deliberate and determine viable mechanisms or processes that link culture and care in a way that produces positive outcomes and advances personal and/or community health (**Figure 1-7**).

Figure 1-7   Cybernetic application of patient values

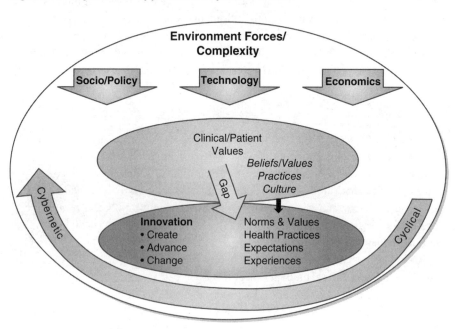

THE CULTURAL FRAMEWORK FOR INNOVATION AND CARE

Innovation is certainly more than the sum of its parts. In every system/organization, innovation occurs because there is both an environment and leadership that generate the context, conditions, and drive for innovation as a way of life (Rivenburgh, 2014). This context provides the vessel within which the vision and values of the system, opportunities for translating vision into action, and commitment of individuals at every level exists as a backdrop to the actions of innovation. Without a particularly definitive context that meets the fundamental criteria supporting innovation, the dynamics associated with innovation simply do not function. Although the contextual foundations are not complex, they are fundamental. When the foundations are not established, innovation is not possible.

Following are some of the critical cultural circumstances essential to providing the frame within which any innovation process is supported (**Figure 1-8**). Herein the relationship between evidence and innovation is affirmed and the continuum that is necessary to sustain both is established and structured as a cultural requirement for each.

Figure 1-8   Culture of care within a culture of innovation

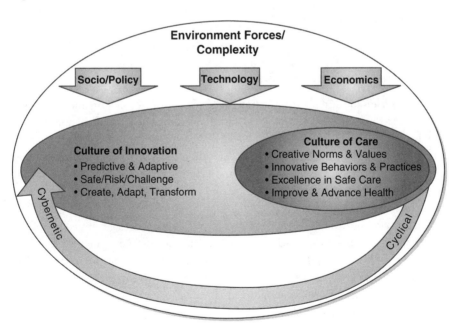

Creative Norms and Values

Leaders who are committed to establishing a strong relationship between evidence and innovation recognize that the organizational culture must demonstrate specific conditions that support innovation as the organization's way of doing business. This means that structure includes processes and mechanisms of shared rules in developing organizational strategies, models of shared decision making, locating the predominant locus of control for decisions and actions at the point of service, and systems of reward for risk taking, out-of-the-box thinking, structural mechanisms that support innovation, and the legal and methodological components associated with the successful processes of innovation.

In addition, leaders recognize the inherent interaction between evidence and innovation, and recognize the indispensable organizational and leadership ingredients that support the associative thinking that links them. These associated mental processes demonstrate the capacity to determine the relationships and intersections among seemingly unrelated interactions, processes, and actions. The structures and culture of the organization and its leaders certify that innovation is embedded in evidence and is demonstrated by organizational members' capacity to merge past practices, protocols, and data generation (all sources of evidence) with different or challenging mental models, new modes of thinking and acting, and new insights and connections, all generated from the evidentiary platform and stimulated by the culture where expectations continually raise the bar (all elements of innovation).

Innovative Behaviors and Practices

Innovation takes life and form at the point of service where 90% of organizational life is experienced. Leaders in innovative organizations recognize that innovation is a collective enterprise, and no successful innovation was ever advanced through unilateral action (Yang, 2015). Culture supporting innovation must give way to behaviors and practices that demonstrate the processes and actions of innovation, ultimately leading to an innovative outcome. After the ground of evidence has been established and serves as the platform for subsequent action, innovative behaviors take precedence. The capacity of individuals to scan and give form to the changes generated out of the environment translate their impact on practice and process and recalibrate their definitive response in recognition of the need for a particular modification/adaptation is essential to organizational sustainability. In a high-intensity environment and milieu of high technological transformation, this innovative cultural overlay becomes an essential driver of organizational life at all levels (Marques, 2014).

Increasingly, of vital importance in this equation in health care is the role of the point-of-service provider. Here this translation from evidence to innovation is incorporated inside the clinical partnership between provider and patient and forms a good part of the substance of this relationship. Ultimately, viable and sustainable innovations must animate here because this is the predominant arena where health scripts are written and lived. Traditional models of vertical control and rigid hierarchical checks and rechecks along with managerial dominance must be realigned into a much stronger collateral, horizontal, and collaborative organizational calibration. Contemporary and mature operating models that promulgate a more adult setting of organizational membership, mutuality, engagement, and ownership, provide exemplars that demonstrate the essential context within which innovative behaviors and practices are stimulated (Nicoletti, 2015). Much of the content of this text includes a focus on the importance in the development of leadership in facilitating the dynamics of innovation.

Excellence and Care

The notion that EBP is demonstrated by rigid parameters, standardization rigidities, deterministic protocols, and judgment-eliminating routines is simply untrue. EBP is grounded in good science and methodology, validated clinical practices, and data-based practices. These characteristics provide the firm foundation that comprise the floor of good practice. In short, they establish the universal platform—measured, analyzed, synthesized, and clarified—upon which all providers stand. However, it is on this evidentiary foundation that the actions of innovation generate. From this place of clarity, the processes of innovation, discernment, creativity, insight, collective wisdom, and clinical practices moved to new heights. Again, evidence establishes the floor of clinical practice, and innovation reaches for its ceiling. Innovation efforts are not simply the act of trying something new, they are the practices and efforts that continually expand the foundational floor of practice and require the same research, diligence, refinement, and scrutiny that is afforded to the EBP process. This is how the discipline of innovation will impact care, practice, cost, outcomes, and organizational structure for better health.

Excellence and best practice is the goal of both evidence and innovation, yet they play different roles. While evidence validates the veracity of the foundations of practice, innovation challenges us on the trajectory toward excellence, obtained through transforming mental models, dialogue and discernment, creative design, and small yet transforming tests of change (Hildrum, 2014). Out of this partnership come new models and methodologies that advance health partnerships, practices, new approaches, and improved service and clinical outcomes. When linked, evidence and innovation together provide the urge for improvement, transformation, and changes in structures and practices that advance the interests and conditions of health for people, populations, and society.

Improving People's Health

No activity in health care has meaning or value if it does not ultimately positively affect the health of those to which it is directed. All the methodologies, practices, and processes that exemplify high levels of service and care are pointless in that there is not a net aggregated positive impact evidenced in continuous evolving and improving levels of health. Evidence-based data suggests definitive, viable, and safe foundations for health; sustainable innovation suggests a continuous trajectory toward ever-increasing levels of excellence that advance health.

There is clearly a sufficient indication of the history of healthcare providers' addiction to trendy or catchy initiatives associated with notions of potential improvement in clinical processes or outcomes. If most of these notions actually demonstrated veracity in transforming sustainable improved outcomes, we would by now have seen a significant inverse trajectory in our contemporary quality–cost equation in American health care. Not only is there a powerful need for a frank and unambiguous framework for health improvement, there is also a need to establish regional and national standards of practice measurement and payment that reflect the definitive data generated from sound EBP and well-validated service and care innovations in the American healthcare system. Contemporary and prospective changes in the value-based effort at bundling care and payment around best practices for episodes of care, specific populations, and communities of care provide strong hope that the definitive and normative practices directed to improve and advance health can be more clearly established and their impact on advancing health more specifically demonstrated (Huang, 2015).

The emerging emphasis on creating networks of health service that will now operate across episodes, populations, and communities gets us all closer to the potential to truly improve and advance health. Besides connecting a particular array of health partners around specific episodes, populations, or communities of health service, the communication and interaction among them will help advance role clarity and contribution to health care. Out of these communities of practice and health partnerships will come growing opportunities for using evidence-based methodologies and approaches to defining healthcare common ground and creating new opportunities for innovating relationships, interactions, processes, and the products of health care. There are most clearly gaps across the continuum of health that require innovation and evidence to close.

Culture and Sustainability

Leaders of evidence and innovation must realize that their predominant role is in creating a supportive culture and structure that sustains EBP and the processes of innovation. This means more than simply establishing continuous (some say endless) initiatives that drive one or many elements of change. Over time, organizations and their people become weary of initiatives. The gimmicks and incentives necessary to generate sufficient interest become increasingly more extreme and ridiculous. Organizations, like all systems, are highly complex and dynamic structures in which the many agencies and forces converge to create the conditions and culture within which people work. The effective leader recognizes the necessity to create a synergy among all these agents whose converging effort is a central constituent of meaningful growth and change (Malaina, 2015). Driven by the organization's values and commitment to advancing health and accelerating the healthcare experience, a clinical leader assures his or her own commitment to discipline-specific measures of excellence. These leaders also recognize a solid and generative interface between the action of individual, discipline, and healthcare partners. This culture of personal and professional accountability, partnership, and shared obligation for health becomes the decisive framework for all choices and actions exercised by organizational members.

In evidence-grounded innovative organizations, the leadership capacity of alignment becomes an increasingly important skill as health systems recalibrate their structures and cultures inside of a value-driven health service environment. The convergence necessary among all stakeholders provides a requisite for leaders to assure that their roles, skills, capacities, relationships, and contributions reflect an alignment and synergy that, upon examination, have a specific and conclusive impact on the quality of health service and the net aggregate level of health. There are many activities that can be associated with improving advancing health service. For the leader, the issue is whether these individual sets of activities, when coalesced around patients and users, are integrated in a way in which the impact is substantive and clearly apparent in the positive results on health service and on a healthy community. If this develops into a healthcare way of life and the provider's way of doing business, it becomes the best evidence of the presence of an effective, supportive, and sustainable culture of care. Without the alignment and coordination of innovation activities, leaders risk further fragmentation, one-off solutions, and disconnected systems and practices that could negatively impact the organization and the care provided to individuals.

CYBERNETIC INTERFACE OF INNOVATION AND EVIDENCE

Innovation is meaningless unless some change occurs. It is informed by purpose, which drives in the center of the innovation process and keeps the activities associated with it focused and directed. The innovation trajectory includes a series of stages that enumerate its various processes, all of which lead from idea to outcome. All innovation begins with the mechanics, metrics, and measures that provide the evidence that serves as the basis out of which any innovation generates.

Evidence and innovation reflect two ends of the same continuum. Grounded in solid metrics, research, culture, and practice, evidence provides the rationale and reason supporting the foundations that indicate the appropriateness associated with the potential trajectory toward innovation represented in any transformation, change, or new product. Elements of the cybernetic process operate across all of its components from knowledge creation, practice expertise, clinical values, culture of care, and impact, outcome, or change. The dynamic itself is always creative and reflects a cause-and-effect relationship demonstrated by a forward advance and resulting in some meaningful and viable change.

Driving each stage of the continuum is a relentless and faithful execution of all the components of the trajectory from vision and values, culture, leadership, data and evidence, process movement and measurement, and finally to the innovation; either for a new product or a transformation. Because the dynamic is continuous and cybernetic, the outcome or product reactivates the knowledge process and the metrics and measurements associated with evaluation of effectiveness and the impetus for the very next thing (Nan, Zmud, & Yetgin, 2014).

As the cybernetic cycle reengages the knowledge creation and generation phase, it further stimulates the organization to look at its own characteristics and culture to demand further assessment of the synergy among its culture, its processes, and its impact on transforming health or producing better means for doing so. This assessment is multilateral and multilayered—multilateral insofar as it involves all agents, components, relationships, structures, and functions in the organization at each level of operation; and multilayered because evaluation addresses decisions and directions from governance to the point of service measuring their effectiveness and synergy at every intersection and interaction in the organization (**Figure 1-9**).

It is at this stage that the entire dynamic is viewed as an integrated whole. Questions related to the efficacy of each of the components in the synergy of all of them is a part of the evidence–innovation continuum and the tools and processes that move the system seamlessly among them. Here questions are related to the effectiveness of the cybernetic process and help drive evaluation of its utility and value:

1. Does the trajectory of the organization tightly reflect the demands and characteristics of the environment within which it exists and thrives?
2. Are the strategic priorities for health consistent with the needs and demands of the community the organization serves, and does it advance its level of health?
3. Is the culture and the character of the organization designed and supported in a way that encourages point-of-service ownership of decisions, actions, evaluation grounded in EBP, and driving innovation?
4. Do the organization and its providers demonstrate a high-level degree of partnership with patients, users, populations, and the community in advancing the health of all?

Figure 1-9 Cybernetic integration of innovation & evidence

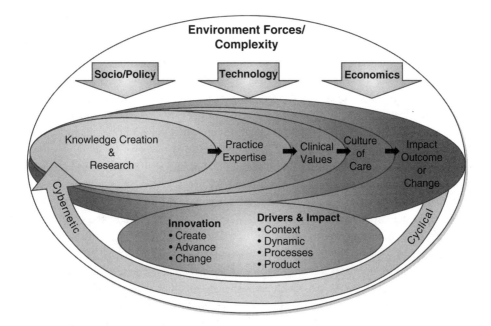

5. Are the values, beliefs, and cultural characteristics of patients and communities incorporated into health relationships and the practices of providers and their partners?
6. Is the health system faithful to its proven and validated evidence-based disciplines and processes, and can it demonstrate improvement and advancement of health as the product of its work?
7. Is the health of the community improving, and can the health system demonstrate a direct relationship between its own evidence-based pratices and innovation?

THE KEY: LEADERSHIP

Most leaders are disappointed by their capacity to stimulate and sustain long-term innovation. McKinsey and Company, in a recent survey of senior executives, found that 65% of them were disappointed in their capacity to stimulate real and sustainable innovation (Barsh, 2008). Although innovation has its unique characteristics, it is still a fundamentally human activity. To understand how to succeed in innovation, leaders need to know what it takes to create a solidly evidence-grounded, successful innovation process.

Innovation, like EBP, is essentially a discipline. It has elements and components, phases and stages, and processes and activities, and it is continually evaluated and adapted to reflect constantly changing realities. Through explication of the cybernetic interface of evidence and innovation model in this chapter, we have specifically pointed out how systematic and cyclical the continuum of evidence and innovation truly is. We also clearly indicated that if it is to be successful, leaders have to create and support a particular culture that is unique to the dynamics of innovation and requires particular leadership skill sets (Mockhber, Wan, & Vakilbashi, 2015).

A priority for leadership should be the understanding that evidence and innovation must be a structured, strategic priority for the organization. In fact, it must be an organizational way of life—a framework for the way it does business. Evidence and innovation depends on structuring the elements and components of the continuum between slices of the cybernetic model discussed in this chapter. Organizing and structuring the strategic activities of the board from environmental scanning to priority setting should be undertaken in a way that reflects the engagement of all stakeholders, from the boardroom to the patient experience. This high degree of inclusion with the right stakeholders signifies that senior leadership has the capacity to set a diverse table around which key stakeholders engage with each other in the processes associated with laying the foundations (evidence) and pushing the walls to create the future (innovation).

After the strategic framework is constructed in the organization, senior leaders must actively create the structures and processes that find and support the often untapped innovation resources at every level of the health system. These creators and innovators, when enabled, act as catalysts for others in the organization and help create a milieu where evidence, creativity, and innovation becomes a normative operating process. By stimulating the culture of innovation, and facilitating innovators and innovative action, leaders begin to create networks that develop around specific innovations and interface with other created agents generating communities of EBP and innovation that, when linked, exemplify a dynamic, engaged, creative milieu.

When the groundwork is laid for creating a culture of dynamic growth and development, evidentiary foundations, and creativity and innovation, a demand for high levels of trust in the organization emerge. People cannot risk, experiment, or stretch in an environment where they do not feel secure or embraced. Creativity and laying the groundwork for evidence and for advancing the elements of innovation is a noisy generative process filled with uncertainties, experimentation, and risk. Engagement in any of these activities will be limited to the extent that there is a sense of comfort and trust that the organization is a safe place for extending oneself and that leadership will support the related necessary innovative behaviors and practices. In this kind of environment, members of the organization feel that their efforts are valued, that the system is structured to support the generation and development of those ideas, and that there will be concerted and collective support throughout the cybernetic and dynamic continuum between evidence and innovation (Zia & Khan, 2014).

Ultimately, the commitment to evidence and innovation is demonstrated in how the leader embeds the dynamics associated with EBP and innovation practices in all the ways in which the organization works. The question for leadership is: how are the characteristics and elements associated with evidence and innovation embedded in board meetings, the senior staff priority setting, regular operational meetings, clinical standards and practices, discipline-specific and interdisciplinary meetings, deliberations, councils, point-of-service models of care, interdisciplinary interactions, and so forth? How do the new models of value-driven transdisciplinary and patient-centered health service delivery demonstrate the ownership and engagement of key creative stakeholders at the point of service? And finally, in truly innovative organizations, how do structures and infrastructure continually support a culture where the engagement of evidence and innovation is the prevailing organizational frame of reference.? The expectation of every member in the organization is that he or she is a part of a continuous innovation dynamic, grounded in evidence and encouraged to continually stretch toward excellence. The ascending determinant of success in all of this will be found in how the health system's basis in evidence, and reach for innovation and excellence results in enhancing the patient experience and advancing the health of the community. Without having done that, none of this will matter.

REFERENCES

Aarons, G., Ehrhart, M., Farahnak, L., & Hurlburt, M. (2015). Leadership and organizational change for implementation: A randomized mixed method pilot study of leadership and organization development intervention for evidence-based practice implementation. *Implementation Science: IS, 10*(11), 1–12.

Barsh, J. (2008, January). Leadership and innovation. *McKinsey Quarterly,* 1–6.

Belar, C. (2014). Transformation through relationships. *Creative Nursing, 20*(2), 75–81.

Bleich, M. (2014). Developing leaders and systems thinkers. *The Journal of Continuing Education in Nursing, 45*(4), 158–159.

Brown, A. (2014). Organizational paradigms and sustainability in excellence: From mechanistic approaches to learning and innovation. *International Journal of Quality and Service Sciences, 6*(2), 181–190.

Brown, C. (2014). The Iowa model of evidence-based practice to promote quality care: An illustrated example in oncology nursing. *Clinical Journal of Oncology Nursing, 18*(2), 157–159.

Costich, J., Scutchfield, F., & Ingram, R. (2015). Population health, public health, and accountable care: Emerging roles and relationships. *American Journal of Public Health, 105*(5), 846–850.

Cristofoli, D., Markovic, J., & Meneguzzo, M. (2014). Governance, management and performance in public networks: How to be successful in shared governance networks. *Journal of Management & Governance, 18*(1), 77–93.

Dalkir, K. (2013). *Knowledge management in theory and practice.* St. Louis, MO: Elsevier.

Damie, N. (2014). Commentary by the American College of Physicians on the "Joint Principles: Integrating behavioral health care into the patient-centered medical home." *Families, Systems & Health: The Journal of Collaborative Family Healthcare, 32*(2), 151–152.

Davis, M. M., Mahanna, E., Joly, B., Zelek, M., & Riley, W. (2014). Creating quality improvement culture in public health agencies. *American Journal of Public Health, 104*(1), 98–104.

De Bruijne, M. (2010). *Managing Professionals.* London, U.K.: Rutledge.

Grant, S., Guthrie, B., Entwistle, V., & Williams, B. (2014). In metal ethnography of organizational culture in primary care medical practice. *Journal of Health Organization and Management, 28*(1), 21–40.

Grimmer, K., Dizon, J., Milanese, S., King, E., & Beaton, K. (2014). Efficient clinical evaluation of guideline quality: Development and testing of a new tool. *BMC Medical Research Methodology, 14*(63), 2–10.

Hansen, M. (2013). *Collaboration: How leaders avoid the traps, create unity, and reap results.* Boston, MA: Harvard Business School Press.

Hildrum, J. (2014). Turning stone into gold and silver into stone: On the importance of studying innovation. *The Innovation Journal, 19*(2), 1–5.

Hofbaur, M., Murawski, C., Karlsson, J., & Freddie, H. (2013). Innovation in orthopedic surgery as it relates to evidence-based practice. *Kneecap Surgery, Sports Traumatology, Arthroscopy, 21*(3), 511–515.

Huang, J. (2015). Bundled payment and enhanced recovery after surgery. *The Journal of Medical Practice Management: MPM, 30*(5), 349–353.

Kaplan, R., Witkowski, M., Abbot, M., Guzman, A., & Higgins, L. (2014). Using time-driven activity-based costing to identify value improvement opportunities in healthcare. *Journal of Healthcare Management, 59*(6), 399–413.

Lubejko, B. (2014). Improving the evidence base of nursing education programs. *The Journal of Continuing Education in Nursing, 45*(8), 336–343.

Malaina, A. (2015). Two complexities: The need to link complex thinking and complex adaptive systems science. *Emergence: Complexity and Organization, 17*(1), 1–9.

Malloch, K., & Porter-O'Grady, T. (2010). *Introduction to evidence-based practice in nursing and health care* (2nd ed.). Sudbury, MA: Jones & Bartlett Learning.

Marques, J. (2014). Closed versus open innovation: Evolution or combination? *International Journal of Business and Management, 9*(3), 196–203.

McNelis, A. M., Ironside, P. M., Zvonar, S., & Ebright, P. (2014). Advancing the science of research in nursing education: Contributions of the critical decision at the. *Journal of Nursing Education, 53*(2), 61–64.

Melnyck, B., & Overholt, E. (2014). *Evidence-based practice in nursing and healthcare: A guide to best practice* (3rd ed.). New York, NY: Wolters Kluwer.

Merry, A. F., & Hamblin, R. (2012). More for less: Best patient outcomes in a time of financial restraint. *Journal of ExtraCorporeal Technology, 44*(4), 178–185.

Mockhber, M., Wan, K. T., & Vakilbashi, A. (2015). Effect of transformational leadership and its components on organizational innovation. *Journal of Management Studies, 8*(2), 221–241.

Morrar, R. (2014). Innovation and services: A literature review. *Technology Innovation Management Review, 4*(4), 6–14.

Nan, N., Zmud, R., & Yetgin, E. (2014). A complex adaptive systems perspective of innovation diffusion: An integrated theory and validated virtual laboratory. *Computational and Mathematical Organization Theory Organization Theory, 20*(1), 52–56.

Nandan, M., & Scott, P. (2014). Interprofessional practice and education: Holistic approaches to complex healthcare challenges. *Journal of Allied Health, 43*(3), 150–156.

Napier, A., Ancarno, C., Butler, B., Calbrese, J., & Charter, A. (2014). Culture and health. *The Lancet, 384*, 1607–1639.

Nicoletti, B. (2015). Optimizing innovation with the lean and digitized innovation process. *Technology Innovation Management Review, 5*(3), 29–38.

Paul, S., Muller, H., Preiser, R., Neto, F., & Marwala, T. (2014). Developing a management decision-making model based on a complexity perspective with reference to the Bee Algorithm. *Emergence: Complexity and Organization, 16*(4), 1–13.

Pickering, A. (2014). Cybernetic futures. *Technology and Culture Innovation Management Review, 55*(1), 245–248.

Pilon, B. (2015). Evidence-based development nurse led interprofessional teams. *Nursing Management, 22*(3), 35–40.

Porter-O'Grady, T., & Malloch, K. (2010). Partnership economics: Creating value through evidence-based workload management. In T. Porter-O'Grady & K. Malloch (Eds.), *Introduction to evidence-based practice in nursing and healthcare* Cambridge, MA. Jones & Bartlett (2nd ed., pp. 181–220).

Porter-O'Grady, T., & Malloch, K. (Eds.). (2014). *Creating and sustaining a culture and an environment for evidence-based practice* (Vol. 3, 3rd ed.). New York, NY: Wolters Kluwer.

Porter-O'Grady, T., & Malloch, K. (2016). *Quantum leadership: Building better partnerships for sustainable health* (3rd ed.). Burlington, MA: Jones & Bartlett Learning.

Quinn, E., Huckel-Schneider, C., Campbell, D., Seale, H., & Milat, A. (2014). How can knowledge exchange portals assist in knowledge management for evidence-informed decision-making in public health? *BMC Public Health, 14,* 443–444.

Rivenburgh, D. (2014). Creating a vibrant, thriving,responsible culture. *The Journal for Quality and Participation, 37*(1), 4–9.

Rook, L. (2013). Mental models, a robust definition. *The Learning Organization, 20*(1), 38–47.

Sarkadi, A., Sampaio, F., Kelly, M., & Feldman, I. (2014). A novel approach using outcome distribution curves to estimate the population level impact of the public health intervention. *Journal of Clinical Epidemiology, 67*(7), 785–792.

Schartinger, D., Miles, I., Saritas, O., Amanatidou, E., & Giesecke, S. (2015). Personal health systems technologies: Critical issues in service innovation and diffusion. *Technology Innovation Management Review, 5*(2), 46–57.

Shaw, F., Asomugha, C., Conway, P. H., & Rain, A. (2014). The Patient Protection and Affordable Care Act: Opportunities for prevention and public health. *The Lancet, 384*(9937), 75–82.

Sheikh, K., George, A., & Gilson, L. (2014). People-centered science: Strengthening the practice of health policy and systems research. *Health Research Policy and Systems, 12*(1), 19–20.

Simpao, A., Ahumada, L., Galvaz, J., & Rehman, M. (2014). A review of analytics and clinical information in health care. *Journal of Medical Systems, 38*(4), 45–51.

Spencer, T., Detrich, R., & Slocum, T. (2012). Evidence-based practice: A framework for making effective decisions. *Education and Treatment of Children, 35*(2), 127–151.

Starck, P., & Rooney, L. (2015). Leadership for the integration of comprehensive care and interprofessional collaboration. *Clinical Scholars Review, 8*(1), 43–48.

Weberg, D. (2013). *Complexity leadership theory and innovation: A new framework for innovation leadership.* (PhD Doctoral), Arizona State Univesity, Phoenix, AZ.

Wills, M. (2013). Decisions through data: Analytics in healthcare. *Journal of Healthcare Management, 54*(4), 254–256.

Yang, U. (2015). Role of task characteristics in the relationship between technological innovation and project success. *International Journal of Innovation, Management and Technology, 6*(2), 100–104.

Yolles, M. (2010). *Organizations as complex systems: An introduction to knowledge cybernetics (managing the complex).* Charlotte, NC: Information Age.

Zia, Y., & Khan, M. (2014). Organizational trust: A cultural perspective. *The Journal of Humanities and Social Sciences, 22*(2), 127–134.

CHAPTER 2

Innovation Leadership Behaviors: Starting the Complexity Journey

Daniel Weberg

CHAPTER OBJECTIVES

Upon completion of this chapter, the reader will be able to:

1. Identify three leadership theory categories and their impact on innovation and evidence-based practice (EBP).
2. Discuss basic foundations of complexity science and complexity leadership.
3. Describe and recognize seven characteristics of innovation leaders.

The creation, implementation, and measurement of innovation backed by evidence requires organizations to reconceptualize the notion of leadership from being embodied and centralized in a single individual to leadership emerging through the interactions among teams. Technology has also enhanced the complexity of the healthcare system and has created a change in the ability of individuals to understand and move the system while operating in silos. The future of healthcare transformation and quality improvement requires innovation practices steeped in evidence-based principles and implemented across silos to improve health outcomes. Change and leadership in complex environments emerge as the result of team behaviors rather than simply the actions of a single administrator or manager working through the hierarchical organizational structure alone. This chapter will describe how leadership emerges from the interactions of team members to move innovation forward in an organization. The chapter will describe organizational pressures impacting innovation and the innovation leadership gap, discuss the inadequacies of antiquated leadership practices in addressing innovation behaviors, and discuss seven behaviors of innovation and how leaders can recognize and apply them to their practice.

ORGANIZATIONAL PRESSURES THAT FACILITATE ADAPTATION

The implementation of an innovation is not a single planned event, but rather the synthesis of multiple interactions and changes that occur as the innovation is introduced into the system (Goldstein, 2008; Hazy, Goldstein & Lichtenstein, 2007; Uhl-Bien & Marion, 2008). This structure affirms that innovation occurs over time as interconnected individuals in the organization adapt, through small changes, to environmental pressures. These pressures may be financial, social, cultural, or market forces that require adaptive changes to the current operating schema of the organization or its workers. According to Plowman and Duchon (2008), these emerging actions are the essence of change: "Change occurs continuously, as minor adaptations, which can accumulate, amplify and become radical" (2008, p. 145).

Organizations are influenced by both external and internal pressures. External pressures occur among industry competitors, systems, and regulatory environments that an organization operates in. For example, federal policy changes, new competitor services or products, and changes in consumer demand, all represent external pressures to the organization that could catalyze changes, innovations, and the need for new evidence to guide practice. Leaders can use external pressures as signposts signaling changes that require their organizations or departments to innovate. One specific example of an external pressure is the consumerism of health care that is sparked by the social–technical revolution of apps, access to data, and fluid user experiences.

Discussion

Health care has traditionally been slow to adopt disruptive technologies, compared to other industries, but consumers are demanding that their experience at the physician's office or hospital mimic their experience at a nice hotel or on Amazon .com. Healthcare teams can look at this consumer shift as a signpost to improve care experiences and interactions with the healthcare system and as a litmus test to decide what work in the organization is no longer needed.

Discuss three consumer-driven shifts you have seen in health care and the leadership behaviors that are driving these shifts. Are the shifts based in evidence or simply a response to consumer demand?

Internal pressures arise from the interactions among people and groups within an organization. Some examples of internal pressures include organizational culture, hierarchy restructuring, employee satisfaction, staffing issues, and budget surplus or deficit. Leaders and teams can facilitate, influence, and impact internal pressures to create conditions for innovation, change, and adaptation to occur. For example, leaders can impact staffing concerns through facilitating a culture of unit-based teams to enable complex problem solving rather than attempting to only individually address staff concerns. Healthcare systems are complex and networked organizations, and both internal and external pressures can cause varying shifts requiring adaptation and leadership from the frontline caregivers to the executive team.

Case Example

External and internal pressures do not act independently on an organization. Because of the complexity of healthcare organizations, external and internal pressures overlap in multifaceted ways. A large integrated healthcare system provides a good case example of how external and internal pressures impact organizations in complex and unpredictable ways.

External pressures include increased competition in the price of insurance, federal legislation increasing the number of insured people, and the creation of Accountable Care Organizations. These pressures have impacted healthcare providers and insurers throughout the United States and, specifically, have created the conditions and opportunities for the executive team in large integrated health system to articulate a new brand strategy focused on affordable and quality care. This new brand strategy catalyzed multiple parts of the organization to shift their innovation and evidence foci to reduce costs while improving quality care outcomes. It especially catalyzed the frontline nurses, technicians, and other care team members. Unit-based teams across the organization's 30-plus hospitals focused their performance improvement efforts to reduce waste in the system. The teams rallied behind the affordability and quality mantra and began implementing small changes that created large impacts.

In this example, the teams were catalyzed by external pressures and leveraged the internal culture and structures to implement changes that resulted in local improvements that influenced national affordability and quality. The health system recently achieved the highest level of Leapfrog quality recognition (http://www.leapfroggroup .org/tophospitals) for 30 of its 36 hospitals.

INNOVATION AND THE LEADERSHIP GAP

The integration of innovation into healthcare organizations is a social practice focused on developing new processes, products, and services to improve quality and reduce costs (Drucker, 1985; Rosing, Frese, & Bausch, 2011). Innovation processes are full of paradoxes and tensions, yet much of the literature reflects innovation as a uniform or linear process. This dichotomy suggests a gap between the current perceptions of how innovation occurs and how innovation is led. The innovation leadership gap originates from a difference between traditional notions of leadership that are grounded in command-and-control and linear assumptions, and the idea of complexity or innovation leadership, which is based on assumptions of teams, network effects, and unpredictability. According to Rosing and colleagues (2011), innovation requires leadership that can facilitate nonlinear and emergent social process that lead to improved organizational outcomes. This can be translated to mean that leaders must facilitate teams that can work together to create novel changes. Because innovation is a nonlinear social process that requires complex and nonlinear leadership behaviors, individual-based problem solving, silo-based conversations, and miss-aligned ideation are not behaviors that will lead to successful innovation. Healthcare leaders who hope to drive organizational success must facilitate teams. Innovation requires different leadership behaviors than those that were successful in the past, and leaders and teams must practice differently to facilitate adaptation and change in health care.

Traditional leadership methods, such as command and control (controlling), leader-centric decision making (autocratic), and a one-size-fits-all (standardized) management style, were negatively associated with acceptance of change and the implementation of innovation. Furthermore, Lotrecchiano (2010) found that innovation is more successfully implemented when progressive leadership behaviors, such as engaging the organizational network and proactively seeking out innovations, are practiced. Leadership is an influencing factor in how innovation occurs in organizations, and, more specifically, traditional leadership behaviors appear to limit innovation in organizations (Howell & Avolio, 1993; Rosing et al., 2011). According to Berwick (2003), healthcare workers need to develop competencies for innovation. Leadership theories and subsequent leadership behaviors and tactics that focus on command and control, standardization, and autocratic tactics are incompatible with the emergent, complex, and social characteristics of innovation in organizations. Before innovation leadership characteristics are introduced, it is helpful to understand the theoretical basis of traditional leadership models.

LEADERSHIP RESEARCH

There are four global conceptual frameworks in the study of leadership theory evolution: trait, style, transformation, and complexity (Bass, 2008; Uhl-Bien & Marion, 2008). Each evolutionary stage has informed the development of the next phase. The role of the leader grew from focusing on individuals running entire enterprises to a broader role of facilitator of employee transformation and ultimately to the catalyst, regulator, and meaning maker of change and innovation. Leadership theory progressed from yielding all organizational power to the individual leader to diffusing the power among the followers or team members. These role and power distribution changes provided

Table 2-1 Description of Leadership Theories Pertaining to Innovation and EBP

Leadership Theory	Innovation	EBP
Trait	Initiated by leader, problem focused	Linear process tied to leader
Style	Congruent with team's style, initiated by leader, problem focused	Leader as champion
Transformational	Vision set by leader, leader empowers and motivates followers	Must be part of vision of leader
Complexity	Responsibility of all agents in the system; leaders create conditions to focus innovation	All users consume evidence, interpret it, and adapt based on it

insight into the future role of leadership and the leadership of innovation. This section will present the history and description of four important conceptual frameworks in leadership theory, beginning with the three traditional frameworks, and discuss how they inform future leadership practices and evidence-based innovation (**Table 2-1**).

TRAIT LEADERSHIP THEORIES

Early leadership theories that focused on individual leaders were called "great man" theories. The great man theories assumed that a leader was born to lead and held traits that were universally tied to good leadership (Bass, 2008). The great man concept, which dominated leadership from 1904 until 1970, was developed during a time of industrial revolution in which the goal of organizations was to increase production and quantity. The leaders' actions focused on productivity, motivating employees to work, and contingent rewards (Bass, 2008).

Nursing and healthcare literature continues to reflect traits as a part of leadership definitions. Yoder-Wise (2007) and Kelly (2008) discussed nursing leadership as one individual using traits and styles to influence others toward goal achievement. These definitions do not account for other factors that may influence goal attainment in organizations, such as collaboration and emergent leadership. Crosby and Shields (2010) attempted to identify effective nurse leader traits and found that behaviors that facilitated collaboration were more prevalent than any innate traits.

The foundations of change and innovation for trait-based leaders were ensconced within the individual leaders, not teams. The goal of organizations was to control resources, avoid uncertainty, and control change (Poole & Van de Ven, 2004). Innovation, under trait-focused leadership, occurred only when embedded routines were broken and novel solutions were implemented by the leader in a problem-focused approach. However, Howell and Avolio (1993) found that leaders who made unilateral decisions were much less successful than collaborative leaders in creating innovation within their organizations. This highlights the fact that individual leaders are less likely to create novel solutions to problems if they act alone.

Equally important is the impact of trait leadership ideals on EBP. Trait leadership theories can manifest EBP as a linear process with a single unidirectional answer that originated from the leader with little input from the team. Examples of this type of EBP practice can be found in outdated clinician-centered models of care in which questioning the expert on care interventions was heavily discouraged and could result in a formal reprimand or humiliation. This type of culture does not support evidence or team-based care and can create organizational cultures that lead to poor quality, uncoordinated care, and cost increases (Wong, Cummings, & Ducharme, 2013).

Trait theories have several limitations. There is a lack of research on women and minority leaders, which created a gap that limits the understanding of the traits of successful leaders (Bass, 2008). Additionally, no universal traits have been linked to a significant number of successful leaders. The lack of cultural discernment creates assumptions and values that center on mechanistic work flow and productivity. Motivation of staff is assumed to be driven by the leader and supported by the organizational operational theories of command and control.

The trait era identified certain aspects the leader needed to achieve success. Anderson, Manno, O'Connor, and Gallagher (2010) linked several traits, such as approachability, conflict management, and honesty, among others, to the improvement of quality measures on nursing units. These studies focused only on the individual leader actions, and the researchers did not investigate the influence of other nurses and health professionals in the system. The lack of evidence confirming a set of universal leader traits that was independent of cultural context led researchers and theorists to change focus from universal traits to leadership style (Northouse, 2015).

STYLE LEADERSHIP THEORIES

As the industrial revolution gave way to more complex organizational forms, and because trait theories did not adequately explain all the facets of leadership, a new group of leadership theories emerged. The style theories contended that leaders emerge when their style fits that of the group from which they are emerging (Bass, 2008; Northouse, 2015). For example, a leader might have an autocratic or democratic style of leadership rather than universal leadership traits. According to the style theory, leaders were successful when their pattern of behavior had a goodness of fit with the group they were leading (Bass, 2008). To maintain power, leaders select followers that fit best with the leader's personal style.

Leadership style theories did not account for all the factors that impacted innovation. Cummings, Midodzi, Wong, and Estabrooks (2010) found that leadership style alone is not connected to patient mortality. Rather, the researchers found that when the organization had a connected and consistent organizational culture, patient mortality was lower. Cummings and colleagues (2010) found that regardless of style, leaders who used relational and transformational styles have better quality outcomes than those who practice autocracy.

In style leadership, innovation typically occurs in response to an identified issue or problem. The leader's approach to innovation is limited based on the style of leadership he or she displays and will be successfully implemented only as long as the approach and solution is congruent with that of the whole team. Leaders that utilize assumptions of style theories as the predominant base of their leadership practice may limit innovation in organizations. Style leaders may have the tendency to select teams of followers based on similarity to the leader's view. This creates homogeneous teams with less diversity, which thus limits the amount of divergent thinking that is a proven catalyst to innovation. Additionally, certain styles of leadership can lead to poor innovation sustainability. For example, teams led by charismatic leaders may have early innovation success, but when the charismatic leader is not present, an innovation void is created because the followers are reliant on the leader for direction and inspiration.

In similar ways, style leadership theory assumptions can also impact EBP. Much like innovation, the sustainability of the EBP interventions may be reliant on the individual leader supporting the process. For example, a charismatic physician champion may support and manage the organizational dynamics to implement a complex fall intervention, but when that physician is absent, the organization moves back to old practices. Other styles, such as autocratic leadership, can support the leader in demanding certain practices, which may cause resentment, rebellion, and frustration in the followers who must implement a practice in which they were not involved in creating (Aarons & Sommerfeld, 2012; Bass, 2008; Porter-O'Grady & Malloch, 2015).

Leaders that practice only a single leadership style or set of assumptions may not be successful in innovation because there are several styles of leadership that were found to be successful depending on the context of the group goals and organizational structure (Cooper & Brady, 1981). The practice of one leadership style places the leader at risk for stagnation and poor adaptability to the constantly changing organizational environment. The discovery of successful styles led other leadership scholars to shift the focus of leadership research to the idea of contextually based leadership. In contextually based leadership theories, leaders change their style to meet the immediate needs of the followers and the organization (Cooper & Brady, 1981; Northouse, 2015). Leadership theories that grew from the contextual assumption are transformational and charismatic leadership (Bass, 2008).

TRANSFORMATIONAL LEADERSHIP THEORIES

The third conceptual framework of leadership theory development includes transformational leadership. Transformational leadership elevated the leader from planner and motivator to a role that lay at the boundaries of the organization (Bass, 2008). No longer did the organizational leader work as a planner and productivity manager, but rather as a vision setter and boundary manager. This elevation of the leader role left a gap between the leader and the point of production in hierarchy-based organizations. To fill this gap, the role of the manager emerged (Bass, 2008). The manager was expected to assume the role of motivator, productivity controller, planner, and supervisor, and it perpetuated the industrial idea of productivity management (Bass, 2008). With the creation of the manager role in the organization, the leader was freed from the day-to-day work and could focus attention on the relationships among organizational stakeholders and followers. The leader, as opposed to the manager, now focused on external pressures, while the manager was left to manage internal pressures. Networking among organizations quickly became the locus of the competitive advantage and was a valued skill for the individual leader.

Transformational leadership theories conceptualize the locus of control originating from the followers rather than the individual leader. This conceptual shift changed the focus of leadership research to focus on the relationships leaders had with their followers and their organization. Networking and relationships became the main focus of the leader role.

Significant research has been conducted on the impact of transactional (trait and style) and transformational leadership styles on organizational quality, innovation, and cost (Avolio & Bass, 2002; Failla & Stichler, 2008; Nielsen, Yarker, Randall, & Munir, 2009; Stordeur, D'hoore, & Vandernberghe, 2001). Gowan, Henegan, and McFadden (2009) found that transformational leadership, when combined with quality management, improved knowledge acquisition in healthcare organizations. Saint and colleagues (2010) studied healthcare leaders around the country and discovered that those with more transformational behaviors fostered cultures that had a lower incidence of hospital-acquired infections. Transformational leadership was found to be preferable and generally to have a more positive impact in terms of staff satisfaction, employee retention, innovation implementation, and organizational success (Failla & Stichler, 2008). These studies also conceptualized the leader as an individual and demonstrated that the main responsibility of the transformational leader was to motivate staff, which is a hierarchal approach to leadership.

Transformational leadership theory purports that the individual leader must help their followers transcend to become extraordinary organizational teams (Northouse, 2015). The impact of transformational leaders on innovation can be mixed. Although transformational leaders focus on empowering their followers to become more adaptable, the underlying assumption of transformational leadership is that followers are powerless to become intrinsically motivated, initiate change themselves, or lead themselves. These assumptions can cause the leader to reject innovations that originate from the front lines because it might not align or represent the vision of the transformational leader. Additionally, leaders who practice transformational leadership might also spend a disproportionate amount of time on setting an organizational vision where the vision can become restrictive and reflective of the individual leader's vision, not that of the organization or the other members of the organization. As we will discuss later in this chapter, misaligned or individual-focused visions actually restrict innovation in organizations. One thing is clear: transformational leadership will create more innovation opportunities than simply practicing reward and punishment styles, such as transactional leadership behaviors (Weberg, 2013).

Transformational leadership has been linked to positive outcomes for the implementation of EBP frameworks in health care (Aarons & Sommerfeld, 2012). The assumptions that transformational leaders appeal to the higher moral values and ethics of the followers may be one reason why transformational leaders can accomplish EBP more effectively, although studies have also shown that transactional leadership has improved EBP adoption (Aarons, 2006). This may suggest that any leadership that focuses on EBP will improve adoption in the short term. Because organizational growth and development are not short-term goals, the focus of innovation and EBP leadership shifts to determine what type of leadership will sustain the practice of EBP and allow the organization to enculturate it rather than treat it as yet another transformational initiative.

OUTCOMES OF TRADITIONAL LEADERSHIP MODELS

Traditional leadership theories and models are limited in their description of leadership behaviors (Plowman & Duchon, 2008). Historically, leadership theory focused on special traits of leaders, situational demands, the interaction of leader traits and situational context, and the dyadic relationship between leader and follower (Bass, 2008). Traditional leadership studies, according to Cherulnik, Donley, Wiewel, and Miller (2001), have studied only two outcomes: how leaders are chosen, and how well leaders function. These research traditions have defined a leader only as an individual who can influence followers through motivation, manipulation, action, reward, or punishment (Bass, 2008). For example, one limitation of transformational leadership research is that the leader is conceptualized as an individual, and the organizational culture and emergence of unpredictable leadership within followers and teams in the organization is ignored. Ignoring organizational culture leads to narrow conclusions regarding why the organizational change occurred (Lord, 2008).

Leadership in the traditional sense is a role rather than a set of behaviors, and it places power in the position rather than in relationships (Plowman & Duchon, 2008). Conger (1998) stated that leaders who assume command-and-control behaviors and operate from the traditional paradigm of leadership damage organizations by creating inefficient and broken systems. Health care has been directly impacted by these leadership traditions.

Boonstra and Broekhuis (2010) cited risk-averse and innovation-naive leadership and resistance to change as major reasons for the slow adoption of electronic medical records (EMR) and possibly EBP. Further, traditional models of leadership are associated with high staff burnout, poor patient care outcomes, high turnover of staff, and negative impact on cost and outcomes (Failla & Stichler, 2008; Kanste, 2008; Kleinman, 2004). Losada (1999) found teams that focused on personal agendas were lower performing than teams that allowed for emergent leadership. Additionally, nursing homes whose managers practiced command-and-control behaviors had worse patient outcomes than facilities whose managers facilitated interconnectedness and open communication (Andersen, Issel, & McDaniel, 2003).

The leader's role from the traditional perspective was developed in an age in which the world was focused on industrialization and production quotas (Bass, 2008). Two of the problems associated with poor quality and traditional leadership assumptions are top-down linear thinking and a focus on individuals.

Traditional Leaders as Top–Down Linear Thinkers

Leadership theories that were developed during the industrial era, on the basis of which many current healthcare leaders were trained, focused on maximizing production through linear processes (Bass, 2008; Porter-O'Grady & Malloch, 2015). Linear models assume that the input to the system will yield a proportional and predictable output. For example, a leader who attempts to reduce budget overruns by simply cutting supplies, staff, or hours is employing linear leadership without taking unpredictable system impacts into account. A focus on linear processes removes the capacity for the system to effectively change and innovate because effective change and innovation take place through relationship building, nonlinear processes, and coevolution (Plowman & Duchon, 2008). The notion of relationships, nonlinearity, and coevolution leading to positive innovation has been empirically confirmed (Losada, 1999; Lotrecchiano, 2010; Wu, Yang, & Chiang, 2011). When interaction and connections are removed from the system, the system becomes weaker and less able to translate information into knowledge for change

(Delia, 2010). According to Uhl-Bien and Marion (2008), leaders who facilitate team members to make strong and meaningful connections within the system can create organizations that can adapt, innovate, and remain sustainable in a complex environment.

By reducing the number and quality of relationships within the organization, the organization voids its alignment with the complexity level of the environment, making the organization reactive rather than proactive (Goldstein, 2008). Leaders can reduce relationships, and consequently the power of the network, by limiting interactions among team members. This may be through leader-focused problem solving, reducing interactions or meetings to discuss department needs, or repeatedly dismissing staff concerns or ideas. The reduction in relationships can take place because of impediments to information flow, poor relationships among team members or departments, lack of diversity in the system, and ineffective communication patterns, among others (Goldstein, 2008; Lord, 2008). Howell and Avolio (1993) found that innovation was successful when leadership engaged the organizational network rather than prescribing solutions through the hierarchy. Therefore, the gap in practice and understanding of leadership behaviors that lead to innovation in healthcare organizations remains a high priority for leaders and scholars.

Leaders using linear thinking contribute to the system inefficiencies in health care today. For example, EMR implementation is now a core concern to healthcare organizations and leaders, yet the first EMR was planned back in 1970 and was launched as a free application by the U.S. Department of Veterans Affairs in 1997 (Kumar & Aldrich, 2010). Now, nearly 20 years later, organizations are scrambling to implement electronic records in massive rollout campaigns that cost millions of dollars and result in years of work in post implementation to optimize the system. Innovations like EMRs require complex systems leadership and adaptive behaviors to be successful. Leading in top–down and linear methodologies results in missing key complexities in implementation, such as training, adoption, user interfaces, and nuances in practice that can result in major inefficiencies in the system.

Leaders as Individuals

Stacey (2007) suggested that leaders who are disconnected from the organizational culture and create visions and plans without input from the team can push the system away from its desired state and thus increase organizational anxiety. Leaders can become disconnected from the organization if they conceptualize leadership as an individual endeavor. All of the leadership theories discussed thus far in this chapter have conceptualized leaders and leadership as originating from individuals instead of from the interactions of groups and teams. Although organizations can be influenced by individuals, leadership that results in organizations adopting new work or adapting to environmental pressures results from many more sources, including the organizational interactions that make up culture.

Schein (2004) suggested that organizational culture is made up of deep assumptions that drive behavior at the subconscious level, values that influence day-to-day work, and physical rituals or objects that define the work, called artifacts. By understanding the impact of leadership behaviors within the organizational culture, the leader can better work with the complex variables of personality, and other people in the system can aid in the development of appropriate solutions and trajectories for the organization.

Box 2-1 What Are Artifacts, Values, and Deep Assumptions?

Artifacts are physical representations of the organization's culture. Signs, banners, decorations, unit setups, and trinkets in a unit or department can give the leader clues about the values of the organizational culture. For example, at the start of each shift, nurses may place yellow sticky notes with their names on mobile computer workstations to claim them as theirs. If others use the claimed workstation, the associated nurse may reprimand the violator and proceed to discuss the many ways the person had disrupted her work flow. This example provides insights into the values of the unit, including poor adaptability to work flow disruption, individual nurse-centered care practices, and potentially a lack of computer resources to carry out work. Just as leaders can use artifacts to gather information about a culture, leaders can also use artifacts to begin to change culture. For example, leaders can post innovation quotes in the break room to support innovation thinking. A more active intervention would be to set up meeting space in a way that enables discussion and discourse rather than classroom-style seating charts.

Values and deep assumptions also underlie an organization's culture. Unlike artifacts, values and deep assumptions are shared by actions, interactions, and discussions among the members of the culture. For example, a care team that is unwelcoming to new or inexperienced staff may signal a value placed on years of service over competency of care. To explore values and deep assumptions, the leader must walk in the shoes of the culture and spend time reflecting and interpreting actions, clarifying their meaning with the members, and experiencing the behaviors of the culture to understand and intervene.

DISCUSSION: What artifacts, values, or deep assumptions exist in your place of work, and what do they tell you about the culture of the department or organization? How do these artifacts, values, or deep assumptions assist or inhibit innovation leadership behaviors?

SUMMARY OF TRADITIONAL LEADERSHIP THEORIES

The progression of leadership theories demonstrates the evolution of the role of the leader from command and control, to transforming followers, to networking and relationships. This progression of theory also moves from simple to more complex ideas regarding what influences leadership. According to trait theory, inborn traits alone create good leaders. As the concept of transformational leadership became more widely studied, the idea of leadership as a dynamic relationship among culture, followers, self, and organization became increasingly accepted. Although transformational leadership began to better explain leadership in organizations, there was still a gap between the individual stakeholders and the emergent leadership that was being seen in organizational culture research (Hatch, 2000; Schein, 2004). Practicing leadership using traditional notions also led to specific problems in healthcare organizations.

A gap also exists between the ways in which leadership scholars and organizational culture scholars conceptualize the creation of innovation and organizational life. Complexity leadership theory provides a lens through which this gap narrows by combining leadership and culture as a dynamic that influences one another rather than being discrete. That having a different lens will lend further insight into the realities of organizational life, something Lord (2008) suggested, was not addressed through existing leadership methodologies.

Discussion

Think about the leadership in your current organization or past organizations. What types of leadership (trait, style, transformational) were practiced? Provide a few examples of behaviors you witnessed to support your answer. How did they impact your practice?

COMPLEXITY LEADERSHIP

Leaders are realizing that the world is filled with uncertainty, interrelationships, and self-organizing that does not align well with the linear thinking of trait and style leadership assumptions. In contrast, complexity leadership challenges the long-held assumptions of linear thinking, emerging as a new paradigm of organizational leadership. Complexity leadership behaviors have been shown to improve team performance, increase the ability of the organization to adapt and innovate, and promote quality outcomes (Losada 1999; Shipton, Armstrong, West, & Dawson, 2008; Uhl-Bien & Marion, 2008). For example, Losada (1999) found that teams displaying complexity leadership behaviors performed better than teams that demonstrated command-and-control characteristics. Additionally, Leykum and colleagues (2007) discovered that organizational

Figure 2-1   Elements of complexity leadership

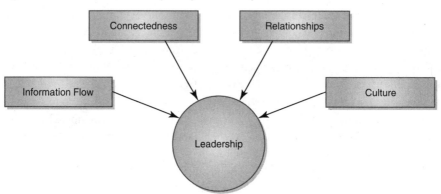

interventions to improve the care of type II diabetes that displayed more complexity characteristics led to better patient outcomes than interventions that were more linear.

The characteristics of complexity leadership theory (CLT) include leadership recognition of interrelationships, emergence, and fostering innovation (Uhl-Bien & Marion, 2008). CLT recognizes the dynamic interactions that take place within organizations as they change, create innovation, and evolve with a focus on complex relationships and network interaction rather than controlling, standardizing, and autocracy (Uhl-Bien & Marion, 2008) (**Figure 2-1**).

For healthcare organizations to accommodate innovations, and EBP to increase quality and shift from volume to value services, leadership must focus on collaboration, self-organization, and construction of strong networks among agents in the system (Uhl-Bien & Marion, 2008).

CLT was developed to address the shortcomings of traditional leadership theory in explaining the way organizations evolve through leadership in the knowledge era (Uhl-Bien & Marion, 2008). CLT focuses on leadership rather than the leader. Leaders are individuals who influence others toward an outcome, and leadership is the process by which agents of a system learn their way out of problems toward adaptive outcomes (Uhl-Bien & Marion, 2008). There are three leadership behaviors within CLT: administrative, adaptive, and enabling.

Administrative leadership is conceptualized as the formal hierarchy of the organization, including the chief executive officer, directors, managers, and other formalized leadership positions (Uhl-Bien & Marion, 2008). The administrative leadership behavior is closely related to the traditional leadership ideas presented earlier in this chapter. Administrative leadership is conceptualized in CLT because of the underlying assumption that organizations cannot exist without some formal structure (Uhl-Bien & Marion, 2008).

Although this framework is similar to traditional notions of leadership, CLT describes administrative leadership as being only one piece of leadership rather than the predominant function of leadership within organizations. Administrative leadership in CLT improves applicability to current organizations by acknowledging their existing structures as a relevant part of leadership and innovation.

The second leadership component is the adaptive leader. According to Uhl-Bien and Marion (2008), adaptive leadership is "an emergent, interactive dynamic that produces adaptive outcomes in a social system" (2008, p. 200). Adaptive leadership differs from administrative leadership in that adaptive leadership is the collective action that emerges from interactive exchanges among agents in the system (Delia, 2010). Uhl-Bien and Marion (2008) argued that adaptive leadership is the source of change in an organization and arises from the diverse opinions, conflict, and heterogeneity of the system.

The third leadership dynamic is enabling leadership. Enabling leadership is a person or group that brings together diverse agents in a system and creates a catalyst for the self-organization and emergent action of adaptive leadership to take place. Enabling leadership is connected to the system in an intimate way and can provide a spark for innovation (Uhl-Bien & Marion, 2008). All three leadership dynamics are entangled and cannot be separated and studied alone (Uhl-Bien & Marion, 2008). As the three complexity leadership behaviors arise in an organization, they shape the complex adaptive system, and in return the complex adaptive system shapes the leadership behaviors.

Burns (2001) surveyed healthcare leaders on their acceptance of the core underpinnings of complexity leadership in relation to creating successful organizations. The results suggested that leaders had intuitive support for the concepts but were uncomfortable with the concepts that required them to give up some control over processes. Specifically, 41% disagreed with the complexity leadership concept that advised leaders to "build a good-enough vision and provide minimum specifications, rather than trying to plan out every little detail" (2001, p. 480). This result suggests that although leaders intuit that complexity leadership is a good practice, they have trouble accepting a loss of direct control that accompanies complexity leadership behaviors.

A study by Hanson and Ford (2010) that used dynamic network analysis, a quantitative complexity analysis tool, demonstrated that the core leaders in a hospital laboratory setting were not formal directors or administrators, but rather customer services representatives—workers on the front line. The study showed through social network analysis methods that the customer service core played an important role in conducting information flow to all others in the lab and had heavy influence among other lab sections. These findings are contrary to what a traditional leader might expect, but from the complexity perspective, to get work done in the lab, an employee would have to interact with customer service workers due to their high influence and information. Hanson and Ford suggested that the assumption that formal leaders hold the core information for operation of the organization is not accurate. Instead, the network of the department was able to accomplish work through distributed power networks rather than strong administrative leadership. Complexity leadership suggests that the network contains significantly more influence, power to change, and capability to accomplish outcomes than any one individual, regardless of that individual's expertise. Departments in which the reliance of work is on one or two individuals have very weak network strength and are at risk of poor adaptability and ultimately failure. For example, if a department relies on a manager to make all decisions—from staffing to supplies to change management—the capability of the unit to function without that manager is very low. This puts the entire unit at risk for chaos when that leader departs. Complexity leaders should focus energy on building strong networks that are able to nimbly adapt to departures, crises, and environmental pressures.

Rowe and Hogarth (2005) used a complex adaptive systems metaphors intervention to facilitate change in public health nursing. The study examined pilot sites that instituted a complex adaptive system tool that was a vehicle for discussion of the strengths and weaknesses of organizational change. This tool was used to facilitate change in behavior and service among public health nurses. According to the researchers, when the formal leaders, from administrators to the nurses on the front line, embraced the movement of decision making and policy setting, an increase in experimentation and innovation arose that led to new service delivery models and to higher levels of responsibility and decision making for the practitioners. This means that when operating under complexity principles, practitioners are more autonomous, make better decisions, and innovate more.

Sweetman (2010) used surveys and social network analysis and found that the characteristics of leadership, innovation, and creativity in organizations were much more decentralized than previously thought. The sample consisted of a 60-person nonprofit that provided a leadership development program to high school and college students. The participants constituted a diverse group: managers, financial services representatives, engineers, and educators. Sweetman (2010) found that innovation was highly correlated with adaptive function ($.59, p < 0.001$), collective creativity ($.67, p < 0.001$), and shared leadership ($.59, p < 0.001$). All three must be present for innovation to occur. Additionally, Sweetman (2010) concluded that one individual is not primarily involved in all innovations and that numerous actors innovate, with innovation occurring across the organization. This finding supports the complexity leadership concept that leadership and innovation can occur at any level and between any individuals in the organization. Sweetman's work was limited to describing specific behaviors of leaders in the decentralized leadership role, or how these behaviors connected with innovation implementation.

Complexity leadership provides a foundation for conceptualizing leaders and leadership differently to facilitate innovation. Additionally, complexity leadership characteristics are congruent with healthcare leaders' ideas of ideal leadership behaviors (self-organizations, emergence, etc.) and improve creativity, lead to more innovation, and engage care providers (Delia, 2010; Rowe & Hogarth, 2005; Sweetman, 2010). The results of these early studies provide evidence that further understanding of the characteristics of complexity leadership in healthcare organizations may provide a new framework to increase innovation, reduce costs, and improve quality.

Innovation in CLT

Complexity leadership suggests that interactions among all agents shape the organizational context and thus deviant or abnormal agents are the result of deeper assumptions in the organization (Uhl-Bien & Marion, 2008). For example, agents in the system may test outdated or irrelevant polices through positive deviant behavior. Positive deviance is behavior that challenges organizational norms to find better ways of working (Jaramillo et al., 2008). When faced with positive deviant behavior, the complexity leader reviews organizational incongruence that may signal needed change (Jaramillo et al., 2008). Behavior that is not consistent with past assumptions may be a sign that innovation is needed rather than considered negative or a threat to stability. The role of leadership as seen through the complexity lens is to help shape a context that is adaptive and evolving and whose energy is focused toward the trajectory of the organization (Marion, 2008). Schwandt (2008) suggested that human actions and interactions are the basis for the emergence of leadership roles.

EBP in CLT

Data and evidence are part of the information flow of the organization and influence how agents in the system act and interact. The role of the leader is to ensure that the information flowing through the system is based on the best evidence and not on rumor, past practices, linear sources, or misinterpretations. It is important that information is not shared without regarding its validity, source, or reliability. In the absence of validated information, agents will begin to make assumptions based on the information at hand. Instilling a culture of EBP in the organization will help remove gaps in information and support more informed adaptations.

Complexity provides a different lens to view interactions and leadership in organizations. Innovation is a core behavior as people adapt based on information flow, interactions, relationships, and organizational culture. Evidence is generated, interpreted, and acted upon across all areas of the system. Leaders should work to build cultures that support interactions, build relationships, and improve information flow to all areas of the organization.

HEALTHCARE QUALITY AND A LACK OF INNOVATION

Traditional and less adequate leadership practices in healthcare systems that lead to practice variation and poor innovation implementation include autocratic, standardized, controlled, and profit-driven behaviors as the means to achieve organizational outcomes. Recent leadership scholars have proposed that the pathway to improving organizational outcomes, and ultimately patient outcomes, may indeed be found in a different leadership model (Delia, 2010; Lord, 2008; Uhl-Bien & Marion, 2008). A leadership practice that is shared among employees, where uncertainty is normative, mutual goals are facilitated, and innovation behaviors are foundational characteristics will support organizations to radically change to meet the challenges of healthcare reform and improved quality (Uhl-Bien & Marion, 2008). In essence, a model in which teams of nurses, physicians, administrators, and other healthcare workers demonstrate leadership behaviors that facilitate change and innovation supported by data and evidence is essential.

Quality issues such as inappropriate variations in care, consumer dissatisfaction, adverse events, medication errors, falls, and surgery mistakes have plagued the United States healthcare system for decades (Nembhard, Alexander, Hoff, & Ramanujam, 2009). Substantial arguments have been made claiming that the lack of improvement in healthcare quality is due to failed innovation implementation and inadequate leadership (Bazzoli, Dynan, Burns, & Yap, 2004; Berwick, 2003; Nembhard et al., 2009). Solutions to many quality issues have been found through innovation in practice supported by evidence, yet implementing, spreading, and sustaining these solutions in practice has been difficult. There is a need to better understand and utilize specific innovation leadership behaviors to improve health care.

Discussion

Lack of innovation leadership is one reason we have a gap in quality health care. Describe one failed implementation you have witnessed and the leadership characteristics that may have hindered the innovation or evidence-based intervention.

LEADERSHIP AS A TEAM DYNAMIC

As information, globalization, and technology continue to grow and impact organizations, the traditional conceptualization of the leader as an individual is no longer adequate. The volume and vastness of evidence available create conditions in which the administrative leaders or healthcare organizations can no longer possess or access enough information to make well-informed decisions (McKelvey, 2008). The same is true not only for administrative leaders, but also for frontline clinicians, managers, directors, and physician leaders.

Table 2-2   New Models of Care

	Old Approach	New Approach
Care	Episodic care	Continuous relationship
Management	Clinician	Clinical team
Decision making	Training and experience	Evidence
Control	Care system	Patient
Variability	Clinician autonomy	Patients preferences, needs
Information flow	Restricted	Encouraged
Safety	Responsibility of the clinician	Responsibility of system
Needs	System reacts	System anticipates
Financial goals	Reduce cost	Reduce waste
Process visibility	Secrecy	Transparency

Data from Kohn, L. T., Corrigan, J. M., & Donaldson, M. S. (Eds.). (2000). *To err is human: Building a safer health system*. Washington, DC: National Academy Press.

Clinical teams and organizations that rely on a disconnected group of individuals to guide evidence and innovation will, over time, fail to meet the dynamic changes that are present in health care. **Table 2-2** demonstrates the dynamic shift in expectations and deliverables present in the healthcare system. Only a small percentage of hospitals, health plans, and physician groups have been able to fully embrace these transitions in transparency, evidence generation, patient-centered care, and innovation despite the national shift to embrace Accountable Care Organization models. The reason only a few organizations have been able to fully adapt is that the majority of organizational leadership and clinical practice is guided by individuals working in silos rather than leveraging the collective knowledge of the larger system.

SEVEN CHARACTERISTICS OF INNOVATION LEADERSHIP

In many cases, the implementation of innovation or EBP is not a single planned event, but rather the synthesis of multiple interactions and changes that occur as the innovation is introduced. This structure is consistent with the work of Goldstein (2008),

Uhl-Bien and Marion (2008), and Hazy and colleagues (2007), who noted that innovation occurs over time as interconnected individuals in the organization adapt, through small changes, to pressures internally and externally by displaying leadership behaviors. Plowman and Duchon (2008) described these emerging actions as the essence of change: "Change occurs continuously, as minor adaptations, which can accumulate, amplify and become radical" (2008, p. 145). The innovation in organizations occurs as information flows through the organization, is processed, and disrupts or shifts the normal operating procedures. These disruptions are reflected as team members challenge their assumptions of how to best complete work and interact, and the organization changes its structure to accommodate the innovation. These structural changes can be in culture, the hierarchical organization, or care delivery.

Leadership behaviors are exhibited by all members of the organization and are not solely expressed by individuals acting alone or those with formal leadership roles. Leadership behaviors are displayed when opportunities are presented in the internal and external environment of the organization. The seven innovation leadership characteristics described in the following sections have been identified as influencing the movement of the organization toward adaption to the changing conditions: boundary spanning, risk taking, visioning, leveraging opportunity, adaptation, coordination of information flow, and facilitation. Each of these seven characteristics will be summarized and discussed in the context of innovation leadership.

Boundary Spanning

In traditional leadership, boundary spanning is reserved for top levels of the organizational hierarchy (Bass, 2008; Poole & Van de Ven, 2004). Boundary spanning is the process of agents in a system making connections to otherwise unconnected groups. Boundary spanning is usually demonstrated by multiple team members regardless of their formal titles. Boundary spanners look for outside guidance, ideas, and relationships to secure resources and increase knowledge within the organization. Boundary spanning activities increase the information flow into the organization and provide other team members with vital data that influences their leadership behaviors and subsequent actions. Boundary spanning also increases the connections and relationships of the organization, effectively building a larger network through which information could be exchanged and used to continually shift the work of the organization.

Boundary spanning is a behavior demonstrated by multiple individuals in the organization. This characteristic emerges as a team recognizes its deficits in knowledge about an innovation or organizational shift. Team members with connections external to the organization seek out information from these sources and introduce this information to the rest of the team to facilitate decision making and innovation integration.

Recognizing Boundary Spanning

CLT provides a framework to better understand boundary spanning by categorizing the administrative, enabling, and adaptive leadership behaviors (Schreiber, 2006; Uhl-Bien & Marion, 2008). Boundary spanning is demonstrated by multiple agents at different times in the innovation process, which is inconsistent with traditional notions of individual-focused leadership (Schreiber, 2006). Recognizing how boundary spanning occurs in organizations may inform how other teams gather external information to facilitate innovation implementation.

Administrative leadership behaviors include boundary spanning across disciplines and individuals to support funding, planning, and space allocations that help introduce resources needed for innovation to enter the system. Administrative leadership is demonstrated by both formal leaders and informal leaders within the system (Uhl-Bien & Marion, 2008).

Enabling leadership behaviors can occur in both formal and informal leaders as they gather external expertise to consult on ideas or projects in which internal capacity was limited. User design experts, technology experts, and even frontline administrative assistants can provide information to build a futuristic innovations and EBP rather than having a single leader plan and design the innovation with his or her individual expertise.

Enabling and administrative behaviors facilitate adaptive leadership behaviors. Adaptive leadership is reflected as team members process the new information gained by the boundary-spanning behaviors and integrate this information into decisions that result in new buildings, new techniques, and shifts in values. For example, team members may process information gathered through boundary spanning and begin to shift their value of their current organizational practices to new, possibly better, practices learned from outside entities. Thus, boundary spanning facilitates allowing team members in the organization to gather enough information to begin challenging assumptions and start taking risks.

Risk Taking

Risk taking is reflected as individuals begin experimenting with untested technologies or practices and gather information about them. Risk taking is dependent on team members actively identifying internal and external pressures and processing the impact and fit with organizational practices and context. A lack of fit creates tension or chaos and provides the needed push to trial new ways of work. This process is congruent with the notion that innovation occurs when organizations are near chaos (Porter-O'Grady & Malloch, 2015; Stacey, 2007; Uhl-Bien & Marion, 2008). Fit finding and testing activities reflect risk-taking behaviors because innovation practices that are tested usually have little evidence supporting them, and there is no blueprint for implementing innovation into the organization. Many risk-taking behaviors focus on trial-and-error efforts that test different technologies and implementation strategies to find the goodness of fit with the organization. The trial-and-error activities challenge the assumption that current practices or methods are adequate and introduce complex technologies and practices to individuals who were not previously comfortable with those technologies and practices. Trial-and-error activity generates information about the innovation that allows team members to assess its value, learn about the functionality, and better understand how to integrate it into the day-to-day activity of workers. Leaders must create a safe environment to support risk taking by using course correction rather than punishment as the norm in dealing with failures. Risk taking also increases the visibility, trialability, and usability of the innovation, which allows others to experience the innovation and create their own assessments of it (Rogers, 2003).

Recognizing Risk Taking

The behaviors of risk taking can also be explained using CLT. Administrative leadership behaviors describe how team members experiment with innovation by remaining open to new teaching modalities and feedback from individuals who are internal and external to the system to help create the future movement of the department. In other words, leaders in the organization should remain open and supportive of risk-taking behaviors.

Enabling leadership behaviors reflects experimentation with an innovation after that innovation was introduced into the organization and its practice was supported through feedback and information flow. Adaptive leadership is demonstrated as the individuals evolve over time, testing the innovation and practice against previous operating schemas and remaining open to adaptive outcomes that differ from the traditional methodology. The adaptive function is a result of the agent's ability to process information and make decisions at the point of service and integrate new practices into his or her work.

Risk-taking behaviors reflect a decision by a team to gather more information about the innovation. Individuals challenge current organizational assumptions, which creates opportunity for change in the organization. Risk taking disrupts the context of the organization and provides an opportunity for other team members to observe the innovation and develop their own assessments of its usefulness. This behavior seems to emerge from the risk taker's focus on maintaining quality of care while adapting to the stresses and opportunities presented by the environment. Risk takers seek out opportunities to test innovations to achieve high-level outcomes based on their professional values and their desire to improve work environments and outcomes.

Visioning

Groups of interconnected agents display the characteristic of visioning in organizations. Visioning is not an individual or isolated activity, and if practiced in a silo, it will lead to dysfunctional and fragmented organizational work. One example occurred in a case study in which faculty members adopted a simulation program into their college. The individual faculty members described their leadership roles as informal, but when these same faculty members described the faculty group as a whole, they described a decision-making body with inherent power. Axelrod and Cohen (2000) suggested that the coevolutionary process of organizations is reflected in the combination of the individual strategy decisions made at the agent level. Uhl-Bien and Marion (2008) suggested that networks of agents work together to create the future. Some decisions may be made in cooperation with other agents, while others are made to further an individual agenda. Both types of decision making—group and individual—occur in organizations and influence the outcomes of the team and the larger departments. The innovative leader must recognize this and learn how to facilitate either process to advance practice and innovation. The visioning process is reflective of the coevolutionary process in which individuals collaborate as a group to create the vision for the team, department, or organization. This dynamic contrasts with many traditional leadership theories that suggest the formal leader must create and vision the future (Bass, 2008). Formal leaders should provide input and suggestions but not create the vision in isolation.

Recognizing Visioning

Visioning reflects the notions of macro-level strategy as described by Dooley and Lichtenstein (2008). Macro leadership behaviors include strategic planning, resource support, gathering funding, and moral support. Leaders who display macro influence and thinking have a disproportionate impact on the organizational trajectory (Dooley & Lichtenstein, 2008; Hazy et al., 2007). For example, agents in a network whose roles are frontline in nature can, through their actions and interactions, create change in the mission of the organization even though leading such change is not within their formal job descriptions. Individuals are able to adjust their behaviors and relationships to translate their day-to-day work to the long-range planning and strategy of the organization as they meet in groups, teams, and cohorts both in formal and informal ways. Collaborative leadership occurs through group interaction and dialogue. Macro leadership behaviors occur through connections and information flow between agents, not through individual decision making and control (Uhl-Bien & Marion, 2008). Leaders and frontline workers, who individually may not carry out strategic planning, come together as a group and exercise macro-level leadership influences that build strategy and inform the organizations vision.

Many professions describe autonomy of decision making as a core value of the professional practice model. This value allows for the professionals to combine autonomous efforts, and create robust strategy and operational standards that are important to the success of the innovation. The traditional notion of managers and directors as planning, leading, and controlling the change process is challenged by recent evidence and complexity research (Weberg, 2013). Rather, formal leaders should view their role as facilitator and influencer. The absence of command-and-control leadership allows for individuals and teams in the organization to develop strategy by connecting the day-to-day work and resulting innovations to the desired outcomes of professional practice, patient outcomes, and organizational success.

Leveraging Opportunity

Leveraging opportunity is a characteristic that is demonstrated by all individuals in an organization. The behavior of leveraging opportunity is reflected in the actions of individuals who look for creative solutions to opportunities that presented themselves in the organization and in the environment. This may be looking for creative funding for innovations, linking current initiatives to support needed changes, or connecting teams working on similar projects to build stronger efforts. For example, the risk-taking behaviors that are adopted in an effort to find a new way to complete work demonstrates a focus on the opportunity rather than on the problem. More specifically, work-arounds, adaptations to EMR templates, and adopting new EBP in complex situations with unclear answers are ways that healthcare workers demonstrate leveraging opportunity.

Recognizing Leveraging Opportunity

Much of the traditional leadership literature highlights problem solving as a key characteristic of formal leaders (Bass, 2008; Plowman & Duchon, 2008; Poole & Van de Ven, 2004). Complexity literature reflects a different focus of leaders in that formal leaders themselves are not equipped to solve all organizational issues and are more effective leaders when they facilitate the team to tackle these issues. Thus, formal leaders should help create and identify the opportunities that teams can leverage in order to innovate. Plowman and Duchon (2008) proposed that conflict and divergence are the first steps in a change process. Further, leaders must be aware of conflict, look for patterns in the disruption, and see the opportunities these disruptions provide for innovation. Leaders who leveraged opportunity displayed enabling and adaptive leadership behaviors (Uhl-Bien & Marion, 2008). Enabling behaviors are reflected in the way opportunities are presented to the others in the organization. Instead of framing the external pressures as problems requiring cuts and reductions, leaders can frame external pressures as opportunities requiring novel solutions. Adaptive behaviors are reflected in the way teams self-adapt and begin implementing new work strategies in response to opportunity and shifts.

Adaptation

The interconnectedness among agents continually restructures as innovation adoption spreads. This is evident as individuals in the organization adapt their roles depending on the opportunities presented by innovation or EBP implementation. For example, in an EMR implementation, some nurses shifted roles from bedside care to solving technology issues and troubleshooting with their colleagues. The technology support role was not part of the formal job expectations, but it was required by the organization to maintain member buy-in for the EMR implementation. These role changes reflect the ability of agents to adapt based on information and need, without requiring a formal hierarchal change or command decision. Many adaptations are based on the drive to implement innovation and more individual-focused human behaviors. Stacey (2007) suggested that complex systems are not predictable because they are impacted by unpredictable human behavior.

Recognizing Adaptation

Individual team members consistently assess their own value to the organization and the need to adapt behavior. When individuals adapt their behaviors from facilitating connections (nursing care) to more managerial work (solving technology issues), the network strength is impacted, resulting in changes to innovation adoption and success. Teams and leaders must recognize the need for coordination in the system and adapt new roles and leadership behaviors to continue the innovation trajectory of the organization.

Usually innovation work ebbs and flows with the connections of the network over time; reduced network coordination results in fragmented innovation. Schreiber and Carley (2008) stated that the collective action of change agents is a source of learning and adaptive response in the system. Further, they described collective change as being fostered by decentralized decision making and strong learning cultures. Both decentralized decision making, in the form of autonomous practice, and a learning culture may help explain how organizations are able to adopt innovation successfully.

Coordination of Information Flow

Individuals and teams in the innovation process should be able to influence how information is shared and interpreted and how agents in the system related to each other in order to implement successful innovation through coordination of information flow. This leadership characteristic helps to evolve the organizational context by using connections and relationships to share new information while making it relevant to the work of the organization. For example, innovation champions may express the successes of innovation to other departments through meetings, one-on-one conversations, and stories. These leadership actions reflect enabling behaviors (Uhl-Bien & Marion, 2008).

Enabling leadership behaviors are demonstrated as the individual team members influence one another by changing how artifacts and values are communicated and by shifting information flow in the organization to influence how other team members perceive an innovation. Strategy documents may be written, and innovation adopters may praise the use of the technique in open forums. Leaders should challenge their own assumptions about the current work and shift their actions and language to convey more positive outcomes of a change in work if there are possible or perceived benefits. This activity gathers buy-in and adds other agents to the network to begin to adapt to the innovation implementation. The actions of value shifting and adaptation align with the work of scholars who described the coevolution of systems toward adaptive outcomes (Axelrod & Cohen, 2000; Hatch, 2000; Hazy et al., 2007; Schein 2004; Uhl-Bien & Marion, 2008; Van de Ven & Hargrave, 2004).

Recognizing Coordination of Information Flow

Leaders can recognize messengers of innovation by looking for evangelists who promote the innovation, examine documents that reflect the underlying response to the innovation, and assess the information that is created about the innovation. For example, innovation champions may promote the use of the innovation and communicate the successes through connections and relationships. Strategy documents can reflect the desire to grow the innovation and to continue to refine and coordinate the efforts when using the innovation. Additionally, formal leaders should continue to assess the organizational context to determine if and when resources or administrative influence is needed to overcome stagnated processes.

Healthcare organizations are complex systems that contain subsystems of a large organization, and leaders must navigate through the bureaucracy by catalyzing change through resource allocation and facilitating a context that values agent autonomy and decentralized decision making. Formal processes such as shared governance, administrative approval processes, and bureaucracy are a normal part of organizational life, but formal leaders can help reduce the restricting impact of these structures on the innovation at the front line of the organization by promoting shared decision making by the end user. As Uhl-Bien and Marion (2008) suggested, leaders can overcome stagnating structures by becoming catalysts and resource gatherers for change. Stacey (2007) described these processes as balancing negative and positive feedback loops in the system to keep it moving at the edge of chaos. Messaging innovation reflects targeted information flow through the organization and results in improving interest in the new techniques.

Facilitation

The role of leaders in influencing information flow centers on helping organizational members to see an innovation as relevant to their work through the characteristic of facilitation. Complexity research shifts the focus of the leader from controlling actions of individuals to influencing and facilitating the information those individuals get and use in the process of decision making. These behaviors influence the system to consider new ways of operating by allowing for professional decision making and innovation. The leadership actions should not be aimed at directing the work of nurses, for example; there should be, instead, a high degree of value placed on professional autonomy. Leaders in the system facilitate and coordinate opportunities for the agents to build connections and relationships with one another and experience the innovation firsthand. Facilitation is displayed in gathering information, making sense of it, and allowing the autonomous agents to integrate it through resource allocation and relationships rather than through command-and-control tactics. In fact, many times, formal leaders may feel they have little direct-line authority to force change on the professional. Their only option is to facilitate and influence innovation.

Recognizing Facilitation

By fostering interactions, facilitating information, and understanding that leadership is a system behavior, leaders can look for the points in the system where their influence is most needed and valued. Developing and facilitating these network interactions helps to build the organizational context that sets the rules of engagement that can lead to emergent displays of leadership without requiring or depending on formal leader input to the system. Facilitation is reflected in practice as team members adopting an innovation aid others to use the new technique through trial and error rather than initially creating perfectly working systems. This process creates a context of ownership around the innovation and allows the team members to develop new skill through utilization of the new technology or practice. Additionally, facilitation allows the team members to customize the innovation to their objectives, which allows them to find the fit between the new technique and their own practice philosophies. This customization improves buy-in to using an innovation and reflects enabling leadership behaviors (Uhl-Bien & Marion, 2008).

Summary of Leadership Characteristics

No one individual reflects the risk taker or the boundary spanner, as is suggested in traditional leadership literature (Bass, 2008). Instead, boundary spanning, risk taking, and the other five leadership characteristics are reflected and practiced through the complex interaction of leadership behaviors by multiple individuals in response to emergent opportunities in the internal and the external environments. Boundary spanning and risk taking reflect the ability of the team to recognize knowledge deficits and seek out external information sources and bring them into the system for processing by other members. Visioning and leveraging opportunities reflect the ability of the team to process information, look for opportunities to integrate the new technique into the organization's context, and create desired outcomes from the information. Adaptation, coordinating information flow, and facilitating reflect the ability of the team to adapt to changing conditions by creating internal emergent structures such as new roles, strategies, and information sharing that facilitate the adoption of the innovation. These characteristics reflect a new framework from which to understand leadership of an innovation—not through the direction of an individual formal leader, but rather as a team focused on achieving the shared outcome of student success.

Leadership of innovation emerges from individual and group interactions. Formal and informal leaders influence information flow by boundary spanning, risk taking, visioning, leveraging opportunity, adaptation, coordination, and facilitation. The system then processes the information through autonomous decision making, collaboration, and formal structures that resulted in an organizational context that guided the implementation of the innovation. Leaders in health care should work to remove barriers to interaction and collaboration, create opportunities to catalyze innovation, and gather resources to further the innovation agenda. Leadership occurs at all levels and ranks in the organization, and the role of leaders of teams and leaders of innovation is that of building alignment and relationships rather than implementing command-and-control tactics.

IMPLICATIONS

The seven behaviors of innovation leadership provide a new understanding of how leaders in health care can facilitate innovation in their organizations. Groups that will benefit most from these implications include nurses and other healthcare professionals, healthcare organizations, healthcare leaders, and researchers. The data and concepts support a new lens to view leadership, organizations, and innovation.

Implications for Nursing and Health Professionals

The seven behaviors of innovation leadership and the underlying CLT framework has several implications for the nursing profession and provides a new lens through which nurses and nursing leaders can facilitate innovation and EBP. Nurses in all roles of the profession can use this framework to begin to build innovation teams to respond to the changing healthcare landscape and align new care innovations with new and existing organizations. Nurses are uniquely positioned to lead the next revolution in health care because they are the hub of care coordination.

Nursing and healthcare leaders can use boundary spanning, risk taking, and messaging to improve information flow into their organizations. Nursing leaders must span beyond their nursing colleagues and the healthcare industry to find novel approaches and technologies to solve the problems of cost and quality facing today's healthcare organizations and nursing workforce. Healthcare professionals at all levels should use risk-taking characteristics to continually test new work flows, technologies, and patient care interventions using early evidence and clinical judgment. This can be done only if information about the changing healthcare landscape, organizational quality metrics, budget, and mission flows to the frontline nursing staff. Without this information, innovation may be restricted or fragmented.

Professional leaders can take risks by helping to recognize the innovative potential of work-arounds and new practices that are unproven but show promise in improving patient care. Leaders can also provide resources and support; additionally, they can facilitate cross-discipline interactions to build these new innovations. Most importantly, formal healthcare leaders can help coordinate the innovation occurring across the organization and facilitate alignment of these innovations with the trajectory of the organization.

Nurses are traditionally the hub of care for patients in hospitals and other places of care. Nurses connect multiple disciplines and coordinate care with a holistic patient focus. Nurses must leverage these connections to build strong collaborative relationships among team members and to design new models of care that are both patient centric and cost effective. They can do so by facilitating learning, exposing the care team to new innovations, and adopting risk-taking behaviors in regard to technology and care innovations.

The proposed leadership behaviors focus on organizational context, which, for nurses, may be of paramount importance. Cultures of nursing, as well as other professions, that are guided by punishment for error, negative attitudes toward young innovators, and the worship of ineffective past practices may lead to stagnated care and worsening quality. This chapter suggests that a culture in which trial and error is welcomed and learning is facilitated leads to new models of work that are more effective than past practices. It is imperative that nursing leaders and frontline nurses take note of the large impact that organizational context has on innovation and change.

Nursing and healthcare professionals have an obligation to the patient to continue to improve care and reduce cost while maintaining the highest ethical principles. Similarly, innovative change can be achieved while maintaining the core values of patient safety and professionalism. This endeavor requires new ways of leading and new definitions of leaders.

Implications for Healthcare Organizations

The described leadership behaviors challenge the traditional hierarchical structures and leadership methodologies present in many healthcare organizations. These traditional structures may be restricting innovation by limiting information flow, restricting connections among agents, and limiting diverse relationships, potentially resulting in fragmented organizational cultures and innovation.

Organizations need to consider restructuring their reporting hierarchy to mimic network relationships and promote information flow to the front line. Additionally, healthcare organizations have to refocus their organizational cultures to promote and support innovation competencies, such as risk taking and boundary spanning, to gain new insights to solve cost and quality problems. Similarly, organizations must focus resources on aligning new ideas with the work of the organization by intentionally crafting innovation messages, facilitating learning about innovations, and creating flexible roles that can adapt to shifting conditions. Proactively seeking innovations to overcome external pressures and working to align the innovation internally with the core mission of the organization are proposed new organizational competencies that are needed to navigate the changing healthcare landscape by facilitating innovation.

Implications for Healthcare Leaders

Healthcare leaders may stand to benefit significantly from the reframing of leadership and leadership behaviors presented in this chapter. The term *leader* refers to all individuals in the organization who administer, enable, and adapt novel solutions to complex situations. Burns (2001) found that healthcare leaders approved of the concepts of complexity leadership and, with the preliminary findings of the proposed framework of this case study, a new leadership framework presents tangible behaviors and characteristics of complexity leadership that healthcare leaders can use to build innovation competency in teams across an organization.

Most importantly, research suggests that formal leaders may be ill equipped to individually promote innovation. Instead, leaders should focus on building teams with the characteristics described in this study to create novel solutions. The focus of leadership should not be on controlling the process, but rather on facilitating the optimization of leadership behaviors across the organization.

Information flow allows the group to have access to and gather needed information to make decisions concerning problem solving and innovation alignment with the organization. Formal leaders can facilitate this process by sharing data and explicating its relevance to the organizational mission. Additionally, formal leaders can eliminate traditional structures that dilute or restrict the sharing of information across groups in the organization. They may do so by reducing the focus on hierarchal reporting structures and individul-focused leadership practices. Adopting a focus on facilitating shared leadership structures may be more advantageous in terms of implementing innovations. All members of an organization can practice risk taking, boundary spanning, and visioning behaviors that aid in challenging less adequate organizational norms, build connections and relationships beyond the walls of the group or organization, and create compelling visions of the future. These behaviors are reflective of complexity leadership and facilitate the recognition of opportunities, improve information flow through the organization, and translate that information into a relevant trajectory for the organization.

Connections and relationships allow a group to access information and share it effectively. Connections without strong relationships reduce information flow and reduce innovation capacity and relevancy. These connections must also be easily changeable as internal and external pressures dictate. This case demonstrates that if resources are not available to solve management-type problems, such as technical issues, the innovation process may stagnate or stop altogether. Leaders in healthcare organizations can reduce this effect by building diverse connections and relationships among teams to leverage unique skill sets as issues arise. For example, if a team is working to implement a technological innovation, building relationships with information technology and electronic media teams may be necessary. Simply connecting these teams is not enough. The teams working toward innovation implementation need to have strong collaborative relationships as well. This means they must be able to move toward a common goal, freely exchange relevant information, and make coordinated decisions to advance the innovation. These relationships can be influenced by leaders in the organization through facilitating shared leadership, improving information flow, and helping build an organizational context that is supportive of teamwork and collaboration.

Organizational context is another factor that influences innovation implementation. Healthcare leaders need to recognize the role this factor plays in facilitating or limiting innovation in organizations. Cultures in which one group dominates decision making, collaboration is not facilitated, and trial and error is punished may be less likely to innovate. For example, a healthcare organization that values only physician leadership without input from nursing and ancillary care providers may result in a culture that restricts information flow about core business practices. This restriction in information flow limits the possible decision options and makes the implemented decisions less relevant to the nonincluded groups. This result leads to maladaptive behaviors and promotes a context of stagnation rather than innovation. An organization that values autonomy of decision making and has a context focused on organizational outcomes can collaborate across specialties to implement an innovation that meets the needs of several different groups.

Formal and informal leaders must recognize the impact and interrelatedness of information flow, connections, relationships, and culture on the innovation work of an organization. By developing new competencies for leadership, removing restrictive organizational context and structures, and facilitating rather than controlling, leaders can build an innovative organization that is ready to adapt and evolve to meet the cost and quality issues that continue to impact the U.S. healthcare system.

REFERENCES

Aarons, G. A. (2006). Transformational transactional leadership: Associations with attitudes toward evidence-based practice. *Psychiatric services, 57*(8), 1162–1169.

Aarons, G. A., & Sommerfeld, D. H. (2012). Leadership, innovation climate, and attitudes toward evidence-based practice during a statewide implementation. *Journal of American Academy of Adolescent Psychiatry, 51*(4), 270–280

Anderson, B. J., Manno, M., O'Connor, P., & Gallagher, E. (2010). Listening to nursing leaders: Using national database of quality indicators data to study excellence in nursing leadership. *Journal of Nursing Administration, 40*(4), 182–187.

Anderson, R. A., Issel, M., & McDaniel, R. R. (2003). Nursing homes as complex adaptive systems: Relationship between management practice and resident outcomes. *Nursing Research, 52*(1), 12–21.

Avolio, B. J., & Bass, B. M. (2002). *Developing potential across a full range of leadership cases on transactional and transformational leadership.* Mahwah, NJ: Lawerence Erlbaum.

Axelrod, R., & Cohen, M. D. (2000). *Harnessing complexity: Implications of a scientific frontier.* New York, NY: Basic Books.

Bass, B. M. (2008). *The Bass handbook of leadership: Theory, research, and managerial applications* (4th ed.). New York, NY: Free Press.

Bazzoli, G. J., Dynan, L., Burns, L. R., & Yap, C. (2004). Two decades of organizational change in health care: What have we learned? *Medical Care Research and Review, 61*(3), 247–331.

Berwick, D. M. (2003). Disseminating innovations in healthcare. *Journal of the American Medical Association, 289*(15), 1969–1975.

Boonstra, A., & Broekhuis, M. (2010). Barriers to the acceptance of electronic medical records by physicians from systematic review to taxonomy and interventions. *BMC Health Services Research, 10*, 231.

Burns, J. P. (2001). Complexity leadership and leadership in healthcare. *Journal of Nursing Administration, 31*(10), 474–482.

Cherulnik, P. D., Donley, K. A., Wiewel, S. R., & Miller, S. R. (2001). Charisma is contagious, the effect of leaders' charisma on observers' affect. *Journal of Applied Social Psychology, 31*(10), 2149–2159.

Conger, J. A. (1998). The dark side of leadership. In G. R. Hickman (Ed.), *Leading organizations: Perspectives for a new era* (pp. 256–277). Thousand Oaks, CA: Sage.

Cooper, J., & Brady, D. W. (1981). Institutional context and leadership style: The house from Cannon to Rayburn. *American Political Science Review, 75*(2), 411–425.

Crosby, F. E., & Shields, C. J. (2010). Preparing the next generation of nurse leaders: An educational needs assessment. *Journal of Continuing Education in Nursing, 41*(8), 363–368.

Cummings, G. G., Midodzi, W. K., Wong, C. A., & Estabrooks, C. A. (2010). The contribution of hospital nursing leadership styles to 30-day patient mortality. *Nursing Research, 59*(5), 331–339.

Delia, E. (2010). *Complexity leadership in industrial innovation teams: A field study of leading, learning, and innovation in heterogeneous teams* (Unpublished doctoral dissertation). Rutgers, Newark, NJ.

Dooley, K., & Lichtenstein, B. (2008). Research methods for studying the dynamics of leadership. In M. Uhl-Bien & R. Marion (Eds.), *Complexity leadership part 1: Conceptual foundations* (pp. 269–290). Charlotte, NC: Information Age.

Drucker, P. (1985). *Innovation and entrepreneurship: Practice and principals.* New York, NY: Harper and Row.

Failla, K., & Stichler, J. (2008). Manager and staff perceptions of the manager's leadership style. *Journal of Nursing Administration, 38*(11), 480–487.

Goldstein, J. (2008). Conceptual foundations of complexity science: Development and main concepts. In M. Uhl-Bien & R. Marion (Eds.), *Complexity leadership part 1: Conceptual foundations* (pp. 17–48). Charlotte, NC: Information Age.

Gowan, C. R., Henegan, S. C., & McFadden, K. L. (2009). Knowledge management as a mediator for the efficacy of transformational leadership and quality management initiatives in U.S. health care. *Health Care Management Review, 34*(2), 129–140.

Hanson, W. R., & Ford, R. (2010). Complexity leadership in healthcare: Leader network awareness. *Procedia Social and Behavioral Sciences, 2,* 6587–6596.

Hatch, M. J. (2000). Dynamics of organizational culture and identity with implications for the leadership of organizational change. In N. Ashkanasy, C. Wilderom, & M. Peterson (Eds.), *The Handbook of Organizational Culture and Climate* (2nd ed., pp. 341–356). Thousand Oaks, CA: Sage.

Hazy, J. K., Goldstein, J. A., & Lichtenstein, B. B. (2007). *Complex systems leadership theory: New perspectives from complexity science on social and organizational effectiveness.* Mansfield, MA: ISCE.

Howell, J. M., & Avolio, B. J. (1993). Transformational leadership, transactional leadership, locus of control, and support for innovation: Key predictors of consolidated-business-unit performance. *Journal of Applied Psychology, 78*(6), 891–902.

Jaramillo, B., Jenkins, C., Kermes, F., Wilson, L. Mazzocco, J., & Longo, T. (2008). Positive deviance: Innovation from the inside out. *Nurse Leader, 6*(2), 30–34.

Kanste, O. (2008). The association between leadership behavior and burnout among nursing personnel in health care. *Vard Nord Utveckl Forsk, 28*(3), 4–8.

Kelly, P. (2008). *Nursing leadership & management* (2nd ed.). Clifton Park, NY: Thomson Delmar Learning.

Kleinman, C. (2004). The relationship between managerial leadership behaviors and staff nurse retention. *Hospital Topics, 82*(4), 3–9.

Kohn, L. T., Corrigan, J. M., & Donaldson, M. S. (Eds.). (2000). *To err is human: Building a safer health system* (Vol. 6). Washington, DC: National Academies Press.

Kumar, S., & Aldrich, K. (2010). Overcoming barriers to electronic medical record (EMR) implementation in the US healthcare system: A comparative study. *Health informatics journal, 16*(4), 306–318.

Leykum, L. K., Pugh, J., Lawrence, V., Parchman, M., Noel, P. H., Cornell, J., & McDaniel, R. R. (2007). Organizational interventions employing principles of complexity science have improved outcomes for patients with type 2 diabetes. *Implementation Science, 2*(28).

Lord, R. (2008). Beyond transactional and transformational leadership: Can leaders still lead when they don't know what to do? In M. Uhl-Bien & R. Marion (Eds.), *Complexity leadership part 1: Conceptual foundations* (pp. 155–184). Charlotte, NC: Information Age.

Losada, M. (1999). The complex dynamics of high performance teams. *Mathematical and computer modeling, 30,* 179–192.

Lotrecchiano, G. R. (2010). Complexity leadership in transdisciplinary learning environments: A knowledge feedback loop. *International Journal of Transdisciplinary Research, 5*(1), 29–63.

Marion, R. (2008). Complexity theory for organizations and organizational leadership. In M. Uhl-Bien & R. Marion (Eds.), *Complexity leadership part 1: Conceptual foundations* (pp. 225–268). Charlotte, NC: Information Age.

McKelvey, B. (2008). Emergent strategy via complexity leadership: Using complexity science and adaptive tension to build distributed intelligence. In M. Uhl-Bien & R. Marion (Eds.), *Complexity leadership part 1: Conceptual foundations* (pp. 225–268). Charlotte, NC: Information Age.

Nembhard, I. M., Alexander, J. A., Hoff, T. J., & Ramanujam, R. (2009). Why does the quality of healthcare continue to lag? Insights from management research. *Academy of Management Perspectives, 23*(1), 24–42.

Nielsen, K., Yarker, J., Randall, R., & Munir, F. (2009). The mediating effects of team and self-efficacy on the relationship between transformational leadership, and job satisfaction and psychological well-being in healthcare professionals: A cross-sectional questionnaire survey. *International Journal of Nursing Studies, 46*(9), 1236–1244.

Northouse, P. G. (2015). *Leadership: Theory and practice.* Thousand Oaks, CA: Sage.

Plowman, D. A., & Duchon, D. (2008). Dispelling the myths about leadership: From cybernetics to emergence. In M. Uhl-Bien & R. Marion (Eds.), *Complexity leadership part 1: Conceptual foundations* (pp. 129–153). Charlotte, NC: Information Age.

Poole, M. S., & Van de Ven, A. H. (2004). *Handbook of organizational change and innovation.* New York, NY: Oxford University Press.

Porter-O'Grady, T., & Malloch, K. (2015). *Quantum leadership: Building better partnerships for sustainable health*. Burlington, MA: Jones & Bartlett Learning.

Rogers, E. M. (2003). *Diffusion of innovations* (5th ed.). New York, NY: Free Press.

Rosing, K., Frese, M., & Bausch, A. (2011). Explaining the heterogeneity of the leadership-innovation relationship: Ambidextrous leadership. *The Leadership Quarterly, 22*(5), 956–974.

Rowe, A., & Hogarth, A. (2005). Use of complex adaptive systems metaphor to achieve professional and organizational change. *Journal of Advanced Nursing, 51*(4), 396–405.

Saint, S., Kowalski, C. P., Banaszak-Holl, J., Forman, J., Damschroder, L., & Krein, S. L. (2010). The importance of leadership in preventing healthcare-associated infection: Results of a multisite qualitative study. *Infection Control and Hospital Epidemiology, 31*(9), 901–907.

Schein, E. H. (2004). *Organizational culture and leadership*. San Francisco, CA: Wiley & Sons.

Schreiber, C. (2006). *Human and organizational risk modeling: Critical personnel and leadership in network organizations*. Carnegie Mellon University, School of Computer Science, Institute for Software Research International. Technical Report, CMU-ISRI-06-120.

Schwandt, D. R. (2008). Individual and collective co-evolution: Leadership as emergent social structuring. In M. Uhl-Bien & R. Marion (Eds.), *Complexity leadership part 1: Conceptual foundations* (pp. 101–127). Charlotte, NC: Information Age.

Schreiber, C., & Carley, K. M. (2008). Dynamic network leadership: Leading for learning and adaptability. In M. Uhl-Bien & R. Marion (Eds.), *Complexity leadership part 1: Conceptual foundations* (pp. 291–332). Charlotte, NC: Information Age.

Shipton, H., Armstrong, C., West, M., & Dawson, J. (2008). The impact of leadership and quality climate on hospital performance. *International Journal for Quality in Health Care, 20*(6), 439–445.

Stacey, R. D. (2007). *Strategic management and organizational dynamics* (5th ed.). New York, NY: Prentice Hall.

Stordeur, S., D'hoore, W., & Vandernberghe, C. (2001). Leadership, organizational stress, and emotional exhaustion among hospital nursing staff. *Journal of Advanced Nursing, 35*(4), 544–542.

Sweetman, D. S. (2010). Exploring the adaptive function in complexity leadership theory: An examination of shared leadership and collective creativity in innovation networks. *Dissertations and Theses from the College of Business Administration*. University of Nebraska-Lincoln.

Uhl-Bien, M., & Marion, R. (2008). *Complexity leadership part 1: Conceptual foundations*. Charlotte, NC: Information Age.

Van de Ven, A. H., & Hargrave, T. J. (2004). Social, technical, institutional change: A literature review and synthesis. In M. S. Poole & A. H. Van de Ven (Eds.), *Handbook of organizational change and innovation* (pp. 259–303). New York, NY: Oxford University Press.

Weberg, D. R. (2013). *Complexity leadership theory and innovation: A new framework for innovation leadership* (Doctoral dissertation, Arizona State University).

Wong, C. A., Cummings, G. G., & Ducharme, L. (2013). The relationship between nursing leadership and patient outcomes: A systematic review update. *Journal of Nursing Management, 21*, 709–724.

Wu, K., Yang, L., & Chiang, I. (2011). Leadership and Six Sigma project success: The role of member cohesiveness and resource management. *Production, Planning & Control, 23*(9), 1–11. doi:10.1080/09537287 .2011.586650

Yoder-Wise, P. S. (2007). Key forecasts shaping nursing's perfect storm. *Nursing Administration Quarterly, 31*(2), 115–119.

CHAPTER 3

Assessing Your Innovation and Evidence Capacity: Essentials for Organizational Infrastructures

Kathy Malloch and Tim Porter-O'Grady

Life is not about waiting for the storms to pass . . . it is about learning how to dance in the rain.

—UNKNOWN

CHAPTER OBJECTIVES

Upon completion of this chapter, the reader will be able to:

1. Examine the challenges and driving forces pushing organizational structure changes.
2. Assess a creative evidentiary approach for organizations transforming their organizations to accountable, evidence-driven systems.
3. Describe key competencies of leaders, managers, and caregivers in an evidentiary model.

INTRODUCTION

The passage of time necessarily brings new ideas, new people, and new expectations for all of us and, in particular, for the work we do in health care. Figuring out what to do to be relevant within a context that moves rapidly and with a mix of digital and manual processes can be overwhelming. What is important in this figuring out process is for each of us to reflect on where we are and where we can now move to as leaders in creating the conditions for the ultimate integration of high levels of evidence and innovative processes.

In this chapter, we discuss the current state of leadership, an overview of the driving forces for changing to higher levels of innovation, the impact of the Internet, new approaches that integrate the evidence-innovation dynamic, and behaviors to transform to the desired organizational infrastructure, with an emphasis on professional accountability. In particular, emphasis is laid on the importance of a dynamic organizational infrastructure that includes defined processes and authority designations, and this is also aligned with desired behaviors to optimize value.

HISTORICAL STATE OF ORGANIZATIONAL LEADERSHIP: SANS EVIDENCE

Historically, there has been a lack of evidentiary thinking and working in organizations. In the past decade, however, much has been made of the high level of judgment and assumptions-based clinical practices that characterize all of the healthcare disciplines (Freshwater & Rolfe, 2004). The attempt to build evidence-based practice has raised a number of significant concerns regarding the foundations of judgment of clinical practitioners (McNamara, 2002). The evidence indicates that much weight has been applied to past practices, individual experiences, and traditional foundations of learning used in the formation of the body of knowledge upon which most practitioners base their own clinical judgments and actions (Smith, 2004). Of course, this foundation for behavior is quite unstable and unreliable—the inadequacies inherent in the dependence on past practice and individual assumptions cannot be understated (McSherry, Simmons, & Abbott, 2002). Even so, for most practitioners, in contemporary clinical situations the past remains the foundation of the vast majority of practice decisions and actions in the present.

This reality of uninformed and evidence-lacking decision making and action, which is readily apparent in clinical practice, is only extended and broadened when we consider leadership and management practices in health care. Indeed, much of management practice is based on an unbounded and wide variation of myth, whim, fancy, fad, and fashion (Malloch & Porter-O'Grady, 1999; Tourish & Hargie, 2004). In no area of human endeavor are there as many nonvalidated assumptions of practice and the management of human behavior as in the arena of management and leadership (Albrecht, 2003). Almost weekly, self-proclaimed management gurus announce new insights regarding leadership and management practice based solely on the expression of their own thinking and fantasy regarding what works and does not work in the leadership of people and organizations. Management and leadership are most bereft of any continuous aggregated and related body of knowledge that would in any way validate the foundations upon which many of the practices of leadership and management are based (Drucker, 2001; Drucker & Stone, 1998; Mintzberg, 1990).

Contemporary notions of accountability would require the resolution of such a difficulty. Yet, new tomes appear weekly on the bookshelves attesting to emerging personal insights with regard to judgments of what makes effective leaders and what produces sustainable outcomes in business and service. At the same time, broad-based evidence of the lack of accountability and ownership with regard to personal decisions and actions in almost every arena is rife both in the United States and on the global stage, demonstrating the paucity of real and effective leadership. This lack of accountability and the corresponding lack of understanding regarding what accountability means underpins much of the problem associated with building an evidentiary foundation to leadership decisions and practices (McDaniel, 2004; Oliver, 2004; Price, 2006).

DRIVING FORCES THAT ARE SHIFTING ORGANIZATIONAL STRUCTURE

The rules of organizational engagement are changing significantly on the basis of the emergence of an informational and technological foundation for human experiences and practices (Trompenaars & Hampden-Turner, 2002). These emerging realities are calling organizations and leaders into a different contextual framework for leadership and the management of work (Wolper, 2004). Goals of improved process times, lower production costs, decreased costs, improved coordination and management of functional interdependencies, and time reductions continue to push organizations forward (Davenport, 2006).

Further, the information age is changing all the rules affecting structure and the processes associated with doing work, achieving outcomes, or producing products (Watkins, 2004). According to Scharmer and Kaufer (2000) and Castells (1998), the changes occurring because of the information age are significant, most notably the Internet. There are now social structures based on networks, an economy tightly linked to information, and cultures steeped in virtual reality. These changes call for rethinking of just about everything a leader does, from visioning to planning to collaborating to implementing to evaluating and on and on.

The new world taking shape before us necessarily impacts the very nature of health care and the ways in which healthcare services are organized, packaged, delivered, and evaluated. Specifically, the availability and sharing of information, the media used for knowledge transfer, the range and types of relationships among providers and patients, and the time required to transfer and share information now require new structures, principles for communication, and outcome expectations for leaders. In particular, the information infrastructure is now able to aggregate huge volumes of data, correlate that information, integrate it, and report it clearly and efficiently.

The changes in how information is communicated, who can access information, real-time availability of information on the Internet, and the availability of digitized media for nearly every bit of information have uniquely impacted traditional organizational structure. These structures serve to define levels of authority, communication pathways, and span of control. The organizational chart at one time defined clear lines of accountability and role relationships believed appropriate for organizational effectiveness and efficiency. Now with the widespread use of the Internet, digital device real-time communication, and self-organizing networks, these boundaries have become blurred at best and nearly invisible in most organizations.

Three areas have significantly changed the nature of work: media communication, location of stakeholders, and time. **Table 3-1** summarizes the description and impact in these areas.

Table 3-1   Comparison of Traditional and Information Age Dimensions

	Traditional	Information Age	Advantages	Disadvantages
Structure for communication and authority designation Who is involved?	Organizational chart Vertical communication	Internet Social networks Open communication	Eliminates silos Increases integration of work products	Uncertainty with open communication Perceived loss of control and power
Media How is knowledge transferred?	Paper, books, video, audio	Digital	Consistency, quality of information	Lack of resources to implement
Space Where does it happen?	Physical buildings/offices Local	Virtual Nonlocal	Space available for open collaboration	Perceived loss of privacy
Time When does it occur?	Business hours	No limits 24 hours/day	Decreases lag time across time zones and between individuals	Blurs the boundaries between work and personal time

Media Communication

The manner of communication among healthcare stakeholders has changed significantly with the availability of transportable and real-time Internet-available information. Communication media have evolved from physical to electronic and from isolated to interactive. The assumptions related to the media or vehicle for transfer of information, including written, oral, and video modalities as the primary vehicles, are challenged in nearly every venue. The availability of text messaging, instant messaging, and social networks has contributed greatly to the new model for organizational structure. Communication with anyone now reflects increasing complexity; communication occurs at any time and in any place. Power relationships are now dramatically reconfigured. Communications between executives, managers, and staff are now horizontal, vertical, and diagonal, rather than up-and-down historical lines of authority and chains of command. According to Bennis, Goleman, and Biederman (2008), the effectiveness of an organization depends on the flow of information. Further, the organization's capacity to compete, solve problems, innovate, meet challenges, and achieve goals requires all the organization's intelligence—and this is directly related to the healthy flow of information. Attempts to formally control and limit communication are no longer effective.

No matter how well text is written, it is not an interactive medium. Paper was once the most reliable form for communication; now digital files are becoming the norm. Audiovisual media have also dramatically decreased the need for travel and physical presence. Physical presence has long been exchanged with a multiuser conference line. As global communication occurs quickly and efficiently with access to the Internet and a video camera, connections with multiple individuals in many locations are commonplace. With the introduction of affordable video conferencing, physical presence is less important. Heavy desktop computers have been replaced with flat-screen monitors and handheld devices. Data storage capacity is significant because sophisticated users have unlimited access to information on the Internet. Leadership roles have evolved to include roles of accessing, filtering, and interpreting information for others. With this rapid and prolific ability to instantly communicate comes further disruption of the organization requiring leaders to embrace the network of communications or attempt to maintain linear order. Both have advantages and disadvantages.

The changes in media availability will alter current work flows in the organization and require new ways to manage the decreased length of processing time, data storage, hardware, and software. Further, although media have been more readily available to others, it is nearly impossible for workers to access, interpret, and manage the information as quickly as it is now available. The limitations are now human personnel availability rather than the timely movement of media. Another interesting phenomenon is the challenges of privacy regulations and how to be compliant with them. In some cases, leaders are restricting access to text, web, and video media and are thus restricting information flow into the organization, reinforcing a linear model of communication rather than the complex reality.

Another example of evolving communication is the creation of social media accounts by most senior leaders, inviting members of the organization to share ideas and feedback continuously. Rather than the traditional, formal face-to-face meeting, leaders are now accessible to employees with Internet access 24 hours a day, 7 days a week. Based on these changes, new assumptions about the structure of organizations are needed. The new infrastructure is now based on openness and minimal lines of authority or divisions of work units. Behaviors and structures that support unconstrained communication and open relationships are redefining the roles and accountabilities of both leaders and staff.

Stakeholder Location

The location of both providers and users of the healthcare system changed dramatically with the introduction of the Internet. Providers are now often remote while providing assessment, observations, and robotic interventions. As a result, the role of physical space and location is changing. The functionality and utility of physical space in many settings has shifted from accommodating both providers and users of the healthcare system to accommodation for the user of the system and the technology to support virtual services. Further, both the provider and user may remain in their own settings while the technology equipment is stored in central locations. Gathering together at common sites is becoming the exception rather than the rule.

In the current context of large and complex facilities, the physical space among individuals, offices, and geographical locations that once resulted in a delay in communication between individuals, as well as a delay in the transmittance of paper documents, is now minimized and in some cases eliminated. The need for individual office space is now questioned regularly. The utility and purpose of individual private office space and the affordability of spaces used that are used less than 10% of the time provide an opportunity for new configurations. Space for teamwork rather than individual work space is preferred. What is not clear is the appropriate mix of face time on-site and off-site in which communication occurs using audiovisual technologies. Even with the best technologies, physical gatherings remain an essential part of the work processes. To be sure, there is nothing better than a welcome hug from a long-time colleague or a welcoming hand extended to a new member of the team. As the organization moves forward, efforts will continue to determine how best to optimize human gatherings and available technology. New consideration about the use of physical space will focus on value, flexibility, and multipurpose use for both individuals and teams. Current examples include the repurposing of waiting areas to healing spaces, multiuser access to examination rooms based on need rather than specific ownership of a room, and multipurpose telemedicine rooms supporting multiple providers. These changes require new approaches in managing virtual workforces and off-site clinicians to assure engagement in the organizational vision and mission while supporting a work–life balance.

Discussion: Media, Space, and Time

The changes from the Internet impact different generations in different ways. Convene a group that includes representatives from as many generations as possible and explore the following topics:

- Ask each person how he or she has been impacted (or not) by the changes in media, space, and time.
- What practice changes have been necessary to accommodate the ready access to individuals and data?
- Are there innovations or changes that could assist all generations with these advances?

Time

Traditionally, work was accomplished at the workplace during specified hours. With the Internet, the time parameters for availability and access to data are forever blurred. Shared files and social networks now make connections possible at any time in any location across the globe. Waiting time for global dialogue is nearly nonexistent and often dependent only on the work and sleep schedules of individuals around the world. No longer is the individual waiting for the mail to arrive—an e-mail is waiting!

Further, traditional shift times and lengths may be even more flexible as virtual care is integrated with physical, on-site care. Research on fatigue of caregivers identified issues of compromised competence near 12.5 hours in a 24-hour period or 40 hours in 1 week (Geiger-Brown et al., 2012; Martin, 2014; Rogers, 2002; Stimpfel, Lake, Barton, Gorman, & Aiken, 2013). Different shift lengths or rest period intervals may be required with increased screen monitoring work.

MORE THOUGHTS ON THE IMPACT OF THE INTERNET

To be sure, the unceremonious dismantling of traditional organizational structures and processes increases the chaos in healthcare organizations. Necessarily, the evolving organizational infrastructure is dynamic rather than static and stable. The available digital world requires leaders to continually challenge the expectations of turnaround time and access to individuals related to organizational communication, interdisciplinary collaboration, the location of providers and patients, and the time frames in which this work can occur.

While these advances are exciting to many individuals, some individuals are resistant to the shifts to the digital world. The resistance is part of the transformation to a new paradigm and necessarily increases chaos and complexity for the leader. The resistance to advancement of an evidentiary paradigm may in fact be driven by the historical absence of focus on evidentiary thinking and processes.

It is important to remember that the role of leaders in an evidence–innovation dynamic is relatively new but critical to organizational effectiveness. Creating evidence to support the evolving organizational structure dynamic is an imperative for successful organizational performance.

If your actions inspire others to dream more, learn more, do more and become more, you are a leader.

—JOHN QUINCY ADAMS

MOVING FORWARD: RETHINKING ORGANIZATIONAL STRUCTURE AND ROLE ACCOUNTABILITIES

The transformational work for leaders begins with an end in mind; a desired state that is believed to achieve value for the users of the organization. An assessment and gap analysis on the basis of organizational context and professional roles begins the process. In the next section of this chapter, new thoughts on the foundational framework for this work and specific changes in role obligations and behaviors are discussed. Necessarily, this work must be fully sensitive to and carefully integrated into the organizational culture—the underlying assumptions, defining values, and artifacts that embody the organization. The behaviors and norms supportive of new expectations include a vision and infrastructure that continually support and develop the capacity to change, the capacity to evaluate and integrate changes resulting from digital innovations, increased communication access, media management, and expedited work flow. **Figure 3-1** reflects the proposed evidentiary dynamic and the intersecting components.

Stability is no longer the goal for the healthcare leader; the goals now support continual evaluation of new ideas while ensuring that competent and safe patient care is provided. The emphasis on high-reliability organizations is now more actively tempered with the notion of focus and accountability on the work being done with the understanding that procedures necessarily will change. The emphasis must not be on

Figure 3-1 Evidentiary organization: Dynamics and intersection components

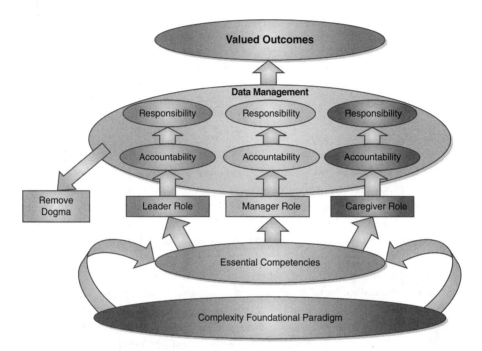

completing high-reliability checklists and redundancies; the emphasis, or time out, needs to focus on defining the team's goal: what is the team doing, and is it the right thing? Are we using the most contemporary, evidence-based approach for the work we are doing?

Now, the challenge for the leader is how to facilitate the development of essential roles, accountabilities, competence, and expectations in team members for excellence in patient care services and simultaneously ensure flexibility and openness to new and emerging processes. The desired healthcare culture is no longer able to solely support cultures of rote performance based on standards, practices, and technology developed yesterday and achieve the optimal outcomes of today and tomorrow. The continual evaluation and introduction of new work processes and technology require higher levels of presence and engagement than ever thought possible.

In addition to the expectations for evolving work processes, an increase in diversity competence is expected. Patients are now from a global, virtual world that is increasingly diverse. Caregiver knowledge of multiple cultural traditions, beliefs, and values is foundational. An increasing challenge is for the caregiver to sublimate personal values in deference to the patient's unique values. Providing patient care services from the perspective of one's social obligation as a provider now assumes more significance in the global world. Preferences for treatment modalities, family involvement, life and death rituals, and so the role of the caregiver vary more widely now, based on the individual patient. Now more than ever the provision of person and family-centered care is essential (Barnsteiner, Disch & Walton, 2014). The best decisions for the patient based on his or her beliefs and values must now be supported by structures and processes in the healthcare system as the norm rather than the exception.

As such, leadership staff is called to skillfully and persistently work to transform the organizational culture to be less reliant on traditional static authority-based communication structures to a more dynamic infrastructure that recognizes interrelated and intersecting roles and communication across complex networks. These changes are only now possible because of our increasing capacity to apprehend organizational complexity brought about by the Internet. Necessarily, the traditional box and line organizational diagrams need to go by the wayside because there is no information to be gained from them. The Internet, as previously noted, has eliminated hierarchies and standard lines of communication, thus the historical diagrams do not provide direction or information for members of the organization.

This endeavor requires a series of steps that begin with personal and organizational reflection and a call to the table of the most senior leaders to generate both a framework and a set of expectations with regard to evidence-based decision making and action taking (Giacco, 2003; Wager, Wickham, & Glaser, 2005). Reflection at the highest levels of the organization and the construction of evidentiary foundations upon which strategy, tactics, performance, and outcome measures can be based, create a foundation from which data that builds evidence-driven practices can emerge. Further, their relationship to positive impacts and outcomes can be established. These steps include transformation to a complexity-driven foundation, creation of clear accountability expectations for role performance, and development of a sophisticated data management infrastructure.

COMPLEXITY: MOVING FROM STATIC TO DYNAMIC PARADIGM

Recognition of the nature of the complexity in organizations is an important step in beginning the transformation. In quantum thinking and within complexity-defined systems, change is a constant, a fundamental dynamic of existence. In this circumstance, change is an existential condition, uncontrolled, beyond human manipulation; it is also a fundamental characteristic and operation of the universe (Blum, 2006). Complexity and complex systems thinking and research have provided a strong contemporary foundation for rethinking and reconfiguring the leadership and management and caregiver roles in complex organizations (Murphy, Ruch, Pepicello, & Murphy, 1997; Shan & Ang, 2008; Suh, 2005; Zimmerman, Lindberg, & Plsek, 1998). Thus, the organizational structure must now be influenced by these complexity attributes.

Accomplishment will prove to be a journey, not a destination.

—DWIGHT D. EISENHOWER

The most important element to shift to an evidentiary framework for the leader is the recognition that past leadership practices have been guided by linear, cognitive, and rational processes that reflect rather predictable changes in processes and outputs. In the new environment, decision making and action must reflect more nonlinear and quantum influences in human dynamics and behavior. The evidence-based leader understands that human (and, therefore, health) behavior, is such that change is better conceptualized, understood, and addressed through the lens of complex adaptive/responsive processes (Ang & Yin, 2008).

The attributes of nonlinearity, self-organization, uncertainty, emergence, interaction, intersection, and limited span of control describe the nature of complex organizations. The complex systems literature has demonstrated the power and influence of self-organization and emergence within organizations (Miller & Scott, 2007). This new research is revising the foundations for understanding leadership practices and behavior and even reconceptualizing the role and application of leadership in organization decision making and actions (Morrison, 2007).

Much of the work on complex systems sciences emerged from the biological, social, and physical sciences. The convergence of those data revealed patterns of behavior that emerged from examples of interacting and intersecting human societies, e-systems, ecosystems, the human brain, and bee colonies, among others (Rouse, 2007). These various exemplars of systems now serve to inform our understanding of the role of the leader and the interactions of leaders with and within the systems of which they are a part (Stacey, 2007).

A larger question related to complex systems is how much control should be exercised by the agent of control (the manager) within systems—in this case, within the healthcare system. We know that varying levels of agency control are evident in a variety of systems. For example, on the Internet, almost no central control is exerted. In contrast, in the military and the solar system, high levels of control are exhibited. In the human body, intermediate interacting levels of control are evidenced.

Degrees of criticalness also influence level of agent control. In highly critical circumstances, where the life of an organism or system is directly and dramatically threatened, high levels of control are necessary to stabilize the system and bring it back into balance. By comparison, in systems with a high level of equilibrium and good responsive interface between external environmental challenges and demands, and internal mechanisms of response, low levels of critical condition exist and, therefore, there is a reduced need for levels of agent control (Solow & Szmerekovsky, 2006).

Within the frame of complexity, there is the understanding that complex adaptive systems represent a highly complex dynamic of interacting and intersecting forces operating externally and internally, constantly affecting the life of the system (Yin & Ang, 2008). For example, the management of a patient in a critical care unit requires much more agent intervention surveillance and intensity than does the management of a patient in a long-term care facility or hospice setting. In many day-to-day nursing activities and work flows, increased control by management can actually inhibit the ability for the frontline care provider to use the best evidence, exercise clinical judgment, or practice at the top of his or her license. Excessive control and micromanagement removes adaptability from the system.

The degree of agent control and manipulation of circumstance and relational variables leads to different agent roles and relationships with respect to the amount of control needed or desired. Evidence-based management perceives this relationship in terms of the complex network of intersections and interactions and the degree of internally generated locus of control or the degree of external management of control. In broad terms, the incidence of emergent leadership and its influence on decision making and action may be directly related to the level of agent control, ranging from highly critical (greatest agent control) to highly self-managed (least agent control). For example, the greatest agent control would be for a leader to assign a project and the project plan to the team complete the work; in the least control situation, the leader would assign problem resolution (outcome) to the team to determine what the process and approach should be to address the problem. The next area of assessment for the leader is assuring the presence of an evidentiary dynamic—a dynamic that fully integrates operations and innovation as well as the transformation between them.

Integrating Operations and Innovation

In current organizations, increasing efforts to address complexity are seen in the establishment of innovation centers or departments to support and assess new products and processes—processes that are congruent with a complexity paradigm in which uncertainty is the norm, and emergence, and highly interacting and intersecting relationships are present. **Box 3-1** includes common strategies currently used by organizations to generate new ideas and processes. The contemporary organization requires an infrastructure that effectively supports both the linear, predictable, evidence-based processes in routine operations alongside the integration of innovations to replace

Box 3-1 Tools to Advance Change and Innovation

- Deep dive: A particular area is selected for observation in multiple ways. Work flows, photos, interviews, and observations are gathered by a team to analyze current processes and brainstorm new ways of doing the current work processes (Kelly, 2005).
- Directed creativity: A situation is proposed to encourage and advance new ideas. For example, individuals are presented with the following scenario and directed to respond: A new unit is being designed for medical–surgical patients. If there were no limits on space, technology, resources, staff, or financial resources, how would you design the unit for the future in a way to dramatically improve the cost and quality of the healthcare experience (Plsek, 1997).
- Mind mapping: Mind mapping is a software tool for collecting, organizing, and synthesizing large amounts of data in layers, with complex relationships. It is a very useful tool for documents connectivity, interdependencies, and emerging phenomena in health care.
- Innovation space: An innovation space is a place or laboratory where inquiring minds collaborate to create a more livable and sustainable world focused on developing products that create market value while serving real societal needs—products that are progressive, possible, and profitable (Boradkar, 2010).
- Brainstorming: A collective exercise process to generate ideas. A good exercise generates 100 ideas. This is different from directed creativity in that brainstorming focuses on suspending judgment and criticism, encourages freewheel thinking and quantity of ideas, and builds on the ideas of others (Endsley, 2010).

outdated operations at the appropriate time as well as an openness to testing and implementing new ideas. Oftentimes, this seems contradictory; however, in an evidentiary dynamic model, both the evidence-based work and the creation of new evidence from innovation must be supported in an ongoing process. Traditional organizational models have segmented innovation from routine operations and limited the flexibility and responsiveness of the organization.

The accelerated velocity of the introduction of new ideas further supports the need for an integrated approach to an advancement of innovation and an emphasis on the transition from innovation to operation. More importantly, there is a need to integrate the work of innovation with the work of each particular role. New ideas should be generated and developed in ways that take into account the perspectives of point-of-care knowledge workers. In a complexity-driven organizational model, the lines among operations, innovations, and transformation become blurred as responsibility and accountability behaviors are elevated and particularized for each role in the organization.

In an evidence-based framework, engagement and involvement inside the innovation process reflect the least intensity of agent control, allowing the greatest freedom in an environment that fosters successful innovation. Ready access to all of the supports, resources, tools, and processes that facilitate the energetic and free-flowing activities of creativity would be essential to innovation. The manager in this case would create conditions and circumstances that permit this more open dynamic to thrive. By contrast, emergence of this type of control would be less likely in a situation where the variables need to be tightly manipulated and managed with narrowly defined but clearly applied manager (agent) control, such as in situations involving employee discipline, critical interventions, system control (such as in a prison), or terrorism. The next section presents a discussion of the transformation of three essential professional roles.

LEADERS, MANAGERS, AND DIRECT CARE PROVIDER ROLES IN AN EVIDENTIARY DYNAMIC

Three major roles are required in an evidentiary organization: leader, manager, and caregiver. Each of these roles has distinct descriptions. **Table 3-2** provides an overview of the essential elements of each role and the supportive accountability, responsibility, and value for each role. Note that each of these roles is considered a knowledge worker's because his or her work is based on knowledge capital and includes nonroutine problem solving and creative thinking (Reinhardt, Schmidt, Sloep & Drachsler, 2011).

First, the leader role is accountable to create the organizational context for value creation—a context that provides the support necessary to ensure that appropriate decisions and actions are undertaken along with adequate resources for the work and desired outcomes. Like all roles, the leader bases decisions on evidence and the importance of creating new evidence where none is available. The leader is aware of the confluence and consonance of interactions among external environmental forces and internal relational, operational, and behavioral responses to an ever-changing set of circumstances (Frandkov, 1999). Members of an evidentiary community reflect attitudes, competencies, and specific role behaviors to support the transformed organization.

The role of leadership in this movement is self-evident. Because leaders have the predominant role in creating the context and providing the supports necessary to ensure that appropriate decisions and actions are undertaken, resourcing and applying structure to these new models are obligations of the leader role. Performing this role effectively requires clarity of the conceptual role, personal knowledge, leadership principles, collaboration, synthesis, knowledge management, and mentoring. Aware and informed healthcare leaders stay abreast of the changing conditions and context for the application of clinical service. Through deliberation and dialogue at the strategic and tactical

Table 3-2   Evidentiary Organization: Key Roles and Accountabilities

	Knowledge Workers[a]		
	Leader Role	**Manager Role**	**Direct Care Provider role**
Accountable for: • **Doing the right work** • **Focusing on the product and results of work; the actual difference the work makes**	• Creates the context for accountability, responsibility, and value creation • Recognizes the action of complexity and the value of establishing new roles responding to current circumstances • Recognizes the confluence and consonance of interaction between external environmental forces and internal relational, operational, and behavioral response to an ever-changing set of circumstances • Assures there is support necessary for appropriate decisions and actions, resourcing • Integrates an evidence-based value set • Creates the data infrastructure	• Facilitates the planning and construction of designs for creating infrastructure and processes that support point of service, evidence-based data integration and translation of its utility into clinical practice • Applies contemporary research and theory of complex systems, and translation and use of this information in the workplace • Develops the infrastructure for evidence-based processes through the analysis of patterns within the system • Applies clinical research and theory of complex systems and translation, and use of this information in the workplace • Manages data relationships – establish the attachment between data and clinical decision making at the point of service; data are available and integrated for effective decisions	• Accountability for performance and achievement of clinical outcomes rests exclusively and solely with the competent practitioner • Seeks out and uses all available evidence/data to make decisions and provide care

(*Continued*)

Table 3-2 **Evidentiary Organization: Key Roles and Accountabilities** *(Continued)*

	Knowledge Workers[a]		
	Leader Role	**Manager Role**	**Direct Care Provider role**
Responsible for: • **Doing the work well**	• Provides effective systems, structures, and resources for the work to be done	• Provides effective infrastructures for patient care recognizing complexity, interrelationships, and current evidence within patient care dynamics	• Provides evidence-based, state-of-the-art patient care that results in the desired value to the patient and family
Valued Outcomes	• Increased health of populations served • Increases evidentiary resources • Goodness of fit between desired outcomes (value) and effective processes associated with obtaining them • Sustainable		

[a] Knowledge worker: An individual whose main capital is knowledge and has an emphasis on nonroutine problem solving that requires a combination of convergent, divergent, and creative thinking.
Data from Reinhardt, W., Schmidt, B., Sloep, P., & Drachsler, H. (2011). Knowledge worker roles and actions: Results of two empirical studies. *Knowledge and Process Management, 18*(3), 150–174. doi:10.1002/kpm.378

levels of the organization, these managers facilitate the planning and construction of designs for creating infrastructure and processes that would support point-of-service, evidence-based data integration and translation of its utility into clinical practice.

The manager represents the contemporary application of the theory and research of the action of complex systems and the translation and use of that understanding in decisions and actions in the workplace. For the manager, just as for the clinician, the development of the infrastructure reflects the application of complexity theory and complex adaptive systems to the work relationships, behaviors, and structures constantly operating to influence clinical practice and outcomes. The manager recognizes the action of complexity and the value of establishing the evolving role factors, including new roles responding to the current circumstances and the activities unfolding within them.

The manager's requisite abilities related to scanning, predictive capacity, and adaptation now come to bear as a critical skill set in the creation of the structures and processes in support of contemporary evidence-based initiatives (Hesselbein, 2002). Indeed, managers represent in their own practice and performance the use of evidentiary strategies and tactics in advising decisions and taking actions related to resource use, demonstrated in their own management of human, fiscal, material, support, and systems accountabilities. The role played by strong, evidence-committed management leaders is enhanced by their willingness to both model and mentor evidentiary dynamics as the appropriate contemporary framework within which all work relationships and clinical performance unfold. Caregivers are accountable for the performance of patient care interventions and the achievement of clinical outcomes using the latest evidence-based interventions. In particular, caregivers are owners of their nontransferable capital and capacity of the application of their work. Their knowledge is mobile and portable; that is, their knowledge goes with them wherever they go.

After the role descriptions are clear for the leader, manager, and direct care giver, the associated accountabilities are identified. These distinctions are necessarily driven from evidence rather than experience and intuition.

ROLE ACCOUNTABILITY, RESPONSIBILITY, AND KNOWLEDGE OWNERSHIP

Each of the described roles have associated behaviors to support a complex system in which evidence and innovation are inexorably interwoven and reflect clear expectations for professional accountability, responsibility, and the management of knowledge.

Accountability

In knowledge work environments such as hospitals and healthcare systems, the notion of accountability takes on special meaning. Knowledge workers own the means of their own capital, and this means is now as significant as any other sources of capital and human-intensive organizations (Reinhart et al., 2011; Sveiby, 1997). Knowledge workers have an individually driven sense of ownership with regard to their knowledge and its demonstration in the applications of work (Hooker & Csikszentmihalvi, 2003). Embedded in this understanding of knowledge work ownership are the mobility and portability of that knowledge because the knowledge worker carries the knowledge wherever he or she operates in the system. This flexibility is another important consideration with regard to accountability. Knowledge workers do not transfer the locus of control for their accountability to institutions, organizations, or others outside their knowledge work community. Accountability for the performance and achievement of outcomes rests exclusively and solely with each role. Accountability for creation of the context of accountability rests with the leader. Accountability for facilitating and designing the infrastructure for practice rests with the manager.

This notion of ownership in relationship to accountability is critical to the professional knowledge worker; it also informs the management of these workers. As such, ownership for the work of practice does not transfer to the management role, and managers cannot be held accountable for the outcomes of practice owned by the caregivers whose capacity and competence are essential to both achieving and sustaining outcomes (Porter-O'Grady, 2000). Because ownership is invested in each role, if the desired outcomes are to be achieved, the role of management is to create an organization and systems context that facilitates, supports, and encourages the ownership and expression of accountability (Albrecht, 2003).

In short, the accountability of management differs in important ways from the accountability of the direct care provider. The effectiveness of work and the achievement of outcomes belongs to the knowledge worker caregiver; the creation of context that frames and supports the work and accountability of staff is the source of accountability for management (Dotlich & Cairo, 2002). The outcome of the knowledge worker management role is the same as that of the knowledge worker staff: effective patient care that leads to positive clinical outcomes. However, accountability for achieving those ends is significantly different in a management role as compared to the knowledge worker staff role. The activities associated with one are differentiated from the activities associated with the other. Yet, both roles are necessary to create the dynamic—the intersection—necessary to sustain performance outcomes.

Discussion

Accountability is a concept often bandied about and misinterpreted. After there is understanding that accountability requires the licensed person to perform interventions as indicated for the patient, there are often challenges from others to modify practice. Consider the following situation:

You are instructed to discontinue protective isolation by the chief executive officer (CEO) because the patient's family has a high profile and does not want to be bothered. Using the principles of accountability, how would you handle this? Can the clinician take directions about patient care from the CEO?

Management accountability relates to the quality and integrity of the direction, and infrastructure of systems, and the degree of integrity of their relationship with the work and performance outcomes of the knowledge worker stakeholders. In partnership with knowledge workers, the leaders of the organization aggregate the efforts of systems and people in a mosaic of intersection and performance that networks strategy, infrastructure, resources, and knowledge work in the configuration (a dance, if you will) of consonance and contribution that advances both the clinical outcomes for patients and the organizational viability of the system (Pidd, 2004).

Indeed, managers represent in their own practice and performance the use of evidentiary strategies and tactics in advising decisions and taking actions related to resource use, demonstrated in their own management of human, fiscal, material, support, and systems accountabilities. The role played by strong, evidence-committed management leaders is enhanced by their willingness to both model and mentor evidentiary dynamics as the appropriate contemporary framework within which all work relationships and clinical performance unfold. As the new context based on complexity emerges within the three foundational roles and accountability expectations, there are four competencies or attitudes that are also essential behaviors within each of these roles.

Competencies

There are four essential competencies or attitudes for all members of the organization: inquisitive, vulnerable, inclusive, and proactive. **Table 3-3** presents the core content of each competency and role expectation for the leader, manager, and direct caregiver. These are often challenging to identify objectively; however, the results of these competencies are evident in the increasingly successful outcomes of the organization at the individual, organization, and community levels.

Inquisitive

Successful individuals are continually inquisitive about the nature of the work, the factors impacting and the evidence supporting current work, and new ideas that are being introduced. In particular, individuals demonstrate a high regard for and value creativity, have an openness to new ideas, are comfortable in challenging assumptions, and can see conflict as diversity. As agents of change, these individuals are continually enhancing their knowledge of innovation and change content, tools, processes, and challenges. Knowing the science and art of innovation is essential.

There are numerous descriptions and definitions of innovation (**Box 3-2**) that guide the work of innovation leaders. As knowledge in innovation leadership emerges, more descriptions will be presented. The skeptic often dismisses innovation with the belief that nothing new ever really occurs; rather it is only new combinations and iterations of existing products and processes that occur. This approach may indeed be an

Table 3-3 Evidentiary Competencies: Basics for Advancing New Work in Complex Organizations

Competency	Core Content	Role: Leader, Manager, Caregiver
Inquisitive	Innovation knowledge Self-knowledge; personal management; self-care	Knowledge system manager Data manager Role knowledge
Vulnerable/courageous	Courageous Challenges practice and assumptions for increased understanding and improvement Open to new ideas	Experimenter and tester of new ideas
Inclusive	Relationship builder	Facilitator of individuals and teams to achieve value; coach, mentor, collaborate Diversity facilitator; conflict embracer/engager Technology versus humanness
Proactive	Synthesizer; strategist	Critical strategist and value creator; business case creator

example of a delaying tactic and does little to address the need for the organization to be contemporary in its work. Becoming tangled in the conceptual precision discussion may serve only to delay meaningful discussion and attention to the future.

Individuals are also inquisitive about their own personal skill sets. Self-knowledge and competence with innovation and change further assist individuals. A clear understanding of one's personal strengths and limitations as they relate to the evidentiary dynamic is essential to create the business case for developing new ideas.

Assessments of decision making, communication, and conflict resolution styles are foundational areas of focus in self-knowledge assessment. The Myers & Briggs (http://www.myersbriggs.org) and DiSC (http://www.profiles4u.com/what-is-disc-profile.asp) assessments are examples of helpful assessment tools for individuals. Although individuals often overemphasize self-assessments to learn about styles, strengths, and limitations, the label or category into which the individual falls should never be the primary focal point. Rather, the information about styles is intended to provide insight into an overall set of behaviors and does not reflect all activities. The ability to understand others and collaborate with multiple styles in multidisciplinary teams are essential competencies.

Box 3-2 Change and Innovation: Common Descriptions

- The implementation of new or altered products, services, processes, systems, organizational structures, or business models as a means of improving one or more domains of health care quality (AHRQ Health Care Innovations Exchange)
- Anything that creates new resources, processes, or values or improves a company's existing resources, processes, or values (Christenson, Anthony & Roth, 2004)
- The power to redefine the industry; the effort to create purposeful focused change in an enterprise's economic or social potential (Drucker, 1985)
- The conversation of knowledge and ideas into a benefit that may be for commercial use or for the public good; the benefit may be new or improved products, processes, or values (Christenson et al., 2004)
- The power to redefine the industry; the effort to create purposeful, focused change in an enterprise's economic or social potential (Drucker, 1985)
- A new patterning of our experiences of being together as new meaning emerges from ordinary, everyday work conversations (Fonesca, 2002)
- The first practical, concerted implementation of an idea done in a way that brings broad-based, extrinsic recognition to an individual or organization (Plsek, 1997)
- A historic and irreversible change in the way of doing things; creative destruction (Schumpeter, 1943)
- Emergent continuity and transformation of patterns of human interactions understood as ongoing ordinary complex responsive processes of human relating in local situations in the living present (Stacey, 2007)
- Innovation is something new, or perceived as new by the population experiencing the innovation, that has the potential to drive change and redefine health care's economic and/or social potential (Weberg, 2010)
- Fresh thinking that leads to value creation (Vaitheeswaran, 2007)

Individuals also assess their information processing and thinking systems styles as a means to excel. The relationship between emotions and intellectual content is important in understanding not only one's personal style, but also the abilities of others. Consideration is also given to understanding rational and experiential information processing styles (Cerni, Curtis, & Colmar, 2008). Rational processing is analytical, intentional, logical, and slower, whereas experiential information processing is holistic, automatic, associative, and faster. Necessarily, both modes of processing are required to be effective. Areas of strength and areas of development opportunities guide professional development and growth.

Self-care is another area the individual focuses on as part of the self-knowledge assessment. The individual's sense of self is well developed along with the importance of maintaining high levels of performance and wellness. The work in an evidentiary organization is demanding and unrelenting, requiring individuals to be healthy, energetic, and resilient. Oftentimes there is a need for a little bit of narcissism—self-care is essential for energy renewal for the innovation leader. Taking time to balance work with one's personal life is essential to sustain high levels of performance and productivity.

Vulnerability

The second competency is about vulnerability—being open and comfortable with uncertainty and being comfortable with the limitations of one's knowledge (Whitehurst, 2015). Vulnerable individuals are comfortable with the fact that one can never know everything and that this perpetual incompleteness is a fundamental trait of all individuals. The essential work is connecting and creating meaningful relationships with others who have different areas of expertise.

Courage is an element of vulnerability in that the individual is willing to discuss sacred cows and challenge long-standing practices and dare to eliminate obsolete healthcare dogma and not being afraid of criticism or ridicule that might result. This courage also guides the innovation leader in facilitating effective and difficult dialogue. When things are not going well, the individual examines and evaluates the situation and facilitates appropriate course correction quickly. This course correction emphasizes learning from experience without ascribing blame to anyone.

Inclusive

The third competency is about being inclusive of multiple individuals and points of view. As a collaborator, individuals demonstrate high-level competence in listening, encouraging feedback, and conflict utilization. Differing perspectives and values are not seen as conflicts to be resolved or mediated, but rather as an expression of diversity. Many obstacles are encountered along the innovation continuum. Individuals, equipment, resources, and time can all be the source of conflict among team members. The innovation leader perceives conflicts as opportunities to learn more about the issues and to gain insight into the values and beliefs of others. The leader avoids efforts to neutralize or minimize the differing opinions until more information is gained. Necessarily, the innovation leader is a master change facilitator and is able to use conflict as an opportunity to gain further insight of pertinent issues.

For individuals in this type of organization, effective collaboration is about moving from a group of assembled individuals to a team of highly interactive, participative, goal-oriented individuals. Individuals thrive in multidisciplinary teams—the fundamental unit in the organization. The individual is always considered incomplete because one can never know all there is to know. Working alone or in single-discipline dialogue is inefficient and ineffective. Transdisciplinary dialogue is the norm to address issues of complexity and innovation. The innovation leader is patient, tolerant, and interested in diverse discussion to facilitate teamwork. In fact, innovation leaders seek out those known for strong opinions, the ability to challenge others, taking risks, and thinking creatively. In addition, the goal of being inclusive is about learning from others to find common ground while avoiding the rubber stamps of prattled conversation. Principles of appreciative inquiry guide interactions.

Teams often include disparate disciplines, such as clinicians, engineers, computer specialists, designers, and representatives from several generations and ethnic cultures. Courageous individuals are role models in the activities of challenging traditional norms and practices, and confronting each other when resistance is evident. As team members, they encourage comments on others' ideas; withholding feedback is considered counterproductive to the entire process. The goal is for sharing feedback to be a core behavior, rather than optional.

Within each role of leader, manager, and caregiver, the attitude of inclusiveness begets facilitation, coaching, and mentoring. Individuals facilitate the development of innovation principles and strategies among colleagues, adult learning, and the importance of system change. Further, individuals work to empower the creative genius in others. Creative genius is that part of each individual that has a possibilities-oriented, can-do attitude and way of being that communicates to everyone that anything is possible; it is about being full of excitement, energy, and ideas (McGlade & Pek, 2008).

These contextual attributes are realized in the dynamic evidentiary organization in which communication is encouraged and permission is not required to collaborate with others across departments and levels in the organization. There is a spirit of candor and a free flow of information without fear of criticism or reprisal. The reality is that some individuals have information at different times, and sharing ideas informally can increase the organization's capacity to solve problems and meet challenges. The goal is to use information to support optimal organizational performance; it is not to gossip or engage in one-upmanship competitions.

The behaviors of all individuals should reflect communication in an unrestricted manner, interest in new ideas, and willingness to challenge long-held assumptions. This open culture requires tolerance for the possibility of error and a climate in which errors can be discussed freely and the underlying causes investigated and corrected quickly (Whittingham, 2003). The successful culture is one in which leaders are competent across organizational operations, transformations, and innovations.

These competencies assume a high level of trust among individuals in the organization. As the culture evolves, greater trust is earned with much effort and consistency of behaviors. The culture is truly brought to life by the leaders of the organization as they role model their competencies. To be sure, this is an iterative process of cultural evolution and development of leader expertise.

Proactive

The fourth competency is about being proactive, about thinking into the future. Individuals want to be actively planning for a better future. The leader moves from reliance on historical knowledge to imagining, intuiting, inspiring, and reflecting the present as the means to the future (Scharmer & Kaufer, 2000).

The proactive individual demonstrates competence as a synthesizer and strategist and thrives with the rapid and continuous introduction of new ideas, processes, technology, and equipment. Managing and gathering large amounts of data to elicit evidentiary adequacy, value, and potential outcomes further exemplifies performance. Information is quickly synthesized from multiple sources to create a comprehensive set of next steps for advancement using the wisdom of all team members and combined into a critical mass of expertise. New ideas are introduced after careful analysis using a business case for innovation. Individuals formulate key data into formal documents to identify the value of new work, the level of current evidence, and its clear relationship to the mission and vision of the organization.

From this proactive, evidence-building approach, creation of the business case becomes powerful. A business case or the rationale for expenditure of resources under certain circumstances is essential to support appropriate resource allocations (Burns, 2005). The elements of a strong business case for innovation include the following:

- A description of the new product or service
- The intended purpose or goal of the innovation
- Projection of costs specific to accomplish the innovation
- Costs excluded from the proposal and rationale for exclusion
- Projected benefits and rationale for valuing of benefits
- A timeline for the project from initiation to benefits realization
- Anticipated profit or loss
- Expected nonfinancial benefits
- Anticipated risks and plans to mediate risks
- Overall summary of both short-term and long-term value to the organization and community (https://www.nibusinessinfo.co.uk/innovationgrowth)

Within these major categories of the innovation business case, information specific to anticipated productivity changes, reductions in cost, market share, patient quality outcomes, new partnerships, and risks for not moving forward, such as losing market share, productivity loss, employee turnover, and profit margin, must be included. Further, information, that identifies how the new work could differentiate the organization from competitors, benefit multiple constituencies in the organization, and extend the life of the organization as a value-producing entity, is an important element of this business case (Merrifield, Calhoun, & Stevens, 2008).

Building the strategic business case for new and untested ideas requires a modified approach from preparing a traditional business plan because of the unknown outcome of the innovation and the inadequacy of operational tools for innovation. Creating a sustainable budget or projection for an innovation requires knowledge about the past, which may be completely irrelevant, and estimations about the future that include cost of materials, technology, and human resources, and expected revenues. Christensen, Kaufman, and Shih (2008) identified the challenges in creating the business case as the lack of good financial tools to understand the market, build brands, find customers, select employees, organize teams, and develop strategies to advance the work. Specifically, when an organization relies on traditional discounted cash flow and net present value to evaluate investment opportunities, the real returns and benefits are often underestimated. Consideration of fixed and sunk costs using traditional models creates an unfair advantage on challengers and inhibits incumbent firms that attempt to respond. Finally, the emphasis on earnings per share as the primary metric for success diverts resources from investments whose payoff occurs at a much later date. According to Christensen and colleagues (2008), although these tools are good for operations, they create a systematic bias against innovation. It is challenging but not impossible to create the case for new work processes and products given the need for improvements in patient safety and quality outcomes. These four competencies are essential areas for growth and development of contemporary healthcare workers as they continue to develop high-level professional accountability. In addition, each role in the evidentiary organization must be able to access and manage the appropriate data for specific role accountabilities.

EVIDENCE-DRIVEN DECISION MAKING AND ANALYSIS: MANAGING DATA AND MORE DATA

In an evidentiary dynamic organization, management of data by all three roles is critical. To be sure, all organizations are awash with data. It is not so much the collection of data that is important, but rather the ability to use those data, analyze them, and make decisions and take action based on what the analysis reveals (Chakravarthy, 2003; Garvin & Roberto, 2001; Porter-O'Grady & Afable, 2003). Without question, in today's information-driven business world, the ability to manage data and use it appropriately is a fundamental management skill set. This love for and attachment to data, including the management of data and the analysis of its impacts, is a central prerequisite and an essential tool in the armamentarium of the good leader (Davenport, 2006). Attachment to data means having competence for gathering, aggregating, translating, interpreting, and applying it in a way that is meaningful and makes a difference in the lives of those who will use the data. It is important to note that knowledge is the lifeblood of innovative and complex organizations. Leaders then help to translate data into knowledge that will assist members of the organization. Data-driven decision making means more than simply relating to the data. It means establishing an intense relationship with data processes so that the structure of data becomes both a facilitating factor and a seamless integration. The data-driven process supports real-time communication and information, and the application of data entails real-time informing, guiding, and solution seeking at the point of decision and action (Ball, 2000; Oostendorp, 2003). Consider three questions posed by Allworth, Wessel, and Levie (2015):

1. What is the job to be done?
2. In a perfect world, what information would help you complete that job?
3. If you had this information, what inside your organization would need to change?

Of real importance is the ability to make this strong attachment or connection to data and analysis a part of the fundamental work experience for each individual in the organization. Translating data management into a real attachment to the use of data by knowledge workers is a formidable undertaking. Nevertheless, if the connection can be made between the value of work and the extent to which it is informed by data-driven decision making and evaluated by data-clarified measures, then leaders can begin to establish an attachment between the use of data and evidence, and the clinical decisions made and actions taken at the point of service. To accomplish this goal, such processes must be seamlessly integrated into the recording, collection, and assessment of information, and directly connected to the decision processes whose value and accuracy depend on both the veracity and the utility of the knowledge produced in real time by such data processes (Goad, 2002). The fluidity, portability, and mobility of data systems and processes as they are incorporated into knowledge worker activity are the keys to accelerating their viability as tools for both informing decisions and evaluating actions. Competent managers now view this approach not as a new way of doing business, but rather as the *only* way to think and do the work effectively.

To create a meaningful attachment or connection to data and the analytics related to creating relevance from it will require that both practitioners and information systems experts and developers focus on the utility of such systems from the users' perspective (Hildreth & Kimble, 2004). To date, much data have been collected in health care, yet much of those data are neither relevant nor valuable to individuals at the point of service, where the ability to establish the evidence of clinical viability is compromised without this input. The heavy, complex, and overwhelming systems for collecting and managing data simply make them untenable in the work life of the knowledge worker, especially given the myriad clinical pressures constraining his or her time. Continuing emphasis on the development of portability through the use of mobile data devices, remote data access, and handheld devices is essential to creating ease-of-use conditions that satisfy the point-of-service user who needs ready access to critical and real-time data. It is the obligation of managers, in their role of creating and enabling context for evidentiary practices, to make sure that such data processes are both available and useful. If the point-of-service utility of data management systems does not advance, the currently great distance between truly effective evidence-based processes and clinical practices will be sustained over a long period of time (Geisler, Krabbendam, & Schuring, 2003).

Building effective analytics calls for organizations to recalibrate the way in which they collect and integrate data. In hospitals, for example, financial, flow, patient, and clinical performance data should not be looked at as separable elements. Instead, they should be viewed as representing distinct components of essentially the same data set. Each of these elements of data affects the others, thereby providing multiple sources of related information for guiding decision making and action (Locsin, 2001). From a purely business perspective, clinical requirements generated from patient assessment have a direct and immediate impact on financial considerations; they influence how hospitals will get paid for those activities because they invariably fall both under and outside of the auspices of third-party payers. This, in turn, has a direct impact on both the patient and the organization—one that can be ignored only at the peril of both. Evidence-based management requires knowing the value of these interfaces, recognizing how the implications of the data may affect both the business and the practices of the organization, and subsequently taking the requisite actions necessary to positively problem solve (Jurewicz & Cutler, 2003). Laying the foundation for analytics as a process for linking and integrating the business of care with the practice of care is essential to generate practitioner-centered values that directly relate to the patients they serve, the decisions they make, and the positive outcomes they attempt to achieve. It is especially important in the transformation to a higher level of digital processes and resources that healthcare work remain a human–relational process that enhances health and well-being and not a robotic process that eliminates the need for human contact, understanding of social situations, and the individual persona. Thoughts on the human–technology interface should necessarily be considered in the creation of a data management infrastructure.

TECHNOLOGY AND HUMAN INTEGRATION

The interface between humans and technology is now of great concern and interest to both patients and healthcare workers. There is great interest in new devices and software that is coupled with concern for health care becoming too impersonal or robotic. Algorithms are emerging to support decision making in new and creative ways (Frick, 2015); however, human judgment must still be the cornerstone for patient care. As new technologies are introduced into the marketplace, individuals are inundated with new devices and software applications believed to enhance the value of healthcare services. Decision making for the addition of software or devices necessarily follows an evidentiary process. Evidence that the additional technology will indeed provide additional value to the organization is often not readily available, in spite of overwhelming enthusiasm about the additional technology from an emotional perspective. The creation of human-centered technologies has assisted many health populations in monitoring diseases such as diabetes, hypertension, patient safety alerts, and stress management sensors. Robots are now entering health care to do many standardized tasks, and some even have artificial intelligence capacity. An essential consideration in choosing technology in a complex organization is how to retain a balance of humanness in a highly technological world. Individuals in highly technological environments must work hard to avoid total reliance on technology and, at the same time, envision a better future.

OVERCOMING DOGMA AND BELIEF

Increasing one's capacity can only be done with the addition of more hours—or with the elimination of nonvalued work. No matter how intensely one wishes to do more with less, that is not possible. It is about doing only work that results in value for the user of the healthcare system. To be sure, the process of eliminating non-value-added work is often blocked by historical dogma and beliefs. Past practice, historical precedent, dogma, belief, and ideology all serve to create a contextual framework that informs action. Professions—most notably, nursing and medicine—have long historical attachments to process in the memories, mythologies, fantasies, and stories that create an idealization of practice and a disconnect from fact and reality (Anderson & Willson, 2008). For example, the traditional attachment to policy and procedure now represents a significant impediment to building evidence-based systems and infrastructure. In fact, policy and procedure are anathema to evidentiary processes representing a mental model and organizational framework that operate with constructs demonstrating a polar difference from the ones that now represent the fluidity of information management and clinical decision making (Birch, 2007; Oostendorp, 2003). Reliance on policy and procedural constructs represents an understanding of practice as being part of a fixed operational and clinical system. Policy and procedural constructs demonstrate a belief that change is external, incremental, and situational—none of which, as we now know, holds true. Individuals now must purposefully give consideration to elimination of existing work that might be duplicative, outmoded, or nonvalue producing. Eliminating duplicative or unnecessary work is one of the more difficult tasks for the team. Too often, emotional attachment or personal interest in tasks becomes the primary rationale for retaining duplicative or ineffective processes. At some point the team needs

> **Box 3-3** Evidence-Based Motivation: Truth
>
> You cannot motivate anyone to do anything! People are already motivated. However, their motivation may not be aligned with group goals. The role of the leader is to create this alignment, not to motivate people.

to work together to collaboratively abandon those processes. Failing to eliminate dogmatic practices and unnecessary work obstructs or negates the new work as it becomes burdensome and perceived as an add-on.

CAVEAT: BEWARE OF MOTIVATION STRATEGIES

There is one final thought about the work in creating and assessing ones' infrastructure for evidence and innovation. If the forces of motivation were understood and the research related to those forces were incorporated into management capacity, managers might spend more of their resources and energy on creating the conditions of alignment (Barry, Murcko, & Brubaker, 2002; Fottler, Ford, & Heaton, 2002). Aligning individual motivations with organizational goals has a much longer history of well-researched validation than do efforts at employee motivation (Gottlieb, 2003; Lencioni, 2002). Creating both the infrastructure and the expectation of alignment of individual behaviors with organizational goals requires a particular set of skills, including ownership, engagement, investment, and strong linked and integrated efforts at performance evaluation and course correction (Malloch & Porter-O'Grady, 2006). Good evidence suggests that efforts in this arena have a direct payoff in terms of accomplishment and outcomes. No such body of evidence has been uncovered for organizational efforts at employee motivation.

Case Example

John Stanton, RN, MBA, is the critical care director for a small healthcare organization in the Midwest. He has reviewed the national driving forces for healthcare reform and believes he has a good understanding of them. He believes changes are needed in his organization, and he is unsure where to start to determine what needs to be changed and where innovation would be needed. John is also uncertain about the innovation competencies of his team members. He believes all the key stakeholders should be involved in this assessment. He would like to have a list of questions to begin the discussion. He formulated the following list to present to the team to begin the process.

Using the valued outcomes diagram as a focal point, John planned to ask individuals to share their perceptions of the level of understanding for each of these concepts:

- Personal knowledge:
  - What does complexity mean to you as a caregiver?
  - Share an innovation experience that you believe was successful.
  - How is your role unique as a member of this unit?
  - What interventions that you do are directly linked to patient improvement?
  - What measures do you think are important to evaluate the quality of your care?
- System perceptions:
  - How ready do you believe the organization is for the full implementation of the Patient Protection and Affordable Care Act?
  - What would our unit need to do to provide 100% fully integrated continuum care?
  - Which care processes or interventions that are provided in our unit result in value to the patient?
  - Which care processes do not result in value and could be considered for elimination?

John is hopeful that if he can understand the current level of team member understanding about the drivers for change, their unique role contributions and the nature of value-based health care, he will be able to develop a plan to make evidence-driven improvements and identify opportunities for innovation in his unit.

Questions

1. Do you think John is on the right track?
2. What will be the obstacles to this process?
3. What suggestions would you make to John?

Case Example

Leaders are continually steeped in complexity and change. Several competencies are essential for survival in the contemporary healthcare organization. After reading this chapter, Melissa Rogers, chief nursing executive of a large Southwest healthcare system, believed a leadership development program focusing on complexity was needed for her leaders. Melissa also reviewed additional leadership literature and believed most leaders were transactional in nature. She engaged the shared governance council to share her ideas.

The goals of this process included the following:

1. Gain an increased understanding of the basic attributes of complexity science to create a common foundation for all leaders.
2. Develop scenarios that reflect the reality of complexity attributes in routing practice to demonstrate the pragmatic value of learning about complexity and the potential impact of outcomes.
3. Describe the differences between complexity leadership and transactional leadership to further illustrate how leadership behaviors could be more facilitative and less directive as a means to increase team engagement.

The council then created and implemented a year-long formal plan to engage leaders in learning new behaviors. The plan included didactic online sessions for each leader and monthly team sessions in which complexity leadership scenarios were discussed.

To evaluate the impact of this work, Melissa believed there would be changes in nurse satisfaction and patient engagement. Using your facility satisfaction surveys for both nurses and patients, what specific items do you believe should improve? Can you link the improvement to a specific complexity principle? For example, is an improvement in staff perception of involvement related to a better understanding of the attribute of interrelatedness?

SUMMARY

Changes in communication modalities, new work flow processes, multivariate evaluation measurement variables, innovative outcome expectations, and the quest for clear and visible value are undeniable for organizations. These evolutions reflect the new realities of space, time, structure, and substance. Effective organizational cultures must now support a more pronounced evidentiary work dynamic that fully integrates the contents and interrelationships of the innovation to evidence continuum. This will necessarily result in more effective operations and the continual creation, evaluation, and introduction of new and better ideas.

REFERENCES

Agency for Healthcare Innovations Exchange. https://innovations.ahrq.gov/
Albrecht, K. (2003). *The power of minds at work: Organizational intelligence in action.* New York: AMACOM.
Allworth, J., Wessel, M., & Levie, A. (2015). 3 questions to get the most out of your company's data. Retrieved from https://hbr.org/2015/01/3-questions-to-get-the-most-out-of-your-companys-data

Anderson, J., & Willson, P. (2008). Clinical decision support systems in nursing: Synthesis of the science for evidence-based practice. *CIN: Computers, Informatics, Nursing, 26*(3), 151–158.

Ang, Y., & Yin, S. (2008). *Intelligent complex adaptive systems*. Chicago, IL: IGI.

Ball, M.J. (2000). *Nursing informatics: Where caring and technology meet* (3rd ed.) New York: Springer.

Barnsteiner, J., Disch, J., & Walton, M. K. (2014). *Person and family centered care*. Indianapolis, IN: Sigma Theta Tau International.

Barry, R., Murcko, A., & Brubaker, C. (2002). *The Six Sigma book for healthcare*. Chicago, IL: Health Administration Press.

Bennis, W., Goleman, D., & Biederman, W. (2008, Fall). Creating a transparent culture. *Leader to Leader, 21*–27.

Birch, D. (2007). *Digital identity management*. Los Angeles, CA: Gower.

Blum, M. (2006). *Continuity, quantum, continuum, and dialectic: The foundational logics of Western historical thinking*. Chicago, IL: Peter Lang.

Boradkar, P. (2010). Transdisciplinary design in the classroom. In T. Porter-O'Grady & K. Malloch (Eds.), *Innovation leadership: Creating the landscape of health care* (pp. 109–133). Sudbury, MA: Jones & Bartlett Learning.

Burns, L. R. (Ed.). (2005). *The business of healthcare innovation*. New York, NY: Cambridge University Press.

Business Case for Innovation. https://www.nibusinessinfo.co.uk/innovationgrowth

Castells, M. (1998). *The information age: Economy, society and culture* (Vol. III). Malden, MA: Blackwell.

Cerni, T., Curtis, G. J., & Colmar, S. H. (2008). Information processing and leadership styles: Constructive thinking and transformational leadership. *Journal of Leadership Studies, 2*(1), 60–73.

Chakravarthy, B. (2003). *Strategy process: Shaping the contours of the field*. Malden, MA: Blackwell.

Christensen, C.M., Anthony, S.P., & Roth, E.A. (2004). *Seeing what's next: Using theories of innovation to predict industry change*. Boston: Harvard Business School Press.

Christensen, C. M., Kaufman, S. P., & Shih, W. C. (2008). Innovation killers: How financial tools destroy your capacity to do new things. *Harvard Business Review, 86*(1), 98–105.

Davenport, T. (2006). Competing on analytics. *Harvard Business Review, 82*(1), 24–36.

Dotlich, D. L., & Cairo, P. C. (2002). *Unnatural leadership: Going against intuition and experience to develop ten new leadership instincts*. San Francisco, CA: Jossey Bass.

Drucker, P.F. (1985), May/June). The discipline of innovation. *Harvard Business Review, 63*, 67–72

Drucker, P. F. (2001). *The essential Drucker: Selections from the management works of Peter F. Drucker*. New York, NY: HarperBusiness.

Drucker, P., & Stone, N. (1998). *On the profession of management*. Boston, MA: Harvard Business School.

Endsley, S. (2010). Innovation in action: A practical system for getting results. In T. Porter-O'Grady & K. Malloch (Eds.), *Innovation leadership: Creating the landscape of health care*, (pp. 59–86). Sudbury, MA: Jones & Bartlett Learning.

Fonseca, J. (2002). *Complexity and innovation in organizations*. London: Routledge.

Fottler, M., Ford, R., & Heaton, C. (2002). *Achieving service excellence*. Chicago, IL: Health Administration Press.

Frandkov, A. (1999). *Nonlinear and adaptive control of complex systems*. New York, NY: Springer.

Freshwater, D., & Rolfe, G. (2004). *Deconstructing evidence based practice*. New York, NY: Routledge.

Frick, W. (2015). Here's why people trust human judgment over algorithms. https://hbr.org/2015/02/heres-why-people-trust-human-judgment-over-algorithms

Garvin, D., & Roberto, M. (2001). What you don't know about making decisions. *Harvard Business Review, 79*(9), 108–118.

Geiger-Brown, J., Rogers, V. E., Trinkoff, A. M., Kane, R. L., Bausell, R. B., & Scharf, S. M. (2012). Sleep, sleepiness, fatigue, and performance of 12-hour-shift nurses. *Chronobiology International, 29*(2), 211–219. doi:10.3109/07420528.2011.645752

Geisler, E., Krabbendam, K., & Schuring, R. (2003). *Technology, health care, and management in the hospital of the future*. Westport, CT: Praeger.

Giacco, A. F. (2003). *Maverick management: Strategies for success*. Newark, NJ: University of Delaware Press.

Goad, T. W. (2002). *Information literacy and workplace performance*. Westport, CT: Quorum Books.

Gottlieb, M. R. (2003). *Managing group process*. Westport, CT: Praeger.

Hesselbein, F. (2002). *Hesselbein on leadership*. San Francisco, CA: Jossey Bass.

Hildreth, P. M., & Kimble, C. (2004). *Knowledge networks: Innovation through communities of practice*. Hershey, PA: Idea Group.

Hooker, C., & Csikszentmihalvi, M. (2003). Rethinking the motivation and structuring of knowledge work. In C. Pearce & J. Conger (Eds.), *Shared leadership: Reframing the hows and whys of leadership* (pp. 217–233). Thousand Oaks, CA: Sage.

Jurewicz, L., & Cutler, T. (2003). *High tech, high touch: Library customer service through technology*. Chicago, IL: American Library Association.

Kelly, T. (2005). *Ten faces of innovation*. New York, NY: Doubleday.

Lencioni, P. (2002). *The five dysfunctions of a team*. San Francisco, CA: Jossey Bass.

Locsin, R. C. (2001). *Advancing technology, caring, and nursing*. Westport, CT: Auburn House.

Malloch, K., & Porter-O'Grady, T. (1999). Partnership economics: Nursing's challenge in a quantum age. *Nursing Economics, 17*(6), 299–307.

Malloch, K., & Porter-O'Grady, T. (2006). *Introduction to evidence-based practice in nursing and health care*. Sudbury, MA: Jones & Bartlett Publishers.

Martin, D. J. (2014). Literature review: Nurse fatigue related to shift length. *Missouri State Board of Nursing Newsletter, 16*(1), 7. Retrieved from http://pr.mo.gov/boards/nursing/publications/newsletters/2014-02-01.pdf

McDaniel, C. (2004). *Organizational ethics: Research and ethical environments*. Burlington, VT: Ashgate.

McGlade, J., & Pek, A. (2008, Summer). Spark your creative genius. *Leader to Leader*, 1–15.

McNamara, O. (2002). *Becoming an evidence based practitioner: A framework for teacher–researchers*. New York, NY: Routledge/Falmer.

McSherry, R., Simmons, M., & Abbott, P. (2002). *Evidence informed nursing: A guide for clinical nurses*. New York, NY: Routledge.

Merrifield, R., Calhoun, J., & Stevens, D. (2008). The next revolution in productivity. *Harvard Business Review, 86*(6), 73–80.

Miller, J., & Scott, P. (2007). *Complex adaptive systems: An introduction to computational models of social life*. Princeton, NJ: Princeton University Press.

Mintzberg, H. (1990). The manager's job: Folklore and fact. *Harvard Business Review, 48*(2), 163–176.

Morrison, K. (2007). *Complexity leadership*. Charlotte, NC: Information Age.

Murphy, E., Ruch, S., Pepicello, J., & Murphy, M. (1997). Managing an increasingly complex system. *Nursing Management, 28*(10), 33–38.

Oliver, R. W. (2004). *What is transparency?* New York: McGraw-Hill.

Oostendorp, H. V. (2003). *Cognition in a digital world*. Mahwah, NJ: Lawrence Erlbaum.

Pidd, M. (2004). *Systems modeling: Theory and practice*. Hoboken, NJ: John Wiley & Sons.

Plsek, P. E. (1997). *Creativity, innovation and quality*. Milwaukee, WI: ASQ Quality Press.

Porter-O'Grady, T. (2000). Interdisciplinary shared governance: A partnership model for high performance in a managed care environment. *Seminars for Nurse Managers, 8*(3), 158–169.

Porter-O'Grady, T., & Afable, R. (2003). The technology of partnership. *Health Progress, 84*(3), 41–52.

Price, T. L. (2006). *Understanding ethical failures in leadership*. New York, NY: Cambridge University Press.

Reinhardt, W., Schmidt, B., Sloep, P., & Drachsler, H. (2011). Knowledge worker roles and actions—results of two empirical studies. *Knowledge and Process Management*, 18(3), 150–174. doi:10.1002/kpm.378

Rogers, A. E. (2002). Sleep deprivation and the ED night shift. *Journal of Emergency Nursing, 28*, 1–2.

Rouse, W. (2007). Complex engineered, organizational and natural systems: Issues underlying the complexity of systems and fundamental research needed to address these issues. *Systems Engineering, 10*(3), 260–271.

Scharmer, O., & Kaufer, K. (2000). Universities as the birthplace for the entrepreneuring human being. Retrieved from http://www.ottoscharmer.com/docs/articles/2000_Uni21us.pdf

Shan, Y., & Ang, Y. (2008). *Applications of complex adaptive systems.* Hershey, PA: IGI.

Shumpeter, J. (1943). *Capitalism, socialism, and democracy.* New York, NY: Harper.

Smith, P. (2004). *Shaping the facts: Evidence based nursing and health care.* New York, NY: Churchill Livingstone.

Solow, D., & Szmerekovsky, J. (2006). The role of leadership: What management science can give back to the study of complex systems. *Emergence: Complexity and Organizations, 8*(4), 52–60.

Stacey, R. (2007). *Complexity and the experience of leading organizations.* New York, NY: Routledge.

Stimpfel, A. W., Lake, E. T., Barton, S., Gorman, K. C., & Aiken, L. H. (2013). How differing shift lengths relate to quality outcomes in pediatrics. *Journal of Nursing Administration, 43*(2), 95–100.

Suh, N. P. (2005). *Complexity: Theory and applications.* New York, NY: Oxford University Press.

Sveiby, K. (1997). *The new organizational wealth.* San Francisco, CA: BerrettKoehler.

Tourish, D., & Hargie, O. (2004). *Key issues in organizational communication.* New York, NY: Routledge.

Trompenaars, A., & Hampden-Turner, C. (2002). *21 leaders for the 21st century: How innovative leaders manage in the digital age.* New York, NY: McGraw-Hill.

Vaitheeswaran, V. (2007, October 11). *A survey of innovation: A discussion with Vijay Vaitheeswaran of* The Economist [Audio podcast]. Retrieved from http://www.economist.com/node/9934754

Wager, K., Wickham, F., & Glaser, J. (2005). *Managing healthcare information systems: A practical approach for healthcare executives.* San Francisco, CA: Jossey Bass.

Watkins, S. (2004). 21st-century corporate governance: The growing pressure on the board toward a corporate solution. In R. P. Gandossy & J.A. Sonnefeld (Eds.), *Leadership and governance from the inside out* (pp. 27–36). New York: John Wiley & Sons.

Weberg, D. (2010). Transformational leadership and staff retention: An evidence review with implications for healthcare systems. *Nursing Administration Quarterly.* 34(3); 246–258.

Whitehurst, J. (2015). Be a leader who can admit mistakes. Retrieved from https://hbr.org/2015/06/be-a-leader-who-can-admit-mistakes

Whittingham, R. B. (2003). *The blame machine: Why human error causes accidents.* Boston, MA: Elsevier.

Wolper, L. F. (2004). *Health care administration: Planning, implementing, and managing organized delivery systems* (4th ed.). Sudbury, MA: Jones and Bartlett Publishers.

Yin, S., & Ang, Y. (2008). *Applications of complex adaptive systems.* Chicago, IL: IGI.

Zimmerman, B., Lindberg, C., & Plsek, P. (1998). *Edgeware.* Irving, TX: VHA.

CHAPTER 4

Patient-Centered Care, Evidence, and Innovation

Daniel Weberg and Sandra Davidson

CHAPTER OBJECTIVES

Upon completion of this chapter, the reader will be able to:

1. Describe foundational elements of patient-centered care.
2. Explore the continuum of patient-centered and relationship-centered care.
3. Describe the skills, knowledge, and values that enable relationship-centered care.
4. Discuss ways in which leaders can support patient-centered care at different levels such as, the individual, team, and system.
5. Apply evidence-based practice (EBP) and innovation leadership principles that support patient-centered and relationship-centered care.

Patient-centered care is often referenced in healthcare organization missions, visions, and values, yet many organizations struggle to implement the principles necessary for practitioners, teams, and systems to deliver patient-centered care. Even in contemporary health care, patients are often treated as powerless and lacking sufficient knowledge to make decisions about care, and they are assumed to be inherently noncompliant (Levesque, Hovey, & Bedos, 2013). The view of patients as unequals in the system perpetuates a strong power dynamic that influences the behavior of patients, the practitioners, and the system. This traditional practitioner-as-expert power dynamic needs to be reconceptualized and facilitated through leadership behaviors that enable meaningful connections between patients and the healthcare system. This chapter will explore the historical evolution of patient-centered care and related healthcare concepts to provide a context for the current state of practice. Specifically, the influences of EBP, technology, and interprofessional practice will be discussed. Relationship-centered care as an additional model for healthcare delivery will be presented. Case studies that exemplify patient-centered care at the organizational, team, and individual levels will be presented and discussed.

ORIGINS AND EVOLUTION OF PATIENT-CENTERED CARE

The concept of patient-centered care first emerged in the 1960s. Prior to this, health care was steeped in the modern biomedical model, which is very much in alignment with positivism and the age of the machine that are reflected in the broader societal trends of the time. Tremendous breakthroughs were occurring in our knowledge of health and illness in the 1950s (such as the polio vaccine, pacemakers, and organ transplants). Medical research was focused on fixing the body. Physicians were regarded as experts, and in the context of the social conventions of the time, the doctor was always right.

In the 1960s and 1970s, large-scale social movements, such as women's liberation and the fight for equality among marginalized groups in society, moved forward and gained prominence. There was also a growing distrust and questioning of authority (e.g., government, big corporations). Health care was not immune to this trend. Practitioners whose clinical expertise was once beyond contestation now began to be questioned and even challenged at times. An example of this is the growing debate around women's reproductive rights (contraception and abortion) in the 1970s. Health care began to move into the biopsychosocial era. There is a growing acknowledgement of the mind–body connection and research establishing the social determinant of health (Syme, 2005) that began to influence the practice and education of healthcare providers. It is in this climate that the concept of patient-centered care emerged. There was a beginning recognition that patients' unique attributes (e.g., lifestyle, values, socioeconomic status, mental state) influence their health. Healthcare providers began to dialogue with patients about their health and illness experiences instead of talking at them or down to them.

In the 1970s, the role and scope of nurses in particular was important in the move to patient-centered care. Nurses embraced and formalized their role as patient advocates. Patient advocacy emerged as a concept alongside the development of patient rights in the early 1970s (Mallik, 1997). George Annas, an American attorney, created the Model Bill of Patient Rights in 1974. The formalization of patient rights arose from the larger social context of the time that was imbued with distrust of authority and power, growing consumerism, and the civil rights movement. Annas believed that nurses were poised optimally in healthcare settings to advocate for patients' rights (Annas & Healey, 1974; Mallik, 1997), and indeed, as history has shown, the role of the nurse as a patient advocate became a cornerstone of nursing practice.

The 1980s and early 1990s saw the trend toward patient-centered care continue and intensify. McWhinney foreshadowed many of the advances and changes to the patient–provider relationship:

*It will focus on the person and his or her environment
and relationships, as strong determinants of health and
disease . . . Sometimes the role of the physician will be to
prescribe, but always it will be to mobilize, by every means
possible, the patient's own healing powers. To do this, physicians
will have to be much more than technologists. They will require
advanced skills in communication and in understanding the
deeper meanings that illness has for patients. (1984, p. 6)*

In the1980s and 1990s, there was growth in fields such as medical anthropology and medical ethics. The principles and practices of phenomenology found their way into health care (Suchman, 2011). Thus, there was a greater focus on understanding the patient experience of health and illness, and with this lens patients were viewed as having significant knowledge, and their ability to share with providers and participate in patient–provider collaboration was enhanced. Clinical decisions were no longer the exclusive domain of the clinical expert, but rather shared decision making emerged between patients and providers as the new standard. However, there were still tensions among the long-held identities and traditions of the provider as expert, the movement toward patient empowerment, and shared decision making. This tension still exists today in many healthcare settings.

New Terminology: Relationship-Centered Care

As McWhinney imagined, by the 1990s the educational preparation of doctors and nurses included an emphasis on therapeutic communication, patient interviewing, and skills for establishing and maintaining relationships with patients. By the mid-1990s, patient-centered care was a widely accepted and practiced model in health care. However, as the patient-centered care model was enacted and lived by both providers and patients, there was a growing awareness that although it was always central to health care, the *relationships* that care providers formed with patients, communities, and other practitioners had not generally been explored or taught explicitly (Tresolini & Pew-Fetzer Task Force, 1994).

Although the biopsychosocial model that had been embraced since the 1970s helped focus attention on the multidimensional nature of illness, it also invited reductionist thinking and isolation of these elements (specialization, for example), further

Figure 4-1 Evolution of patient-centered care

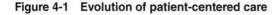

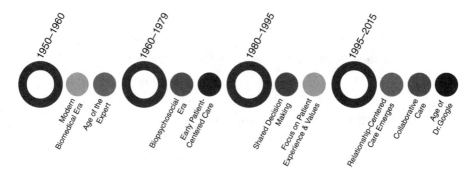

objectifying the patient and the illness experience (Tresolini & Pew-Fetzer Task Force, 1994). Likewise, although the patient-centered care model promoted a more holistic approach, it did not explicitly embrace the larger constellation of relationships and interactions beyond the provider and patient. As such, the new term *relationship-centered care* was introduced into the healthcare vernacular with the Pew-Fetzer Task Force report in 1994 (Tresolini & Pew-Fetzer Task Force, 1994).

The focus on relationships as a central feature of health care built on many traditions in the nursing profession. It also retained many of the foundational concepts found in the biopsychosocial and patient-centered care models. However, the new phrase *relationship-centered care* affirmed the centrality of relationships in contemporary health care and their importance in health and healing. Relationship-centered care will be explored more fully in a subsequent section of this chapter. **Figure 4-1** is a diagram of the evolution of patient-centered care.

From the 1990s to the 2010s there has been an emergence, evolution, and finessing of terminology that relates to the basic concept of collaboration in health care. The terms *multidisciplinary, interdisciplinary*, and *transdisciplinary* are peppered throughout the literature. Often these terms are ambiguously defined and used interchangeably (Choi & Pak, 2006), which contributes to a conceptual fog where we lack clarity about how we should best organize and carry out our work together in health care. Based on an extensive review of the literature and existing definitions, Choi and Pak (2006) proposed the following definitions:

- Multidisciplinary: Draws on knowledge from different disciplines but stays within the boundaries of those fields.
- Interdisciplinarity: Analyzes, synthesizes and harmonizes links between disciplines into a coordinated and coherent whole.

Figure 4-2 Comparing collaboration

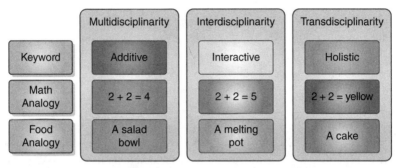

Data from Choi, B. K., & Pak, A. P. (2006). Multidisciplinarity, interdisciplinarity and transdisciplinarity in health research, services, education and policy: 1. Definitions, objectives, and evidence of effectiveness. *Clinical & Investigative Medicine, 29*(6), 351–364.

- Transdisciplinarity: Integrates the natural, social and health sciences in a humanities context, and in so doing transcends each of their traditional boundaries (Choi & Pak, 2006, p. 359).

Further, Choi and Pak offered some useful conceptual analogies to differentiate the various types of collaboration (**Figure 4-2**). In an effort to minimize future confusion and misconceptions about these three types of collaboration, they also advocated for the use of the more generic term *multiple disciplinary* when the level and nature of collaboration among multiple disciplines is unknown or not specified (Choi & Pak, 2006).

In any form of collaborative, multiple-disciplinary care, the patient is the *raison d'être*.

Patient-centered care can be enacted using any of the previous models of collaboration. The level and type of participation that the patient may have in each model will vary, similarly to the nature of the collaboration among disciplines. The next section explores another element that shapes and defines the nature of the practitioner–patient relationship in health care. The knowledge era and increased accessibility to vast amounts of information via the World Wide Web has forever changed patient-centered care.

PATIENT-CENTERED CARE IN THE KNOWLEDGE ERA

In the past several decades, we have seen the rise of the knowledge era. New knowledge is created at an unprecedented rate, and most of it is widely and easily accessible via the

World Wide Web. The Web has democratized knowledge and information. As the old adage goes, knowledge is power. Previously, knowledge was privileged to those who had the means to access it. In the 19th century, this included those with the means to access and read books and/or attend school to access knowledge. This is in alignment with the age of the expert in health care, where health-related knowledge was accessible only to those who entered training programs (physicians, nurses, pharmacists, etc.). This perpetuated the long-held power dynamics in which healthcare experts held power over patients, who had little access to specialized health information.

Today, health-related information is available to anyone with access to an Internet connection. This means that patients have access to an ever-expanding amount of health information. From a pure access perspective, the Web has changed the power dynamic by providing patients with access to health-related information. With this access comes new opportunities and challenges.

The concept of health literacy has been a topic of discussion in health care since the 1970s. With the dawn of the knowledge era, *e-health literacy* has emerged as a new form of literacy that forms the basis of informed healthcare decision making and meaningful patient participation in their own health care. E-health literacy is defined as "the ability to seek, find, understand, and appraise health information from electronic sources and apply the knowledge gained to addressing or solving a health problem" (Norman & Skinner, 2006, p. 3). E-health literacy combines components from different literacy skill sets and applies them to e-health promotion and care. Norman & Skinner (2006) described six core skills (or literacies) that are inherent in e-health literacy: traditional literacy, health literacy, information literacy, scientific literacy, media literacy, and computer literacy. From this list, it is easy to see that e-health literacy is a complex competency that requires ongoing engagement and continuous learning on the part of both patients and practitioners.

Dr. Google

The name of the Internet search engine Google has become a verb. It is commonplace that when a have a question to which we do not know the answer, we "google it." In the context of healthcare information and in response to questions such as, "I have (these symptoms), what's wrong with me?" the phenomenon known as Dr. Google has emerged (see Box 4-1).

The Urban Dictionary (2015) defines Dr. Google as "a person medically qualified by Google's search engine to diagnose symptoms of sickness."

In an era when information is freely accessible and ubiquitous, patients are able to be more informed about their symptoms and care. Websites such as WebMD, PatientsLikeMe, and Google provide access to detailed, and sometimes inaccurate, information about potential diagnoses, treatments and their risks, and home remedies. This information dynamically changes the patient–provider relationship as patients enter the clinic armed with expectations, treatment recommendations, and potential

---

Box 4-1 Dr. Google in Action

Mr. Jones: My son has the plague. I looked up his symptoms on Google.

Dr. McCarthy: Your son has the plague? Well, send him to the emergency room.

Dr. McCarthy: *Note to self—his son is fine, but Mr. Jones has a case of Dr. Google.

---

diagnoses before the care provider even does an assessment. To traditional biomedical care providers, this dynamic may be seen as disrespectful and contrary to the medical expert model of care. In fact, some providers have advocated that patients not discuss their own research until the provider has finished an assessment to not wrongly influence the differential diagnosis.

Instead of rejecting or delaying patient-driven evidence during the encounter, providers and organizations may deploy tactics to facilitate the patient in accessing more relevant information to inform their decision making. For example, health systems can set up websites that contain vetted lists of mobile apps, informational content, and tools to facilitate provider–patient discussions. By helping create the context for information gathering, organizations and providers can be better prepared for incorporating patient evidence into the care continuum. By offering information resources to the patient, the provider or organization is strengthening the relationship with the patient and helping the patient build his or her own external network of support. Even with greater involvement of providers and organizations in developing and providing reputable and evidence-based patient resources, there is still no replacement for high-quality and patient-centered interactions with care providers. **Box 4-2** reiterates the difficulties and dangers of the Dr. Google phenomenon.

Kemper & Mettler (2002) developed the concept of an *information prescription* as a way to constructively leverage information to enhance the relationship between providers and patients. Practitioners create an information prescription based on the patient's needs and health situation. The care provider is able to ensure that the prescription is filled with evidence-based information that will provide the patient with high-quality resources. In some cases, providers work with informatics specialists or health librarians to fill these prescriptions (Gavgani & Mahami, 2012), and in other settings a practitioner may use a handheld device and the Internet to provide the patient with reputable and high-quality links to resources on the Web (Woolf et al., 2005). The information prescription, or what Kemper & Mettler (2002) described as information therapy, is one example of how providers can leverage technology to engage patients and their families in patient-centered and evidence-based health care.

Box 4-2 Online Symptom Checkers? Seek a Second Opinion

In a recent study by Semigran, Linder, Gidengil, and Mehrotra (2015), standardized patient symptoms were input in 23 symptom checker web applications to determine accuracy of diagnosis. The symptom checkers, many from reputable organizations, accurately provided the correct diagnosis only 34% of the time and had the correct diagnosis listed in the top 20 only 58% of the time.

Many EBP models include patient preference as a core behavior in the evidence and intervention process. Melnyk & Fineout-Overholt's EBP model (**Figure 4-3**) is one example of purposefully integrating patient preference and the process of shared decision making between patients and providers. Indeed, the concept of informed choice comes into play here. In light of our conversation about e-health literacy and Dr. Google in the context of patient-centered care, it becomes clear that patients who have access to high-quality evidence and health information, and who also possess e-health literacy skills to make sense of it, can most meaningfully engage in shared decision making about their care.

Figure 4-3   Merging the art and science: EBP in a context of caring

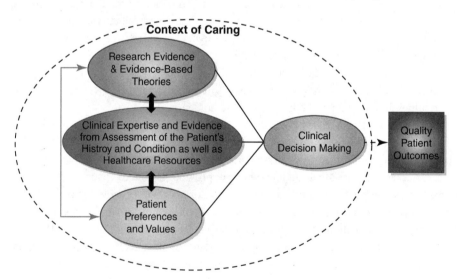

Reproduced from Melnyk, B., & Fineout-Overholt, E. (2005). *Evidence-based practice in nursing and healthcare.* Philadelphia, PA: Lippincott Williams & Wilkins. (Chapter 1, p. 15).

TOOLS TO ENGAGE PATIENTS IN INNOVATION AND EBP

The term *evidence-based innovation* seems counterintuitive. If innovation is something new that drives significant change in the social and economic workings of the organization, and evidence takes 17 years to reach implementation, how can innovation be evidence based (Melnyk, 2014; Weberg, 2013)? Through a linear lens, evidence would appear to limit the ability for organizations to create disruptive patient-centered innovation. In essence, traditional notions of evidence are too slow to support rapid cycle change.

One tool for linking evidence, innovation, and patient-centered care is the user-centered design methodology, which is used to define many different methodologies of engaging the end user in the creation of a product, process, or innovation (Kelly & Litman, 2001). User-centered design is meant to solve difficult problems by extensively studying user habits, presenting users with early product iterations for review, and building processes and products in rapid iteration cycles driven by the feedback loops of users and their needs (Muller & Thoring, 2012). There are many tools to implement user-centered design in practice, including journey mapping, hassle maps, brainstorming, rapid prototyping, and others. Many of these tools can be found online. The key for the healthcare leader who is attempting to implement patient-centered care is that he or she understands that the organization needs to tap the expertise and experiences of the users they serve and reliably incorporate that information back into the creation of their patient-centered care tool kit.

By shifting the lens to view the system as a complex adaptive dynamic we can conceptualize user-driven evidence to be an essential aspect of the innovation process. According to Porter-O'Grady and Malloch (2007), identifying the problem and understanding the systemic impacts is the first part of any successful innovation framework. Problem identification cannot take place in a leadership silo; studies and practical experience have shown that user-centered design methodologies allow innovation teams to create a link between the best clinical evidence and the needs of the patients or end users (Dykes et al., 2014). From this viewpoint, traditional research provides innovators with evidence to set the foundation of any given problem; however, evidence can also come in the form of real-time data, in-depth process mapping, and data from technologies such as real-time location systems and electronic medical records. By combining these diverse and complex sources of data, innovators can better understand the problem and speed up the innovation process. Additionally, the resulting solution is informed by the end user rather than a separate team trying to anticipate needs.

User-centered design is not as easy as it sounds. One cannot simply ask patients about their experience and label the resulting solution as a patient-centered implementation. User-centered design is a rigorous process that takes trained experts, ethnographers, and an organizational will to truly inform complex processes with user-generated input. The rigor of user-centered design does not mean, however, that leaders need to hire expensive design firms and consultants to incorporate information into their patient-centered innovation processes. Simple tools exist to aid users in starting the journey. One tool is discovery interviews to gain insights into the user experience and how it might be different from assumptions by those outside the process.

User-Centered Design Tool: Discovery Interviews

Description
Design challenges are often based on real or perceived deficits in service or performance. As previously noted, gap analysis can help clarify where the greatest opportunities for innovation may lie. Equally important, however, is the exploration of the aspects of health care that providers and patients experience in the delivery process, especially those aspects that bring delight and satisfaction to the users. Discovery interviews are rooted in the work of appreciative inquiry. Discovery involves interviews with users of the healthcare system, service, or product and is focused on eliciting their experiences.

Use
1. Identify the users to interview.
2. Construct the interview guide.
3. Conduct the interviews.
4. Analyze the themes that emerge.
5. Group themes into affinity groups.

Users that are chosen should reflect the full spectrum of the experience. They should include patients and families, physicians and nursing staff, and other professional staff.

The interview guide should be a brief, one-page outline of key questions. The questions should be open ended and solicit the stories of the users. For example, some questions might be as follows:

- "Tell me what it is like being a [patient, provider] . . ."
- "What do you value most about being a [patient, provider] at this . . ."
- "What do you find unique about being a [patient, provider] at this . . ."

- "Describe your best experience being a [patient, provider] at this . . ."
- "If you had three wishes to make this a better experience as a [patient, provider], what would they be?"
- "If you could redesign one aspect of this experience as a [patient, provider], what would you redesign?"
- "In 5 years, this [name of healthcare setting or service] is being honored for its excellence. Why?"

Arrange for a specific time and place to conduct the discovery interview. Begin by introducing the purpose of the interview and offer an invitation for participants to tell their stories. Ask about their general experience to focus on what brings value and delight. Ask additional deeper questions around themes that are raised, such as "Tell me more about how you get timely and useful information from your doctor." Write down statements as close to verbatim as possible. If you are conducting the interview in the care environment, try to also take notes on the environment and the journey the user is experiencing as you gather information.

After each interview, summarize what you identify as the themes and get feedback from the interviewee. Following completion of the discovery interviews, list all the themes that have emerged across the interviews. The themes, specific problem points, and user insights can be used to design the first prototype of the new process or product. The discovery interviews can also be used as new iterations of the process or product rolled out to elicit new insights and test directional correctness.

User-centered design is a methodology that allows for the incorporation of user-generated evidence into innovation, process design, and product creation within organizations. Leaders should use user-centered design whenever possible, especially when creating patient-centered care practices and processes to ensure that these innovations are built on user need, not on misguided assumptions. Many user-centered design tools exist, but discovery interview is a simple tool to gather user input for an innovative problem-solving effort.

CONTEMPORARY PATIENT-CENTERED CARE

On the surface, patient-centered care seems obvious. Center all interventions, experiences, and interactions a patient has with the healthcare system on his or her personal values and preferences. The literature largely supports this description as well. Foundational literature on patient-centered care has described several common foundations, yet there is no universally accepted definition (Kitson, Marshall, Bassett, & Zeitz, 2013) (**Figure 4-4**).

Morgan & Yoder (2012) conducted a concept analysis of patient-centered care and determined that what constitutes patient-centered care depends on the care environment. This means that patient-centered care is contextually dependent and requires

Box 4-3 Evidence-Based Innovation in Action

One example of how evidence-based innovation led to significant changes that redefined the social and economic potential of an organization started with a time-in-motion study. In an innovative data collection process, location tags were connected to nurses, and the nurses were mapped during a typical shift and the activities they performed were recorded. The findings provided clarity around several assumptions nursing leaders had made about how nurses spend their time. A significant portion of time was spent on documentation and other care delivery tasks, but more than 30% was spent on finding people, equipment, or supplies to carry out the work. Prior to this study, innovative solutions were sometimes selected based on faulty assumptions about the work or simply by subjective descriptions of problems. Now innovation was enhanced by evidence. The gap in what nurses could be doing versus what they were actually doing was finally illuminated. This innovative evidence soon catalyzed several innovation projects.

From the Kaiser Permanente Innovation Consultancy, a in-house IDEO-type organization focused on innovating through design thinking, came a project called Ready Room. Based on data, experience, and work flow analysis from the time-in-motion study, the team discovered that fragmented and siloed data was causing significant issues in patient throughput from the operating room, through the postanesthesia care unit, to the medical-surgical units. By building on evidence from the study and gathering more real-time evidence through process mapping and interviews, the team created a solution with the front lines that unlocked data to aid in decision making that ultimately could improve the hospital functions and nursing, housekeeping, and bed management satisfaction. Evidence, in this case, sparked an idea that was supported by evidence and led to an innovation that was designed by frontline workers to solve a proven need in the organization.

From the design and data elements that came from the project team, it was possible to improve the interaction between previously siloed groups (social change). Prior to this work, teams had easy access only to data in their departments. The operating room managed the operating room, the medical-surgical team managed the medical-surgical unit and the status of rooms; the movement of patients and readiness of staff was fragmented to these groups. By leveraging real-time data and making it easily accessible in meaningful ways, groups could collaborate better, share information faster, and make better decisions. Better efficiency could then impact the financial indicators for the organization. Simply connecting groups with better data to enable better decisions had the potential to decrease wasted time in the expensive operating rooms and improve patient experience.

Reprinted from *The Permanente Journal, 12*(3), 25. Hendrich, A., Chow, M. P., Skierczynski, B. A., & Lu, Z. (2008). A 36-hospital time and motion study: How do medical-surgical nurses spend their time? Copyright 2008, with permission from The Permanenet Press. www.kp.org/permanentejournal

Figure 4-4   Elements of patient-centered care

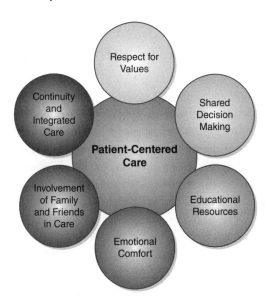

flexibility and adaptability in implementing the foundational elements across a healthcare system. For example, patient-centered care may look very different in a primary care office that schedules 15-minute appointments than in a chemotherapy infusion center that sees patients for hours a day. The concept analysis also suggested that patient-centered care in healthcare organizations is the result of three structures. First, the organization must have a vision and commitment (culture) that supports practitioners to collaborate with patients. Second, the teams and team members must have attitudes and behaviors that support patient-centered care. This may be reflected in a stronger focus on the patient relationships than on completing individual tasks. Third, the organization must have shared governance structures that allow for distributed decision making. Distributed decision making removes care decisions from a manager and places them at the point of care. Here, patients and practitioners can be supported to make collaborative decisions based on evidence, preference, and relevancy.

CHALLENGES IN ACHIEVING PATIENT-CENTERED CARE

In the many parts of the healthcare system there are massive power inequities between patients and practitioners. Patients are often described as powerless, noncompliant, and passive actors in their own health. This power dynamic creates challenges in the system, and tensions that must be addressed before patient-centered care can actually support EBP and innovation work.

Tension One: Evidence or Patient Preference

The source of this tension is the result of how practitioners view the distribution of decision-making power between themselves and the patient (Levesque et al., 2013).

Provider content knowledge may overpower patient values and care. The same struggle occurs with the implementation of EBP and innovation. One must sometimes unlearn in order to adapt, adopt, and evolve. The inability for someone to separate the perceived expertise and individually desired outcomes, and submit to a cocreation process in which outcomes, treatments, and decisions are negotiated, stands in stark contrast to many medical models of care. In essence, relying solely on individual knowledge and expertise will subvert the ability for organizations to adopt patient-centered care, EBP, and innovation. Additionally, this tension may cause significant and severe cultural conflicts if either the practitioner or the patient have serious objections to care decisions.

Tension Two: Reality versus Patient Expectations

Many times the desired outcome of creating an organization that supports patient-centered care is to achieve better patient satisfaction, better patient outcomes, and improved organizational outcomes (Rathert, Wyrwich, & Boren, 2012). Moderating the journey from patient-centered care to achieving outcomes is patient condition and patient expectations. Mediating the process is patient activation and patient adherence to treatments. These mediating and moderating variables ensure that patient-centered care is not a linear process but requires leaders, practitioners, and patients to find a dynamic equilibrium between what is really achievable and what the expectations of the outcome might be. For example, a patient with type II diabetes might have an expectation to cure him-or herself through exercise and diet changes, but adherence, family support, and financial hurdles may not allow the patient to meet those expectations. In this example, the patient may be less satisfied with the medical treatment, have poorer outcomes, and impact the organization's overall goal of diabetic treatment despite the organization having significant patient-centered care implementation. Frontline care providers who might face similar challenges need to reflect on their ability to work with the patient to create a mutual understanding of the disease, the possible outcomes, and the impacts that life choices may have on expectations. This process is mutual, and patients should be able to set realistic expectations of treatment goals with their provider. Generally, across all studies in a systematic review of patient-centered care, patient-centered care was linked to improving satisfaction and well-being of patients (Rathert et al., 2012).

Tension Three: Care Environment Impacts or Standardized Experiences

Morgan and Yoder (2012) determined that the care setting has a significant impact on how patient-centered care is conceptualized and implemented. For example, patient-centered care behaviors will be much different in a primary care office restricted to 15-minute visits than in a hospital in which the nurse has 12 hours with the patient. Although the core principles will be the same, the behaviors of both the patient and the care team will need to adapt to remain relevant. This also means that standardizing the whole patient-centered care process in a complex organization may be detrimental to implementation. By focusing on standardizing process instead of principles, the organization may remove the ability for the team to adapt behaviors based on contextual factors and deploy less adequate processes instead. On the other hand, allowing for professional autonomy and decision making in regards to patient-centered care according to individual care environments may lead to an inconsistent brand experience and variations in interactions. By using a complexity lens, one can conceptualize these two extremes on the stability to chaos continuum.

Patients as Sources of Evidence

Patient-centered care is integral to the evidence and innovation work of organizations. In EBP much of the discussion about sources of evidence focuses on research efforts. Another source of evidence is emerging from patients themselves and goes beyond reported symptoms and diagnostic data. As leaders and practitioners work to build patient-centered care capabilities in their system and organizations, new sources of data are needed to both facilitate patient-centered care practice and patient-centered care interventions.

Patient-centered innovation is founded on the principles of user-centered design, in which solutions are cocreated with the users to build sustainable and relevant iterations. Both patient preference and user-centered design concepts described in EBP and innovation literature are complementary to the patient-centered care research. Patient-centered care is a constant in the healthcare innovation process; together, the patient and practitioner cocreate the interventions to achieve a desired outcome. However, patient-centered care is fraught with unpredictability and is enacted in complex and overlapping contexts. As such, there are no hard-and-fast or one-size-fits-all rules about how to create a patient-centric healthcare environment. Rather, the process can be informed by foundational principles that allow leaders, practitioners, patients, and organizations to have guide rails that help to focus behaviors, structures, and decision making that can result in a cocreated, patient-centered care culture (Kitson et al., 2013).

PATIENT-CENTERED LEADERSHIP

Patient-centered care is a vehicle for cocreating innovation and EBP within a system and requires leaders to be adaptable, flexible, and collaborative to overcome the tensions described earlier. Leaders must be able to see the complex system as a whole and translate actions and information from the individual, team, and organizational lens.

Patients as Leaders

In the patient-centered care cultures and in complexity leadership principles, leadership is displayed by all agents in the system (Uhl-Bien & Marion, 2008). Therefore, patients are considered leaders in their care and must also practice leadership behaviors. According to Bernabeo & Holmboe (2013), patients should define the relationship with their provider, clearly articulate health goals and problems, share relevant information about their condition, and actively negotiate decision making. The display of these patient leader behaviors will be impacted by the organizational culture and the relationship the care teams establish with the patient. To partner with the patient, the care providers, organization, and healthcare system must work together to build relationships, provide evidence, share in decision making, and involve the team.

Build Relationships

Leadership is 90% relationships and 10% actions (Porter-O'Grady & Malloch, 2007). At the core of patient-centered care are strong relationships among members of the care team, the patient, and the organization. These relationships will provide linkages in the network to share information, understand values and preferences, engage the family and the care team, and support respect. Each part of the network must participate to build strong relationships.

The patient is responsible for defining and communicating his or her desired care relationship. Whether this is done overtly through specific conversations or covertly through behaviors, body language, and other less direct methods, the source of context for relationships in the care starts with the patient. Direct care providers that are interacting with the patient can facilitate the discovery of the patient's desired relationship and be observant for the covert actions that might also provide insight. From these conversations and actions, the care provider can assist in cocreating the relationship with the patient.

Organizations and the healthcare system as a whole also play a role in facilitating care and team–patient relationship building. Organizations can provide time, support, and resources for care teams and patients to interact and build relationships (Bernabeo & Holmboe, 2013). This may be done through less intimidating care environments, supporting longer patient visits, or building a culture that holds care teams and patients accountable for building relationships. Additionally, the healthcare system can be influenced to support stronger relationships. This could be through reimbursement models, care delivery redesign, and supporting cross-functional care teams to interact with the patient.

Discussion

List several barriers you have seen in your practice to building strong patient relationships. How might you remove these barriers? Describe specific leadership actions that might facilitate relationship building.

Provide Evidence

EBP is another foundational function that supports patient-centered care. Patient preference is at the core of EBP practice, and patients are also robust sources of data for evidence-based decisions. Patients provide evidence by articulating their health concerns, goals, and the associated relevant information. Care team members should be astute in translating the information provided by patients into relevant evidence that will inform treatment options that can be used in shared decision making. While patients provide evidence in the process of diagnoses and treatment, the care provider must also provide evidence by reviewing patient preferences and context, and then present relevant information and options that are clear and transparent to the patient (Kitson et al., 2013). This exchange will also help build a trusting relationship between the team and the patient.

To support evidence in decision making, organizations and systems can provide technology tools that enable point-of-care decision making and evidence-based data. This can be done through electronic medical records supported with clinical decision support tools that link patient information directly to relevant research and treatment options. These systems can speed up and ease the burden of lengthy EBP processes and also catalyze conversations during short patient visits. Additionally, influencing the healthcare system to change reimbursement models to support evidence and patient preference based interventions and treatments could help in building a culture of patient-centered care.

Shared Decision Making

At the core of shared decision making in patient-centered care is the need to rebalance the power distribution between the patient and the provider, or system (Levesque et al., 2013). The patient can help level the power imbalance by being informed about his or her condition and by including family and friends in the decision-making process. Essentially, the patient can help form an individual support network that can better access, interpret, and convey information to the care team. The patient's own network adds power to his or her corner and can help balance the provider experts and intimidating system. Providers can also support the patient network by openly conversing and accepting information from the additional stakeholders. This may mean accepting second opinions and challenges to care plans or facilitating crucial conversations with the patient's network.

Organizations can also provide support for shared decision making. This can be through accountability and culture building efforts or by creating spaces for the shared decision to occur. For example, allowing unrestricted visiting hours may allow the patient's support network to advocate and participate in care decisions more often. Additionally, organizations can utilize technology solutions, such as video calls, to engage family members in discussions if they are not based locally. Leaders can also influence healthcare system changes that create information that can be linked to family members, shift regulations for more open discussion of critical care decisions, and build care environments that support the patient's network in engaging with the care team easily and openly (Kitson et al., 2013; Morgan & Yoder, 2012).

Involve the Team

Patient-centered care is reliant on team-based care concepts in which the patient's network and the care team can collaborate easily and effectively (Bernabeo & Holmboe, 2013; Morgan & Yoder, 2012). Patients must act as if they are part of the team, and providers must allow patients and their networks to participate in the teamwork. Providers must also work collaboratively with the care team by cooperating with other providers, roles, and organizations to facilitate patient-centered care. This may require reflecting on and eliminating barriers such as ego, professional stigmas, cultural biases, and unnecessary competition among departments. Focusing teams on the desired outcomes of satisfaction, quality patient care, and organizational success may help in removing some barriers (Rathert et al., 2012). Additionally, organizations and systems can support team involvement by integrating systems, building accountability models that reward teams above individuals, and supporting information systems that make team care easy and relevant. **Table 4-1** summarizes patient-centered care leadership behaviors.

Table 4-1   Summary of Patient-Centered Care Leadership Behaviors

Leadership Behavior	Patient	Care Provider	Organization	System
Build relationships	Define and communicate desired relationship	Openly partner with patient in care	Provide time/ support for relationship building	Support patient– provider interaction
Provide evidence	Articulate health goals and concerns, share relevant information	Review preferences and present evidence in clear and unbiased way	Ensure access to best evidence for patient and provider	Restructure reimbursement to support patient preference
Shared decision making	Involve family and friends as needed and desired	Support family and friends in decision-making process	Unlimited visiting hours, teleconference support for family meetings, proxy access to medical information	New information systems, redesign care environments
Involve the team	Share information from all sources (multiple providers, Google, family)	Collaborate across roles, scopes of practice, and specialties	Facilitate cooperation between providers and team	Support team-based care, top of license scope

Patient-centered care is a useful construct for organizing how we go about our work in health care. In patient-centered care, as the name suggests, the focus is on the patient— his or her values, preferences, health outcomes, experiences, and needs. A fitting analogy is how we describe our solar system. Just as the sun is the center of our solar system, the patient is the center of healthcare organizations in this model. Other aspects of health care are described in relation to the patient; in the solar system analogy, planets, meteors, and stars are described based on their position relative to the sun.

Another model that is increasingly applied to health care arises from quantum physics and complexity science: the holographic universe. Holography posits that a complete pattern is represented in any component (a fractal) of a system regardless of the size or location of that component (Porter-O'Grady & Malloch, 2007). From the smallest structure or interaction to the largest and most complex aspects of an organization, the same patterns are present and reflected again and again. *Relationship* is the fractal that we will use in this analogy. In relationship-centered care, the non reducible unit of service of high-quality care is composed of both technical and *relational* elements (Malloch, Slutyer & Moore, 2000). The next sections explore relationship-centered care.

> There is only one corner of the universe you can be certain of
> improving, and that's your own self.
>
> —ALDOUS HUXLEY

RELATIONSHIP-CENTERED CARE

As introduced in the beginning section of this chapter, relationship-centered care is a more recent development that integrates patient-centered care and multiple disciplinary interactions that take place amidst a complex healthcare system. The new term *relationship-centered care* is deliberate in that the principles and practices associated with this new movement would not be lumped together with existing practices that seem to perpetuate the linear, mechanistic, and reductionist legacy of the biomedical model. The Pew-Fetzer Task Force report (Tresolini & Pew-Fetzer Task Force, 1994) was the first widely acknowledged monograph about relationship-centered care. In it, the task force acknowledged that health care was on the verge of a new era, and there was reason for optimism. They also suggested that the preferred future of health care would not manifest without attending specifically to the day-to-day work of practitioners and the education required to do that work (Tresolini & Pew-Fetzer Task Force, 1994).

Tresolini and the Pew-Fetzer Task Force warned that

> health care often is based on an individual, disease-oriented,
> subspecialty-focused model that has led to a focus on cure at
> all costs, resulting in care that is fragmented, episodic, and
> often unsatisfying for both patients and practitioners. We are
> at risk, in a new healthcare system, of reproducing the same
> attenuated patient-practitioner relationships and professional
> isolation. (1994, p. 16)

Because the relationship is the central organizing feature of this model of care, three different relationships are highlighted as integral for development and maintenance in relationship-centered care.

First is the provider–patient relationship. **Table 4-2** summarizes the knowledge, skills, and values to be cultivated by the practitioner to sustain patient–provider relationships.

Table 4-2   Areas of Knowledge, Skills, and Values for the Patient–Practitioner Relationship

Area	Knowledge	Skills	Values
Self-awareness	Knowledge of self Understanding self as a resource to others	Reflection on self and work	Importance of self-awareness, self-care, self-growth
Patient experience of health and illness	Role of family, culture, community in development Multiple component of health Multiple threats and contributors to health as dimensions of one reality	Recognize patient's life story and its meaning View health and illness as part of human development	Appreciation of the patient as a whole person Appreciation of the patient's life story and the meaning of the health–illness condition
Developing and maintaining caring relationships	Understanding of threats to the integrity of the relationship (e.g., power inequalities) Understanding of potential for conflict and abuse	Attend fully to the patient Accept and respond to distress in patient and self Respond to moral and ethical challenges Facilitate hope, trust, and faith	Respect for patient's dignity, uniqueness, and integrity (mind–body–spirit unity) Resect for self-determination Respect for person's own power and self-healing processes
Effective communication	Elements of effective communication	Listen Impart information Learn Facilitate learning of others Promote and accept patient's emotions	Importance of being open and nonjudgmental

Second is the practitioner–community relationship. Many health concerns that individuals bring to the patient–practitioner relationship also exist in communities and their institutions. By working to solve community problems that are not associated with one particular patient, healthcare practitioners can have a broader positive impact on the health of many, and indeed prevent future individual health concerns (Tresolini & Pew-Fetzer Task Force, 1994). To this end, practitioners should seek to understand and interact with communities. Using concepts from sociology and cultural anthropology, along with complexity thinking and the concepts of social justice, practitioners can develop an understanding of community dynamics. Coming to know a community also entails paying attention to demographic, political, economic, and business trends that affect community life.

Third are practitioner–practitioner relationships. The quality of the relationships among members of the practitioner community greatly affects the capacity of all those within it to form effective relationships with patients and communities (Tresolini & Pew-Fetzer Task Force, 1994). Comprehensive care depends on the contributions of multiple healthcare providers from a wide range of professions. Effective and satisfying provider-to-provider relationships begin with the foundational skills of being able to listen openly, communicate effectively, and learn cooperatively. Disciplinary diversity must be acknowledged, valued, and leveraged. Different professional traditions of knowledge, cognitive styles, and ways of perceiving are examples of the diversity that must be embraced. Providers may also vary in their degrees of readiness to learn and function as team members. Remaining open to others' ideas, displaying an attitude of humility, mutual trust, support, and empathy are key attributes of members within a thriving provider community (Tresolini & Pew-Fetzer Task Force, 1994).

Another useful development in relationship-centered care are the four principles articulated by Beach & Inui (2006, p. S4):

1. *Relationships in health care ought to include the personhood of participants.*
   "The patient and the practitioner are both unique individuals with their own sets of experiences, values, and perspectives. In RCC [relationship-centered care] practitioners are aware of their own emotions, reactions, and biases, and monitor their own behavior in light of this awareness" (Beach & Inui, 2006, p. S4).
2. *Affect and emotion are important components of relationships in health care.*
   "In RCC, emotional support is given to patients through the emotional presence of the clinician. Relationship-centered care therefore challenges the notion of detached concern, in which stepping back to maintain affective neutrality breaks the bond that holds people together" (Beach & Inui 2006, p. S4).
3. *All healthcare relationships occur in the context of reciprocal influence.*
   Health-related actions do not occur in isolation but are related to one another in time, space, and content. The smallest unit of measure in RCC is a single

person to person interaction. Providers undoubtedly benefit from the opportunity to come to know their patients, and RCC encourages clinicians to grow as a result; providers benefit in serving their patients (human to human).

4. *Relationship-centered care has a moral foundation.*
   Genuine relationships are morally desirable because it is through these relationships that clinicians are capable of generating the interest and investment that one must possess in order to serve others, and to be renewed from that serving (Beach & Inui 2006). As fully human and authentic participants in care interactions, care providers behave more genuinely than if they were acting out a role. This sort of authenticity is morally desirable as an end in itself.

Learning Activity

1. Read the following case example.
2. Use Table 4-2 to identify elements of relationship-centered care that you see being enacted in the case.
3. Compare your thoughts and ideas with a peer.

Case Example: Patient–provider

Jon, a patient in a hospital, is dying of cancer. This case study details one interaction that he has with the nurse who is caring for him. The descriptive narrative is told from the nurse's point of view. The interaction is grounded in relationship-centered care. The case study aims to illustrate that by developing self-awareness and purposefully reflecting upon our day-to-day interactions, it is possible to develop our skills in relationship-centered care. This case study also illustrates many aspects of relationship-centered care, such as authentic caring, genuine relationships, importance of affect and emotion, and the power of reciprocal influence.

I enter the room and see him there, in the bed. A man, 68 years old. His face appears peaceful with his eyes closed. I try to turn to leave, but his dark eyes open and meet mine. "I'm sorry," I say. "I did not want to wake you." "That's okay," he replies. "I wasn't sleeping anyway."

"Jon, how is your pain?" I ask. I observe his face and his body as he seemingly processes my question, searching for an acceptable response. His fists clench the cuff of his sheets. His brow forms a furrow of concern, and his mouth flattens into a thin, terse line. There is silence between us. I sense the tension as the silence persists for several moments.

He is not looking at me; rather, his eyes are cast downward. I feel myself wanting to ask another question or make a comment—anything to ease my discomfort. But then I remind myself that I am not concerned with my discomfort—I had asked about his. I stay silent. I stay in the moment with him, even though it is uncomfortable and awkward.

Finally he whispers, "I'm not good." My mind immediately begins to search my internal database of past similar experiences, even back to how I was taught to respond in nursing school. I so badly want to ease my own discomfort, and his. I catch myself searching for a response that has been successful in the past. I stop. I enter again into the moment with Jon. He is looking at me now, his eyes brimming with tears.

I move toward him and sit in the chair beside his bed because this is what feels right at this moment. In a hushed tone I say, "Tell me more." Again we enter into an abyss of silence. I begin to sense that just being there to endure the silence is what I need to do. The awkwardness and discomfort begin to melt away, and we are together in the silence—just being. He sighs, almost in relief, and then speaks. "I saw my daughter today. I haven't seen or spoken to her in 5 years. It is funny how dying of cancer suddenly brings things into perspective."

My mind begins to fire questions. What could have caused this man and his daughter to not speak for 5 years? How would I feel if I were dying of cancer? Did he answer my question about pain? Again, I catch myself. Even though it has been only a nanosecond, I still feel guilty for letting my mind carry me away from the moment. He continues, "I have so much that I wanted to say to her, but she seemed so angry and I . . . I hesitated." "What do you want to tell her?" I ask. "Oh!" he exclaims—"Everything . . . and nothing! I want to tell her that she has grown up into such a confident and beautiful woman—and how proud I am of her. I want to tell her that I am sorry for things that I have done that I know have hurt her. Mostly, I just want to tell her that I love her."

I sense calmness and peace as it begins to fill to room, and Jon once again enters into silence. I am simply there. I focus on just being there as a healing presence, in the moment with him. We are silent for several minutes. Gradually, his brow softens and all the muscles of his face seem to relax. He loosens his grip on the bed sheets and he sighs again. "Thank you," he says. I am startled by his words, and reply "For what?" "For taking the time to be with me," he says. "I think I can go to sleep now." He begins to lower the head of his bed using the control on the side rail. I rise from the chair and he smiles at me. I smile back. I turn off his lights as he turns on his side to face the window.

He sleeps.

Discussion

In life, it is often the case that the small acts or moments have the greatest impact on people. This is perhaps most evident in situations where we have a heightened awareness of life and death. In many clinical settings this heightened awareness exists. Let us not forget that life and death are themselves often viewed as paradox. In this patient–provider case study it is not so much a life-or-death situation, but rather the struggle of transition from life into death—a paradox in process. The timescale in the case study is also paradoxical. Although the entire interaction takes place in 10 minutes, the layers of relational caring are deep and rich.

In the transition from life toward death, time takes on new meaning for many. Perhaps it is not so much new meaning as a shift in perspective about the concept of time. Stacey, Griffin and Shaw (2000) discussed the difference between the macro-temporal and micro-temporal structures of time. Most of us tend to operate in the macro-temporal structure (past to present to future). The micro-temporal structure opens up the here and now and invites us to examine and make meaning of the experience of the present moment (Stacey et al., 2000). These authors further suggest that this focus on the nature of detailed (micro) interactions can result in the potential for transformation. Practitioner–patient interactions from a relationship-centered care perspective can be enhanced when the practitioner strives to be present in the moment with a patient.

In the case study, we see the nurse striving to stay in the here and now with the patient, and in the end the patient is able to express and move past issues of regret related to his interaction with his daughter. Had the nurse been operating in the macro-temporal time frame, she may have been tempted to use a textbook response, or she may have been too busy planning the patient's care to pay attention and respond authentically to the gestures (verbal and nonverbal) of the patient and situation in the here and now (Stacey et al., 2000).

Dimensions of Personhood and Role

In the case study (as told from the nurse's perspective) we can see her engaging her sense of self-awareness in a way that illuminates how she brings her personhood (nurse as person) to the interaction. She is acutely aware of her own emotions and reactions to the situation as she strives to engage with the patient in an authentic way (Beach & Inui, 2006). It is clear that she is not just playing the part of concerned nurse but that she is truly concerned for Jon.

Affect and Emotion

After the nurse chose to be in the here and now with Jon, the experience changed. The nurse was not simply a detached observer, and she consciously resisted the urge to revert to the neutral, detached professional stance that she was taught in her nursing education. She was emotionally present and therefore more attuned to the details of the verbal and nonverbal cueing in the interaction. Instead of implementing a canned response to the patient's cues, she responded in the micro present with a novel approach; she did what she felt was right, based on the present experience (sat down beside the client, used silence). Put simply, emotional support is provided to the patient through the emotional presence of the provider (Beach & Inui, 2006).

Reciprocal Influence

The nurse's intention to be present as a healing presence shaped the transformation of the patient and indeed the nurse herself. Although the nurse did not know at the beginning of the interaction what the outcome would be (unknowable future), she sensed something familiar about how to behave and respond to the patient in the moment. As she entered into the authentic experience of conversation with Jon, the unknown and known future was changed by their chosen coaction toward the future. Beach and Inui (2006) suggested that relationship-centered care creates an opportunity wherein the patient and provider "develop each other's character, and assist in the attainment of moral virtue" (2006, p. S4). In the case study, for example, the nurse's experience of silence changed. It moved from being very uncomfortable and awkward for the nurse to being peaceful and comfortable. For Jon, the nurse's growing comfort with silence created the time and space for him to express and share his emotions in a way that reduced his pain and fear. Another possible change (albeit more gradual) may be the nurse's growing comfort and confidence in her ability to engage in relationship-centered nurse–patient conversations. The nurse's growing sense of self-efficacy may increase the likelihood that the nurse will continue to practice relationship-centered care. Of course, in both patient- and relationship-centered health care, the patient's goals and needs are the primary focus. However, relationship-centered care opens the potential for providers to grow and develop in the process of caring for patients.

Moral Foundations

Relationship-centered care challenges the traditional ideal in health care that providers should assume a stance of neutrality and detachment. As Griffin (2002) discussed, the notion of seeing yourself outside an interaction, rather than as a participant in the process of cocreating the interaction, is where the breakdown of the mechanistic biomedical model occurs. Watson concurred: "This totalizing of self and other, this turning away from the mystery of our shared humanity . . . can be an act of cruelty to self and others; an inhumane act" (2003, p. 199). The ethics of caring and intentionality (Watson, 2003) fit well with relationship-centered care. Watson (2003) makes reference to the work of Knud Logstrup, a Danish philosopher. She described his work as ethics of hand:

Holding another person's life in one's hand, endows this metaphor with a certain emotional power . . . that we have the power to determine the direction of something in another person's life . . . we're to a large extent inescapably dependent upon one another . . . we are mutually and in a most immediate sense in one another's power. (Logstrup, as cited in Watson, 2003, pp. 198–199)

The ethics of caring (Watson, 2003) reminds us that we are dependent on each other and have a duty to choose goodness and caring for ourselves and each other. The case study illustrates this ethics of hand and caring ethic. The nurse chose not to turn away and see herself as separate from Jon's situation. Rather, she entered into the process with him and for him.

Case Example: Cancer Treatment Centers of America

In this section we explore another case example highlighting a healthcare organization that was founded on patient- and relationship-centered care principles and practices. In addition to calling attention to the patient–provider relationship dynamics, this case will also explore the provider–provider relationship and the provider–community relationship.

Cancer Treatment Centers of America (CTCA) is a group of private, for-profit cancer specialty hospitals that specialize in providing individualized care to patients with advanced stage and complex cancers (Drexler, Davidson, Cimini & Kharoufeh, 2013; Kanter & Bird, 2011). CTCA was founded in 1988 by Richard Stephenson. Mr. Stephenson's impetus for creating CTCA was his personal experience of witnessing his mother's battle with bladder cancer, which she ultimately lost in 1982. The experience left Mr. Stephenson deeply disenchanted with the state of cancer care. The treatment was impersonal, and physicians focused on the disease instead of the patient as a person. Practitioners did not collaborate and seemed to operate in silos of specialization. As a result, the patient was shuffled between various practitioners, and there was an absence of any holistic understanding of the person's medical condition and wants (Kanter & Bird, 2011).

Stephenson wanted to create the kind of care model that he wished would have been available to his own mother. As a result, CTCA employees (who are called stakeholders) at the five hospitals all strive to deliver the Mother Standard of Care. Simply put, this means providing every patient who visits a CTCA facility the same care and compassion that we would wish for our own family. Stephenson's mantra, "It's always and only about the patient," is well known and often quoted by stakeholders across the organization (Kanter & Bird, 2011).

Patient–Provider Relationship

As evidenced by the organization-wide mantra, it is clear that CTCA is truly patient centered. The relationships among providers and patients and their families are authentic, caring, and honest. This is reflected in the CTCA Promise (**Box 4-4**), which is recited by all stakeholders at the beginning of each day or shift as a reminder and reaffirmation of their commitment to provide this kind of care. Each stakeholder (whether a physician or a housekeeper) is empowered to go above and beyond to ensure that the Mother Standard of Care is achieved. As alluded to earlier, the Mother Standard of Care is contingent on integrated and collaborative relationships among all members of the care team.

Provider–Provider Relationships

The stakeholder culture at CTCA is such that the traditional medical hierarchy is minimized. The diversity of care provider roles and perspectives is honored and valued. There is a recognition that no one care provider can do it all, and indeed the integrative

---

Box 4-4 CTCA Promise

You and your healing are at the center of our hearts, minds and actions, every day.

We rally our team around you, delivering compassionate, integrative cancer care for your body, mind and spirit.

We offer clear information, powerful and thorough treatment options, all based on your needs.

We honor your courage, respect your decisions, and offer to share your journey of healing and hope.

Reproduced from Cancer Treatment Centers of America. (2015). About Us: Mission. Retrieved from http://www.cancercenter.com/about-us/mission

multiple disciplinary approach is a cornerstone of this patient-centric approach. To this end, CTCA has designed a specific approach called Patient-Empowered Care (PEC). The approach operates on the Copernican principle that instead of patients and their families being shuffled back and forth from department to department, care providers should revolve around them (Kanter & Bird, 2011). Implementing the model also required a shift in organizational structure, processes, and even physical architecture. In the outpatient clinic, care providers were reorganized into teams consisting of a nurse navigator, clinical nurse, medical oncologist, naturopathic physician, and nutritionist that are all assigned to the same group of patients. When it is time to see the patients, the team members rotate into and out of patient rooms and are able to debrief and collaborate in an adjacent desk area (Kanter & Bird, 2011.)

The PEC model was actualized on the inpatient unit by adopting and implementing an Acuity Adaptable Unit (AAU) model of care. CTCA's Western Regional Medical Center in Goodyear, Arizona, was the pilot site for the Acuity Adaptable Oncology inpatient unit. In this model, hospitalized patients are admitted to one room and are cared for by the same group of care providers throughout their stay. In other words, the care providers adapt to meet the patient needs (Drexler et al., 2013).

In a traditional inpatient model, if a patient's health status becomes more critical, they are transferred from a medical unit to an intensive care unit. In the AAU model, the unit staff (nurses and physicians) adapt to the patient's change in condition. Enabled by acuity-adaptable architecture, the inpatient unit rooms can also accommodate a necessary influx of patient monitoring and treatment equipment. The nurses on the unit have a unique blend of experience and skills that allow them to adapt to a wide range of patient conditions, from intensive care to palliation. Other disciplines on the unit (e.g., pharmacists, respiratory therapists, social workers, and dieticians) also remain constant. In this model, medical errors typically associated with transfers and hand-offs are dramatically decreased, and patient and family satisfaction is high (Drexler et al., 2013). Most importantly, the relationships among providers and between the patients and their providers remain stable and strong.

As you can imagine, the emotional investment in care is enormous, and the relationships the providers develop with patients and their families are close and deeply caring. The potential for emotional distress and burnout are high. Supports for the emotional well-being of providers is critical. Again, the unique provider–provider relationship was leveraged to sustain the well-being of the team. With the guidance and leadership of social work, clinical education, and spiritual care colleagues, a program called Tea for the Soul was developed. This created time and space for providers to express emotions and remembrances about patients who had passed away. It was facilitated by a counsellor and a chaplain. One example of an activity in this program is the creation of memory book for the family that includes sentiments from the providers that had cared for the patient (Drexler et al., 2013).

Provider–Community Relationships

As articulated by Tresolini and the Pew-Fetzer Task Force (1994), the provider relationship with the larger community they care for is a hallmark of relationship-centered care. CTCA as an organization exemplifies this in several notable ways. CTCA acknowledges the high importance that patients living with cancer place on finding new, more effective treatments and the movement toward a cure for the disease. As such, CTCA covers all operating costs for Gateway for Cancer Research, a nonprofit research organization that is committed to funding innovative cancer research to help people living with cancer to feel better, live longer, and beat cancer (Kanter & Bird, 2011). CTCA has also partnered with Stand Up 2 Cancer (SU2C), an organization that seeks to reshape approaches to cancer research and accelerate the delivery of new treatment options (Kanter & Bird, 2011).

ONWARD TO INNOVATIONS IN CARE

In this chapter, we have provided an overview of where we have come from in terms of our thinking and structures of health care over time. We have recounted the evolution from very mechanistic and biomedical models of care towards more holistic and patient centered approaches. Relationship-centered care is presented as an additional lens through which providers and patient can co-create new approaches to care. Information technology, e-health literacy, multiple disciplinary care have also been highlighted as contextual aspects that shape our current (and future) healthcare. systems. Throughout the chapter, we have provided examples, case studies and tools that we hope readers will find useful as they continue to lead innovation and transformation in health care. In terms of EBP, patients should be engaged in the process of examining evidence and also viewed as sources of evidence themselves. Patient centered care is also patient engaged care. Extending the notion of the care team beyond the clinicians to include the patient and their support systems is a critical shift in the structure and process of care. Only then will EBP and innovation intersect to truly transform health care. Without patient involvement, transformation activities and EBP simply fall short of effectiveness.

We encourage you to think big, and pose future forming questions to your peers, patients and communities. "I wonder..." and "What would it look like if..." are two examples of phrases that can invite others into generative conversations about what we can aspire to create together. Innovation is a team sport. High performing teams are characterized by the strong and constructive relationships between all team members. Great teams also pay attention to diversity and ensure that they include a rich array of perspectives and talents. We hope the ideas and examples shared in this chapter will help you to build your own healthcare dream team. . .patients included.

REFERENCES

Annas, G., & Healey, J. (1974). The patient rights advocate. *Journal of Nursing Administration, 4*(3), 25–31.

Beach, M. C., & Inui, T. S. (2006). Relationship-centered care: A constructive reframing. *Journal of General Internal Medicine, 21* (Suppl.1), S3–S8.

Bernabeo, E., & Holmboe, E. S. (2013). Patients, providers, and systems need to acquire a specific set of competencies to achieve truly patient-centered care. *Health Affairs, 32*(2), 250–258.

Cancer Treatment Centers of America (2015). Our promise [webpage]. Retrieved from http://www .cancercenter.com/about-us/mission/

Choi, B. K., & Pak, A. P. (2006). Multidisciplinarity, interdisciplinarity and transdisciplinarity in health research, services, education and policy: 1. Definitions, objectives, and evidence of effectiveness. *Clinical & Investigative Medicine, 29*(6), 351–364.

Drexler, D., Davidson, S., Cimini, W., & Kharoufeh, M. (2013). Integrating evidence, innovation, and outcomes: The oncology acuity-adaptable unit. *Nurse Leader, 11*(2), 26–31. doi:10.1016/j.mnl.2012.12.009

Dykes, P. C., Stade, D., Chang, F., Dalal, A., Getty, G., Kandala, R., . . . Collins, S. (2014). Participatory design and development of a patient-centered toolkit to engage hospitalized patients and care partners in their plan of care. *AMIA Annual Symposium Proceedings* (Vol. 2014, p. 486). American Medical Informatics Association.

Gavgani, V. Z. & Mahami, M. (2012). The assessment of information prescription service to patients with heart valve disease: Applying users' satisfaction study. *Library Philosophy and Practice (e-journal)*. Paper 862. Retrieved from http://digitalcommons.unl.edu/libphilprac/862

Griffin, D. (2002). *The emergence of leadership: Linking self-organization and ethics*. London, U.K.: Routledge.

Hendrich, A., Chow, M. P., Skierczynski, B. A., & Lu, Z. (2008). A 36-hospital time and motion study: How do medical-surgical nurses spend their time? *The Permanente Journal, 12*(3), 25.

Kanter, R. M., & Bird, M. (2011, December). Cancer Treatment Centers of America: Scaling the Mother Standard of Care. *Harvard Business School Case*, 312–073. Retrieved from https://hbr.org/product/ cancer-treatment-centers-of-america-scaling-the-mother-standard-of-care/312073-PDF-ENG

Kelly, T., & Littman, J. (2001). *The art of innovation*. New York, NY: Broadway Business.

Kemper, D. W., & Mettler, M. (2002). Information therapy: Prescribing the right information to the right person at the right time. *Managed Care Quarterly, 10*(4), 43–46.

Kitson, A., Marshall, A., Bassett, K., & Zeitz, K. (2013). What are the core elements of patient-centered care? A narrative review and synthesis of the literature from health policy, medicine and nursing. *Journal of Advanced Nursing, 69*(1), 4–15.

Levesque, M., Hovey, R., & Bedos, C. (2013). Advancing patient-centered care through transformative educational leadership: A critical review of health care professional preparation for patient-centered care. *Journal of Healthcare Leadership, 5*, 35–46.

Mallik, M. (1997). Advocacy in nursing—a review of the literature. *Journal of Advanced Nursing, 25*(1), 130–138. doi:10.1046/j.1365-2648.1997.1997025130.x

Malloch, K., Sluyter, D., & Moore, N. (2000). Relationship-centered care: Achieving true value in healthcare. *Journal of Nursing Administration, 30*(7/8), 379–385.

McWhinney, I. R. (1984). Changing models: The impact of Kuhn's theory on medicine. *Family Practice, 1*(1), 3–8. doi:10.1093/fampra/1.1.3

Melnyk, B., & Fineout-Overholt, E. (2005). *Evidence-based practice in nursing and healthcare*. Philadelphia, PA: Lippincott, Williams & Wilkins

Melnyk, B. M. (2014). Speeding the translation of research into evidence-based practice and conducting projects that impact healthcare quality, patient outcomes and costs: The "so what" outcome factors. *Worldviews on Evidence-Based Nursing, 11*(1), 1–4.

Morgan, S., & Yoder, L. H. (2012). A concept analysis of person-centered care. *Journal of Holistic Nursing, 30*(1), 6–15.

Müller, R. M., & Thoring, K. (2012). Design thinking vs. lean startup: A comparison of two user-driven innovation strategies. *Leading Through Design*, 151. Retrieved from http://www.researchgate.net/profile/ Erik_Bohemia/publication/233801554_Leading_Innovation_through_Design_Proceedings_of_the_ DMI_2012_International_Research_Conference/links/0fcfd50ba3d8153431000000.pdf#page=181

Norman, C. D., & Skinner, H. A. (2006). Ehealth literacy: essential skills for consumer health in a networked world. *Journal of Medical Internet Research, 8*(2), e9. doi:10.2196/jmir.8.2.e9

Porter-O'Grady, T., & Malloch, K. (2007). *Quantum leadership: A resource for health care innovation* (2nd ed.). Sudbury, MA: Jones and Bartlett Publishers.

Rathert, C., Wyrwich, M. D., & Boren, S. A. (2012). Patient-centered care and outcomes: A systematic review of the literature. *Medical Care Research and Review, 70*(4) 351–379

Semigran, H. L., Linder, J. A., Gidengil, C., & Mehrotra, A. (2015). Evaluation of symptom checkers for self diagnosis and triage: Audit study. 351: h3480. Retrieved from http://www.bmj.com/content/351/bmj .h3480.full.pdf+html

Stacey, R. D., Griffin, D., & Shaw, P. (2000). *Complexity and management: Fad or radical challenge to systems thinking*. London, U.K.: Routledge.

Suchman, A. L. (2011). Relationship-centered care and administration. In A. L. Suchman, D. J. Sluyter & P. R. Williamson (Eds.), *Leading change in healthcare: Transforming organizations using complexity, positive psychology and relationship-centered care* (pp. 35–42). London, U.K.: Radcliffe.

Syme, S. L. (2005). Historical perspective: The social determinants of disease—some roots of the movement. *Epidemiologic Perspectives & Innovations : EP+I, 2*(2). doi:10.1186/1742-5573-2-2

Tresolini, C. P., & Pew-Fetzer Task Force. (1994). *Health professions education and relationship-centered care.* [Report]. San Francisco, CA: Pew Health Professions Commission. Retrieved from http://www.rccswmi .org/uploads/PewFetzerRCCreport.pdf

Uhl-Bien, M., & Marion, R. (2008). *Complexity leadership part 1: Conceptual foundations.* Charlotte, NC: Information Age.

Urban Dictionary. (2015). Dr. Google. Retrieved from http://www.urbandictionary.com/define.php?term= Dr+Google

Watson, J. (2003). Love and caring: Ethics of face and hand—an invitation to return to the heart and soul of nursing and our deep humanity. *Nursing Administration Quarterly, 27*(3), 197–202.

Weberg, D. R. (2013). *Complexity leadership theory and innovation: A new framework for innovation leadership* (Doctoral dissertation, Arizona State University).

Woolf, S. H., Chan, E. Y., Harris, R., Sheridan, S. L., Braddock, I. H., Kaplan, R. M., . . . Tunis, S. (2005). Promoting informed choice: Transforming health care to dispense knowledge for decision making. *Annals of Internal Medicine, 143*(4), 293–300.

Supporting Innovation through Evidence

Incorporating New Evidence from Big Data, Emerging Technology, and Disruptive Practices into Your Innovation Ecosystem

Rayne Soriano and Daniel Weberg

CHAPTER OBJECTIVES

Upon completion of this chapter, the reader will be able to:

1. Describe emerging sources of data to inform evidence-based practice (EBP).
2. Discuss leadership competencies to support new sources of evidence.
3. Describe impacts new evidence has on healthcare practices.

INTRODUCTION

In the backdrop of healthcare challenges and linking hospital reimbursements to the quality of care, the need to efficiently access information to maintain and improve quality measures is heightened by benchmarking across organizations and public reporting by hospitals to consumers, insurers, and regulatory bodies (Centers for Medicaid and Medicare Services, 2014; Chassin, Loeb, Schmaltz, & Wachter, 2010; National Quality Forum, 2014; The Joint Commission, 2014). Drivers to improve the quality, safety, and value in the U.S. healthcare system have focused on transformational efforts through channels such as accessing and utilizing data as a staple for health learning (Institute of Medicine, 2010), improving systems for safety (Institute of Medicine, 2000), achieving high-reliability organizations (Chassin & Loeb, 2011), and adopting health information technology (HIT) (Institute of Medicine, 2000, 2012) through groundbreaking and widespread efforts like the implementation of electronic medical records (EMR), thus producing exponentially more data for using complex mathematical algorithms to find answers in big data sets and using those sources of evidence to employ disruptive practices to improve outcomes.

INFORMATION AT THE CAREGIVERS' FINGERTIPS

Traditional sources of evidence for EBP methodologies have focused on comprehensive systematic reviews, randomized control trials (RCT), peer-reviewed journals, and other formal research (Melnyk & Fineout-Overholt, 2011). As technology becomes more and more integrated in health care, new sources of data are available in near real time at the fingertips of caregivers, just like new sources of data are available to consumers through Internet in mobile devices, to help augment more traditional sources of data. These new sources of data serve as a platform allowing frontline clinicians to innovate at the point of care in near real time, thus completely disrupting the current EBP timelines of 17 years from research to practice. In the backdrop of complex and busy environments in health care, whether in acute care hospital settings or crowded primary care clinics, the onus is on HIT vendors in partnership with clinical informatics, and innovation teams to develop seamless and contextual solutions to access information and avoid adding to the information fatigue resulting from growing technology in health care.

Cross-industry, department, and system collaboration requires different leadership behaviors than the pure operational work that many nursing and healthcare leaders focus on. The development and implementation of solutions that bring new sources of data to the bedside in real time, and the cultural and staff support that is required to adopt and sustain such efforts, calls for the ability to view and translate complex systems, understand and enable nonlinear work flows, and understand that all data is not created equal.

NEW SOURCES OF DATA IN HEALTH CARE

As more health information technologies are implemented in healthcare settings across the continuum of care, emerging sources of data have also grown, surrounded with the promise of interoperable systems, portable health information, and improvements in information access leading to better quality care. There are three broad categories of data that are providing new sources of evidence for disruptive practices in health care and shifting the paradigm of EBP to instantly available, accurately curated information that enables the frontline caregivers and organizational leaders to more quickly make decisions, intervene for better outcomes, and potentially control costs and quality in more dynamic and innovative ways.

The first source of new evidence is the ubiquitous use of EMRs to gather, sort, and display data about patients. The second source of new evidence is the emerging categories of wearable devices that collect social and physiological data on individuals and send that data wirelessly to healthcare providers. The third source of new evidence comes from the output of complex mathematical algorithms that can churn and process massive data sets and find patterns, linkages, and visualizations that lend new insights to previously buried information. This chapter will discuss these new sources of evidence, their impact on innovation, and the leadership competencies needed to use new sources of data to implement disruptive strategies.

EMRs as a Source of Evidence and Innovation

The U.S. healthcare environment is complex, with challenges in quality, safety, efficiency, and value. Furthermore, healthcare spending in the United States is greater than in any other industrialized country (Squires, 2012). Despite the mounting financial investment in health care (Robert Wood Johnson Foundation, 2008), the system is plagued with issues that continue to deteriorate the quality of care, such as medical errors (Van Den Bos et al., 2011), overtreatment, failures of care coordination, failures in execution of care processes, administrative complexity, pricing failures, fraud, and abuse (Berwick & Hackbarth, 2012). In the backdrop of ongoing incidences of patient falls, hospital-acquired pressure ulcers, and medication errors in the acute care environment, a critical focus of hospital quality is on nurse-sensitive measures that are indicators of assuring that nursing care is carried out in a safe and evidence-based manner.

New Data Contribution

As a tool to support real-time access to information needed for quality monitoring in general, and for nurse-sensitive quality measures in particular, the EMR has been implemented in many hospitals as part of a mandate under the Health Information Technology for Economic and Clinical Health (HITECH) Act. The U.S. Department of Health and Human Services (2013) defined the EMR as real-time, patient-centered records that make information available instantly, bringing together everything about a patient's health in one place. Beyond the implementation of EMR systems, the meaningful use initiative was developed as an incentive program to assure that EMRs are used according to standards that achieve quality, safety, and efficiency measures (Centers for Medicare and Medicaid Services, 2013).

One of the most significant structural developments for reinforcing information access has been the implementation of EMRs in hospitals. Evaluating caregiver experiences in using EMRs, is important for highlighting opportunities and challenges in utilizing the tool for accessing information to enable quality monitoring. The features and applications within EMRs can also facilitate their use. Studies examining the applications and features of technology in health care have evolved from focusing on specific work functions to focusing on measures of EMR functionality for driving meaningful use in increasing quality, safety, and efficiency. Studies that have examined the features and applications of technology in the healthcare setting have looked at specific functions and various roles, such as continuous patient monitoring by nurses

(Jeskey et al., 2011); data gathering and quality monitoring for operational leaders (Bradley et al., 2003); electronic information systems for planning, organizing, and staffing for managers (Lammintakanen, Saranto, & Kivinen, 2010); and EMRs. Under EMRs, specific functions that were studied include the use of electronic patient support materials and ordering tests, procedures, and drugs (DesRoches, Donelan, Buerhaus, & Zhonghe, 2008); and electronic documentation of medications, vital signs, ongoing assessment data, and progress notes (Kossman and Scheidenhelm, 2008; Moody, Slocumb, Berg, & Jackson, 2004). Findings from these studies have shown that using the EMR must be facilitated through the availability of useful applications and features, such as the ability to document clinical care efficiently and retrieve data for monitoring patient care. With the quality, safety, and efficiency drivers of using EMRs, meaningful use has set the bar for EMR features to higher standards for achieving these outcomes. This raises questions as to how clinicians develop the skill sets to access information using these features in light of the challenges with preparation and training, as well as the structural challenges, and barriers to EMR adoption.

Challenges to Utilization

Despite significant evidence-based interventions and innovations to address major healthcare quality issues such as falls and pressure ulcers, the translation and implementation of that evidence to the frontline caregivers remains a significant problem. Even with the installation and use of EMR systems, clinical decision support remains fragmented from the complex work flows that govern patient care. This fragmentation of information and work flow began with the first EMR systems because these early systems were merely databases and billing support systems that contained clinical notes. As the systems evolved, teams of information technology professionals in healthcare organizations have attempted to optimize the user interface, data structures, and data linking in relevant ways to support care and the care team members. As these optimizations have continued, it has become possible to link evidence-based information that has been vetted through the EBP process directly to care interventions that nurses, physicians, and other care providers are implementing at the point of care. For example, partnerships among third-party content vendors that serve as clinical practice guidelines for nursing plans of care can be integrated into the EMR and activated via decision support engines to highlight the required assessments and interventions based on the most current evidence.

The literature suggests that EMRs as a source of information may be underutilized, with reports of structural and system challenges (Agno & Guo, 2013; Ash & Bates, 2005; Berner & Moss, 2005; DesRoches et al., 2008; Grabenbauer, Skinner, & Windle, 2011; Kossman, 2006; Kossman & Scheidenhelm, 2008; Moody et al., 2004; Rogers, Sockolow, Bowles, Hand, & George, 2013) and process work-arounds that have led to increased complexity and challenges for providers in accessing information due to the persistence of paper documentation and nonintegrated systems (Ash & Bates, 2005; Keenan, Yakel, Dunn Lopez, Tschannen, & Ford, 2013).

In light of the benefits and features of EMRs for improving access to information for quality measures, there is an emerging body of literature from hospital settings with varying sample sizes that reveals that EMR use is problematic for caregivers based on national surveys, large federal and academic health systems, and users from individual hospitals. Structural challenges with accessing information in the EMR include problems filtering information (Berner & Moss, 2005; Grabenbauer et al., 2011); lack of context-sensitive decision support and issues with the usefulness of the data (Berner & Moss, 2005); lack of usable functionality (DesRoches et al., 2008; Rogers et al., 2013); lack of interoperability (Ash & Bates, 2005); lack of technical support (Agno & Guo, 2013); slow system response, need for multiple screens and overuse of check boxes and copy-and-paste documentation (Kossman, 2006; Kossman & Scheidenhelm, 2008); and various system interface challenges (Moody et al., 2004).

Despite the availability of functions that enable automation of work tasks and meaningful use, studies have emerged showing that technology can also be a source of increasing complexity in health care and may not be easy to use, leading to potentially negative implications for all, including healthcare leaders (Flanagan, Saleem, Millitello, Russ, and Doebelling, 2013; Grabenbauer et al., 2011; Kossman & Scheidenhelm, 2008; Moody et al., 2004; Saleem et al., 2009; Whittaker, Aufdenkamp, & Tinley, 2009). To highlight the effects of technology in healthcare environments, Alexander and Kroposki (2001) performed a longitudinal study comparing technology over a 10-year period and found a significant change in the complexity of technology on three dimensions: instability, uncertainty, and variability. As a result of this complexity, a study of electronic information system use by nurse leaders revealed participants described their concerns with information technology addiction and that system outages would lead to stoppages of clinical processes due to the overreliance of technology (Lammintakanen et al., 2010). Two studies also found perceptions that technology increases the workload for staff (Kossman & Scheidenhelm, 2008; Lammintakanen, Kivinen, Saranto, & Kinnunen, 2009), leading nurse leaders to defer from using the systems themselves and delegating any computerized work to those with training in computers and information processing (Lin, Wu, Huang, Tseng, & Lawler, 2007).

Studies of practices related to using electronic databases found that there needs to be a focus on system usability and work processes to support the use of information systems (Lammintakanen et al., 2010); integrated systems are needed for information flow to assist users with efficiently accessing information and guiding them with decision support (Effken, Brewer, Logue, Gephart, and Verran, 2011); and information access and processing skills need to be developed beyond basic computer skills (Syoubuzawa, Yamanouchi, & Takeda, 2006).

Summary of EMRs as a Data Source

The EMR has been an impressive innovation that has facilitated transformations in care through digital documentation. New data that has been generated by EMRs has allowed nurses and other team members to collaborate, share information, and alert one another about care variations, patient needs, and assessment information. Challenges still remain in the implementation of EMRs and the structuring of data contained within them. Leaders need to facilitate processes that match the work flow to documentation systems and support new informatics competencies to fully utilize this rich source of new evidence.

Wearables and Patient-Entered Data

With consumerism of health care growing, there is an emerging trend wherein healthcare organizations are taking advantage of the ubiquity of mobile devices, the Internet, and social media to affect healthy behaviors through virtual means via partnerships with the retail industry. The wearable and patient-entered data revolution has democratized data and freed it from the bowels of paper charts, inefficiently designed mainframe EMRs, and the back office medical practices, and placed it into the uberaccessible Internet cloud. Here the data can be accessed by the whole care team and across systems, crunched by complex algorithms, and used to link personal data to clinical diagnoses, treatment outcomes, and preventive care. But even with the ability to quantify health through these technologies, self-efficacy and motivation remain ongoing challenges.

Discussion

What can be done to integrate and sustain wearable technologies in consumers' lives? Where is the balance between privacy and linking health behaviors to avenues like social media?

Beginning with fitness and diet applications that consumers use to track their health goals, healthcare organizations and application vendors are expanding these tools to quantify overall health, and even utilize gamification and fashion to motivate people to sustain the use of these wearable technologies (Chan et al., 2012; Dobkin, 2013). Patient-entered data is collected and aggregated in many different ways. Wearables are a category of devices that people can wear on and that both actively and passively collect data. Examples of wearables include activity trackers like Fitbit, wirelessly connected insulin pumps, and U.S. Food and Drug Administration (FDA) cleared vital sign monitors like Withings products, among others.

New Data Additions

Wearables are capable of capturing and continuously transmitting millions of data points to create a quantified picture of an individual's activity, habits, vital signs, and body metrics. These discrete and massive data sets have never before been possible in medicine, and they disrupt the very foundations on which diagnosis, treatment, and interventions are founded. They also bring incredible capabilities out of critical care units and into the home. Steinhubl, Muse, and Topol (2015) described some wearables that can optically assess cell microvasculature to continually and accurately measure blood pressure. It is now possible to see every step, every heartbeat, and every brain wave a patient may have in the course of a day and link that data, through complex algorithms, to measures of stress, anxiety, cardiac health, and more. This is in stark contrast to the point-in-time data practitioners received in the past. The wearable revolution provides new sources of evidence to gain new insights into care.

Banaee, Ahmed, and Loutffi (2013) suggested that wearable data will provide the fuel to support big data analytics to mine physiological data and determine new patterns, relationships, and anomalies. Uncovering these new anomalies provides new insights to care, frees evidence from RCT studies, and opens data up to real-time assessment by frontline caregivers. From this freedom of data, practitioners can potentially change care interventions instantly while simultaneously viewing instant impacts to the patient's physiology. Wearable data may provide a new modality for real-time EBP implementation.

Another way wearables are changing how evidence is consumed in care is by freeing once-siloed data from the hands of clinicians and into the view of patients. No longer is vital sign data held in a paper folder in the file room—now real-time trending of activity, diet, and physiology are available at any time to the patient. This freedom of data is impacting how patients self-manage chronic conditions. Fox and Duggan (2013) found that 62% of patients with two or more chronic conditions track their health either by paper or in their heads. Aitken and Gauntlett (2013) suggested that patients who track their health metrics via a mobile app would have an increased compliance percentage. Chiauzzi, Rodarte, and DasMahapatra (2015) suggested that using monitoring devices can make a direct and real-time impact on self-management of patients with chronic conditions. Patients who received data from their monitoring efforts were more likely to change behaviors related to lifestyle. Wearable data is providing a real-time feedback loop to practitioners and patients to support change and adaptation. Now patients, along with the care team, can monitor for abnormalities and patterns in the data and work together to alert one another to issues or successes with treatments.

With the expansion of wearable and mobile technologies, healthcare organizations and third-party vendors are exploring ways to filter and leverage the data from these devices to integrate them into their preventive health plans and provide caregivers with insights about their patients' adherence to care plans and prescriptions. Examples include applying wearable devices in the surgical environment to improve efficiencies and safety (Shantz & Veillette, 2014) to utilizing wearable technologies for assessing daily activity, and fall risk for older adults (Najafi, Armstrong, & Mohler, 2013). As wearable technologies continue to develop in the clinical arena, healthcare providers and organizations will need to form strategies to embrace the new data from these sources so it can be meaningfully used in their patients' care.

Challenges of Wearables

Along with the potential of wearable technologies to impact clinical outcomes and patient engagement, challenges are emerging. The struggles of extracting and utilizing meaningful insights from information systems today is compounded by the introduction of new sources of data. This makes the role of caregivers even more stressful and hard to carry out as more and more data is sent to already overloaded practitioners.

Another area of concern includes increasing regulatory oversight and compliance (Chan et al., 2012). Many devices on the market today are focused on consumers, not specifically on health care. Consumer-grade devices may not be as accurate in data collection, and they cannot be used for clinical diagnosis unless they are FDA approved. Devices used for general wellness, such as weight tracking, fitness, and relaxation, are not currently regulated by the FDA. On the other hand, devices that make specific claims about treating a recognized disease or medical condition will require FDA approval. This approval process also creates a barrier for many companies that have limited funding.

There are social factors that can also impact the validity of the data. Patients who obsess over their own body metrics and instant interventions for any abnormal value, regardless of clinical validity, can hamper adoption of the technology by care teams and insurers (Swan, 2013). There are also questions about the validity and motivation to track personal data to meet treatment goals. Some patients may inaccurately report data or place the wearable on a family member or friend to get data that might be acceptable to the clinician and avoid confrontation about the lack of adherence to treatment plans.

These social, regulatory, and logistic issues related to patient-entered data require leaders to continue to innovate and iterate on solutions for the best use of the data. There is no doubt that the wearable revolution is a new source of data for EBP and innovation in health care. Samples of very early but innovative programs have begun to crop up in the industry, and they are supported by large consumer companies that allow the technology and mechanisms for adoption to remain inexpensive and easy to use.

Case Example

One example of a program that is using wearables as a source of data and evidence for treatments, centers on diabetes management. Data from wireless glucometers is transmitted directly to the complex care case manager, who can review trends over days and months and intervene faster than with the traditional chart review method or patient-reported levels. Data is making the care more efficient and is streamlining work flows.

This diabetic program demonstrates the synthesis of traditional EBP interventions enhanced by unproven and innovative sources of data to improve outcomes in patients. It is just a matter of time before data points from activity and other wearable data will be linked to clinical outcomes and decision support tools to rapidly improve the care that teams can deliver.

Summary of Wearable Evidence

Wearable data sources are dynamically shifting the sources of evidence that patients and providers have to intervene in their own health journey. Advantages including longitudinal data, continuous monitoring, and information feedback loops. There are challenges with validity, the quantity of data, and processing large amounts of data. Healthcare leaders must continue to innovate and explore new ways of using this evidence to change practice and treatment, and also be open to gaining insights from the patients themselves as they recognize patterns drawn from monitoring their everyday life.

Big Data Analytics

With new sources of data from EMR and wearable technologies, organizations are driven to invest in analytical tools and infrastructure to process and utilize vast amounts of data to deliver efficient, effective, and affordable care. Big data analytics has become the engine driving organizations toward becoming learning institutions through means such as the following: improving decision support at the bedside that is underpinned by data; developing clinical and operational dashboards; supporting predictive analytics for early warning of preventable conditions; and serving as a foundation for research and new partnerships to perform studies that were never possible before the emergence of big data.

Big data is defined by Mayer-Schonberger and Cukier (2013) as the application of math to data sets so large that they cannot be managed by traditional data management tools. By applying complex mathematics, the big data systems process variables across massive data sets to infer probabilities of linkages to one another. Big data is not the creation of artificial intelligence or machine learning, although big data is part of the process that supports those endeavors. Everyday examples of big data can be seen in how driverless cars avoid collisions by processing millions of data points from sensors and translate them into speed and breaking pressures to adjust the car with respect to its surroundings. Google and Amazon use big data to determine search patterns, infer desires, and present the most relevant search findings to the user. How might we use big data in health care and leadership?

New Data Additions

As caregivers enter more data into EMR systems, electronic histories and preferences are being built for patients as their digital footprints grow in health care. With this wealth of information in electronic systems, clinicians are beginning to leverage the data through real-time decision support systems that pull from variables such as allergies, medication histories, and patient goals and preferences. Through these tools, not only are clinical outcomes improved by giving providers better insights and situational contexts before engaging patients for the first time, but overall service and patient satisfaction are also improved through the personalization of health care (Bates, Saria, Ohno-Machado, Shah, & Escobar, 2014).

The contribution of big data to health care can be seen in several categories. Research is benefiting from big data through the use of predictive modeling to assess clinical trial attrition rates and improve research and development times. Public health is benefiting by analyzing disease patterns and transmissions across large data sets. They are using that data to more accurately target vaccines and provide services during outbreaks. Additionally, big data is supporting EBP by combining and analyzing data from multiple systems, such as EMRs, insurance databases, genomic data, and unstructured narratives, to infer insights into disease risk and care efficiencies (Raghupathi & Raghupathi, 2014).

To better describe how big data is impacting care environments and operations, we will present two case examples. One case study addresses how big data provides decision support and guidance to nurses for nurse-sensitive quality measures. The other case study describes how data and predictive models are helping to support hospital patient throughput operations.

Case Example: Nurse-sensitive quality measures and big data

Nurse-sensitive quality measures are well established through the National Database of Nursing Quality Indicators (NDNQI), a proprietary database of the American Nurses Association (2014), which collects and evaluates unit-specific nurse-sensitive data from acute care hospitals; the National Quality Forum (2004), a not-for-profit, nonpartisan, membership-based organization that works to catalyze improvements in health care; and the Collaborative Alliance for Nursing Outcomes (CALNOC; 2014), which was a state pilot site that ultimately contributed to the development of the American Nurses Association NDNQI.

Hospital falls are a prime example of the importance of nurse-sensitive quality measures. Each fall costs an average of $13,316 per incident (Wong et al., 2011), and between 700,000 and 1 million people in the United States fall in the hospital each year (Ganz et al., 2013). As of 2008, the Centers for Medicaid and Medicare Services no longer reimburses hospitals when certain types of injuries occur while the patient is hospitalized, and many of these injuries occur after a fall. Nurses are primarily responsible for the assessment, intervention, and documentation for fall prevention as part of their care planning process, and organizations are responsible for implementing a fall prevention program that includes monitoring, communication, and collaboration (Ganz et al., 2013).

From the data entered into EMRs based on risk assessments and medication administration, alerts and banners warn clinicians of patients who are at high risk for falls, delirium, and other conditions that may lead to their deterioration. Big data technology is able to scan massive amounts of records, run them through complex statistical algorithms, and produce suggested relationships among seemingly disparate data points.

Electronic data care plans and interventions are more collaborative among care team members beyond physicians and nurses because the transparency of information and system alerts and referrals are built to include team members from pharmacy, laboratory, radiology, and behavioral health services to assure that everyone is at the table to support patients.

Case Example: Big data to oversee care and operations

Above and beyond the use of data at the point of care, organizations are starting to build dashboards and electronic reports to help provide insights into population trends and allow organizations to use information to prioritize care and shift resources in areas with the most need. Within the infrastructure consisting of manual processes and multiple applications that sometimes produce redundant information, it is vital that organizations provide resources and support to operational leaders, for them to integrate competencies in information knowledge and skills to oversee the quality of care.

One example of how big data is supporting operations is in the use of command centers and predictive census solutions. Historically, hospital census has been estimated by looking at several past years' numbers and averaging the model to estimate the daily average census on any given day. Very few other data points, aside from historical data, are usually taken into account. With the creation of powerful data analysis tools, such as Tableau and others, data analysts are able to take significantly more data points, such as weather, sporting event schedules, regional data points, and other indicators, to create accurate predictions of emergency department visits, surgery cancellations, and admissions that contribute to a real census. From this data, leaders can more efficiently engage staff departments, allocate resources, and plan for overflow events.

Challenges of Big Data

Much of the discussion of big data is centered on the possibilities and potential rather than specific measured results. Raghupathi and Raghupathi (2014) stated that big data is an evolving science with great potential, yet there are many challenges to overcome. Among those challenges they listed are data management practices, ease of use, scalability of platforms, and privacy and security concerns. Recently, several large healthcare organizations have been hacked, resulting in massive data breaches. As big data continues to grow in capability and adoption, security must be of upmost priority.

Summary of Big Data

There are many insights and capabilities that big data and analytics can provide healthcare leaders and care team members. Predictive modeling can help with hospital operations and public health problems. Compiling data from multiple fragmented systems also provides promise of new patterns and connections that can be made. Although there is significant promise in big data capabilities, leaders should be aware of data management and security risks as they deploy these systems. Additionally, leaders should seek to augment decision making with big data technology and not try to replace clinical judgment or critical thinking.

Summary of New Sources of Data in Health Care

As new evidence sources emerge and are continually refined to become more accurate, leaders must be open to unlearning past practices, like staffing from historical data, and develop innovative plans to better use resources that may contrast with past practices. EMRs are providing digitized records that lay the foundation of data for multiple systems to pull from. Wearable technology is providing new sources of patient information that, through big data analytics, will provide care teams with linkages and treatment recommendations never seen before. Big data is an emerging science that shows promise to help leaders, patients, and practitioners connect disparate dots and uncover new meanings among mountains of variables. The new insights generated by new sources of evidence will require a reconfiguration of traditional care and organizational management techniques. Data-driven decision making will become easier to access and implement. Leaders will need new competencies to work in the age of super information. In part, the healthcare leader must exhibit new competencies in informatics and innovation to be successful at optimizing care, and leading in highly complex organizations.

THE DISRUPTION OF EVIDENCE MODEL

Technology is disrupting the ways evidence is being sourced, consumed, and interpreted in health care. In general, the foundation of evidence (data) is being decentralized from large organizational labs, data centers, and healthcare practitioner offices to the homes of the patients. Industry and innovators are sponsoring this dramatic shift with billions of dollars given to healthcare entrepreneurs for novel solutions and industry-funded competitions to build future technologies. One example is a competition to create a working Star Trek tricorder, a single handheld device that can gather vital signs and other data, that a patient can use without the need for clinical expertise or training. Scanadu Scout has developed such a tool in a hockey-puck-sized device that accurately measures blood pressure, pulse, temperature, and oxygen saturation simply by holding the device to one's forehead.

The gathering of clinically accurate data from patients in their everyday life is very different from how medicine captured data in the past. From these new tools will come massive amounts of data into the system, and leaders will need to create new ways of interpreting and linking this data into real-time evidence for clinicians to use. For practitioners and healthcare organizations to stay relevant, they must be aware of the democratization of data and develop ways to leverage it for better care and new organizational structures (**Table 5-1**).

Table 5-1   Sources and Challenges of New Evidence

Tool	New Evidence	Challenges
EMRs	• Digital records • Analytics • Linked decision support • Instant information access • Relevant data alerts	• Underutilized tool • Inefficient systems • Not designed for clinical workflow • Lack of technical support • Interpretation of unstructured data
Wearable technology and sensors	• Continuous monitoring of patient data (vital signs, activity, etc.) • Longitudinal data sets • Data while patient is away from care team	• Too much data • Reliability concerns • Relevancy of data to diagnosis and treatments • Security and accuracy of data • Accuracy of tools to collect data
Big data	• New links among variables • Predictive analytics • Population health insights • Pragmatic intervention recommendations	• Privacy • Emerging field • Technical support and relevancy

EMERGING TECHNOLOGY AND OTHER SOURCES OF NEW EVIDENCE

In addition to EMRs, wearable data sources, and big data analytic capabilities, several emerging technologies are disrupting how data and evidence are collected by patients and providers. According to Wang (2015), investments in health technology related start-up companies topped $4.1 billion in 2014. Wang observed that

> *the top six categories that accounted for 44% of all digital health funding in 2014 were analytics and big data, healthcare consumer engagement, digital medical devices, telemedicine, personalized medicine, and population health management. Personalized medicine, defined as software used to support the practice of medicine customized to an individual's genetics, slid into the top six for the very first time this year. (Wang, 2015)*

Among these start-ups are innovative solutions that are changing the landscape of health care and health data. Two case examples provide evidence of disruptive technology that is changing how data and evidence is collected and consumed.

Hype Versus Value

With any emerging, unproven technology, one must determine if the risk of piloting a new innovation will add value to the system. Many times this determination is impossible to predict without some level of testing, pilot program, proof-of-concept work, or evidence from other organizations' efforts. However, leaders can use a few tools to assess technologies and determine if they are worth placing bets on.

The first tool is the Gartner Hype Cycle. Gartner is a technology research and consulting firm that has developed a report to assess the usefulness and hype factor of emerging technologies in several industries, including health care (Gartner Hype Cycle, 2015). Technologies are assessed and placed along a hype continuum that can provide a starting point for assessing value. Emerging technologies that are just entering the market are said to be at the Innovation Trigger point. Technologies in that area are virtually untested but show theoretical or early stage success in disrupting the market.

As Innovation Trigger technologies move along the continuum over time, they reach the Peak of Inflated Expectations. At the peak, technologies have accumulated significant discussion about the possibilities and disruptive potential they might offer. For example, when Google Glass, a computer that projects data onto a lens that you wear like glasses, was introduced, early adopters were clamoring to get their hands on one. Healthcare thought leaders hypothesized that Google Glass would be a solution for hands-free documentation, operating room emergency checklists, and even real-time telemedicine consults. After several tests, start-up company solutions, and pilots, Google Glass has only started to catch on. Issues with ergonomics, data reliability, and privacy have slowed its adoption. Technologies at the peak should be considered very carefully with significant due diligence in how they might actually deliver value. Small tests of change are recommended to help with assessments at this stage.

After technologies move through the peak of hype, they slide into the Trough of Disillusionment. This happens as adopters use hyped technology and discover that it may not deliver on all the capabilities that were promised. At this stage, adopters are quickly brought back to reality and must further analyze the value to determine if the technology will deliver on expected outcomes. The trough is a good point to assess if pilots should continue or stop for reassessment. An example of a technology that slid into the trough is EMRs. After the hype and promises that EMRs would streamline work flows, liberate data, and make health care easier and more affordable, the technology slowly declined into the trough as end users realized that work flow, documentation, and data was significantly disrupted and made more complex in the early years after adoption. As realization dawned that they are well worth the investment of dollars, optimization, and time, EMRs have moved to the next stage on the hype curve, the Slope of Enlightenment.

Technologies that have begun to climb the Slope of Enlightenment are moving out of the trough and are showing value to the adopters. Although the value is in the early stage, these technologies might have clinical data or other research to support their value claims. More risk-averse organizations should look to technologies in this phase to begin value assessments and pilots. Wearable technology for use in health care is a good example of this phase. Although it has not been fully validated, wearable technology is showing early promise in impacting health outcomes in research studies.

Finally, technologies will reach the Plateau of Productivity. Here technologies have user and research validation, and have proven and demonstrated value to the industry. Expectations and values are closely aligned, and adoption has spread significantly. Innovation leaders should look to this phase of technology as a valid solution for implementation. Technologies that have reached the plateau are telemedicine and speech recognition.

Using the Gartner Hype Cycle as a framework for innovation assessment will allow the innovation leader to determine a baseline for adoption (**Table 5-2**). It helps the user determine how much time and investment might be needed to prove the value of a technology or determine if the technology is worth pursuing at all. It is important to reflect on what problem you are trying to solve and if technology will enable the solution.

Table 5-2 Hype Cycle and Innovation Leadership Linkages

Hype Cycle Phase	Description	Innovation Leadership Actions
Technology trigger	First introduction to the market	Assess technology for potential value; high risk for failure; extra due diligence required
Peak of inflated expectations	Media hype begins, activity beyond early adopters starts	Be aware of overhyped technology; relate tech solution to problem you are trying to solve; try small pilots to assess value or wait for others to publish results
Trough of disillusionment	Negative press begins; capabilities do not match hype; adoption slows	Assess technology's unhyped capabilities and future road map; determine value and ability to meet needs; good time to assess and pilot technologies
Slope of enlightenment	Value and hype are more aligned; adoption increases and realistic expectations are set	Good time for more risk-averse organizations to assess technology; look for expanding capabilities in technology
Plateau of productivity	High adoption rate; hype and expectations are close	Look for rapid adoption and fast-track pilots; evidence and value should support technology near this phase; do not spend significant time proving technology, instead focus on work flow integration and value to specific problem

Evidence-Based Assessment of New Data Sources

Assessing technology and new sources of evidence on the Gartner Hype Cycle is only one way to determine innovation value. Leaders who are looking to try new innovations to improve evidence-based care should also critically examine the proposed technology against an EBP framework as well. The Institute for Healthcare Improvement (IHI)

Box 5-1 Track Emerging Technology

Assessing technology is everyone's responsibility. One way to continually stay on top of emerging technology is to set up informal meetings to discuss the latest trends and determine their hype. Engage staff, early adopters, and others in the discussion to get a well-rounded view of technology and its potential.

has developed a framework for assessing technology and the resulting evidence it produces (Ostrovsky, Deen, Simon, & Mate, 2013).

The authors provide a framework that combines Triple Aim focus areas, level of supporting evidence, investment level, technology type, and end-user criteria. The Triple Aim focus allows leaders to categorize technologies related to what system-level problem they are trying to solve (i.e., patient experience, population health, per capita cost of care). The level of evidence criteria allows the team to compare the support for new technologies in the literature. Technologies can be evidence based, evidence informed, or emerging. Technology type and investment level help the team further determine the cost to implement the technology, and further define the technology solution. Finally, the end-user criteria helps the team identify who should be included in assessments and pilots of the technology.

By combining the IHI and Gartner tools, organizations will have a consumer- and evidence-based framework to assess technologies, and the evidence supporting those technologies. Emerging technology requires leaders to combine tools and frameworks to create assessments because many emerging technologies have little to no formal research supporting them. Leaders must adapt new ways of assessment and interpretation to foster evidence-based innovation. After technologies are selected and implemented, leaders will need to interpret, manage, and communicate information flowing from the devices and systems. Leaders will need specific informatics competencies, which are described in the next section.

INFORMATICS COMPETENCIES FOR LEADERS

To address the emerging advances in health care through HIT, it is important to identify competencies of clinicians in utilizing HIT. The American Nurses Association (2009) published informatics competencies for various levels of nursing leaders, including chief nurses and administrators, as well as operational leaders, to provide guidance to organizations so they can prepare key leaders for the growing use of information and analytics in operations, administration, and financial aspects of their roles. Similarly, the Quality and Safety Education for Nurses (QSEN) organization has developed informatics curricula to bring these competencies to life. Three Delphi studies have emerged that identified informatics competencies for nurses at different levels (Staggers, Gassert, & Curran, 2002) and for nurse leaders (Hart, 2010; Westra & Delaney, 2008). Although many experts in informatics and nursing leadership have contributed their opinions to identify the informatics knowledge, skills, and abilities needed for nurses, and nurse or clinical leaders, further studies are needed to tailor the competencies to the actual practices of caregivers. The nurse or clinical leader role spans a wide array of clinical and administrative responsibilities, and they need to attain the needed competencies to successfully fulfill their duties, including those that address the use of electronic systems for accessing information. There is a paucity in empirical knowledge about the approaches and strategies that clinical leaders employ, within their already complex and stressful roles, to integrate these competencies to work in today's growing digital healthcare environment.

This section will describe informatics competencies needed by leaders at the front line and at the system level. Without skills in interpreting, communicating, and accessing information from multiple systems, leaders will not be prepared for innovative adaptations or EBP.

Frontline Manager Informatics Competencies

The nurse manager role is multifaceted, and the duties and information-needs span a range of operational areas that include financial (Kang et al., 2012; McCallin & Frankson, 2010; Pillay, 2010), staffing (Kleinman, 2003; Pillay, 2010; Thorpe & Loo, 2003), human resources (Kang et al., 2012; Kleinman, 2003; Lin et al., 2007), and staff and patient safety (Armstrong & Laschinger, 2006). The American Nurses Association (2009) provides a comprehensive, but not exhaustive, list of role characteristics that shows their complex nature. Nurse manager priorities are greatly sensitive to external regulatory bodies and benchmarks (Effken et al., 2011), which include state and federal nurse-sensitive quality drivers (American Nurses Association, 2014; CALNOC, 2014; National Quality Forum, 2014). Given the impact of the nurse manager on retention (Raup, 2008; Vesterinen, Isola, & Paasivaara, 2009), satisfaction (Azaare & Gross, 2011; Failla and Stichler, 2008; Rouse, 2009), productivity (Thorpe & Loo, 2003), and outcomes (Casida & Parker, 2011; Pillay, 2010), studies are needed to explore how they access information to support staff retention and satisfaction, productivity measures, and quality outcomes.

Data from electronic sources allows managers to facilitate and grow an evidence-based care environment by enabling three core functions: monitor documentation, monitor practice, and investigate errors through root cause analysis. Competency in these functions allows the manager to enable care teams to gather information in useful ways, translate evidence into practice, and determine where errors in the system might be and facilitate resolution. Managers must rely on several sources to gather information and context for decision making. Electronic methods such as EMR and other electronic systems can help. Additionally, leaders must rely on their ability to develop relationships with team members to gather information verbally and through observation. Combining these information sources allows managers to understand the context of care, the content of care, and the culture of the team environment (**Table 5-3**).

Table 5-3   Quality Monitoring Information Sources and Actions

Sources of Information	Electronic (EMR)	Electronic (non-EMR)	Verbal	Observation	Paper
Monitoring documentation	Procedures Assessments Tasks Regulatory	Electronic reports	Discussion with staff	Documentation rounds	Paper notes
Monitoring practice	Dashboard Chart auditing tools	Electronic reports	Verbal feedback	Evidence-based bundle interventions Infection prevention Procedures Rounds	Paper audit checklists
Investigating or performing a root cause analysis	Assessments Labs Medications Radiology Notes	Electronic reports	Discussion with staff	Practice variations	Patient complaints

Monitoring Documentation

Monitoring documentation reflects the nurse manager's role in validating that documentation; and also reflects care that is actually provided and that is timely, accurate, and in compliance with regulatory requirements.

Types and Sources of Information Needed to Monitor Documentation

The EMR is the primary source of information used to monitor documentation. The types of EMR documentation monitored include nursing procedures (e.g., restraints, blood administration), assessments (e.g., vital signs, fall risk), nursing tasks (e.g., ambulation), and regulatory mandates (e.g., advance directives). In one study, participants described accessing EMR information from reports they generate and then going into the EMR to monitor documentation by clicking into the various areas of EMR information (Soriano, 2015). Some managers performed these activities, and others delegated some or all of these activities to assistant managers or charge nurses who would report the results back to the manager via e-mail or a paper audit checklist.

Participants also reported performing documentation rounds by walking around their units and engaging nurses to review their documentation in the EMR.

It is important to note that the intent, for innovative leaders, is not to demand compliance by monitoring documentation, but to facilitate accurate information flow into the system. The difference lies in how managers act on the information they receive from audits, observations, and electronic reports. Leaders with a competency to understand electronic data and personal cues from the team will be able to facilitate learning, feedback loops, and sustained practice changes by building relationships with staff, and supporting change with data from electronic means. Using the information from monitoring documentation in more transactional ways (i.e., punishing only noncompliance) will result in staff burnout and turnover (Weberg, 2013).

Monitoring Practice

Monitoring practice reflects the nurse manager's role in validating that care actually happened, in general, beyond the information documented by nurses.

Types and Sources of Information Needed to Monitor Practice

Managers can gather information about the care practices of the team through several sources, including e-mails, electronic reports, direct observation and rounding, and communication with staff and patients. E-mails and electronic reports can be received both automatically and in response to the managers' requests for information from various departments in the hospital, including the quality department, risk management, infection control, pharmacy, and lab. E-mails and electronic reports include information about care practice trends and areas needing improvement, such as (1) scan reports from the pharmacy indicating the use of bar codes to avoid medication identification errors; and (2) catheter-associated infection reports from infection control departments, indicating when catheters have been in place longer than recommended. Additionally, leaders can gather information by performing rounds to monitor these areas, including observation of evidence-based interventions for quality bundles that include groups of evidence-based interventions for quality measures, such as fall prevention, hospital-acquired pressure ulcer (HAPU) prevention, ventilator-associated pneumonia, catheter-associated urinary tract infections (CAUTI), and central-line-associated blood stream infections (CLABSI). Leaders can build team relationships by rounding or walking through their units to access information directly by communicating with staff and patients. For example, nurse managers can talk with staff directly about turning patients at risk for pressure ulcers or making sure that medications were scanned prior to administration.

Monitoring practice is an important role for leaders. Data from electronic sources provide the context for intervention by the leader. For example, if reports show increases in falls, pressure ulcers, or other quality issues, leaders can use that information to interact with staff to improve care. Monitoring practice should not be a parental endeavor; instead, it should be used by the leader to gather information to identify areas where EBP might improve care or in situations and problems that might require innovative solutions. From this information the leader can facilitate change with the team.

Investigating Incidents

Performing investigations reflects the nurse manager's role in investigating incidents, such as patient falls, HAPU, CAUTI, and medication errors or discrepancies.

Types and Sources of Information Needed to Investigate Incidents

The information needed to perform investigations was accessed from the EMR, electronic reports of fallouts (areas that need improvement) produced by various departments, reports from incident reporting systems, verbal reports from nursing staff or assistant managers regarding incidents that occurred during the shift, and verbal or written patient complaints. Using the EMR to perform these investigations in combination with getting verbal or written input from staff is essential to understand the context and system inputs. Information accessed in the EMR includes nursing documentation, physician notes, lab results, radiologic results, and medications. This information accessed from the EMR can be used to connect the dots regarding the incident and facilitate a systems view rather than looking for a singular cause.

Incidents involving patient care can be complex and stressful. Leaders and team members should partner to create a culture of growth and learning when errors occur. Leaders can use electronic data to look for patterns in the interactions and systems of care to help find breakdowns that influence error occurrence. Additionally, gathering informal data from team members can also lend insight. Leaders must be competent in both electronic data interpretation and staff relationships to facilitate solutions and more robust, error-free environments of care.

Summary of Frontline Manager Informatics Competencies

As part of their roles in quality monitoring and improvement, nurse managers are required to access comprehensive information from various sources as a basis for assessment, planning, and interventions in their various areas of responsibility (American Nurses Association, 2009). Studies in hospital and individual unit settings have emerged highlighting that the information needs of nurse managers include financial data, supply management data, regulatory standards for quality and safety, patient information for rounds, satisfaction scores, scheduling and staffing data, human resource information (Baker et al., 2012; Effken et al., 2011), and information about the healthcare climate and population needs for developing and managing projects (Macphee & Suryaprakash, 2012). The sources of information can be overwhelming for leaders in health care, but becoming competent in researching, validating, and interpreting this information is a core competency of future leaders. Frontline managers can use data to interpret the context of care and to facilitate innovation and EBP activities to improve quality (**Table 5-4**).

Table 5-4   Examples of EMR Data to Monitor Practice

Role Component	Monitoring Documentation (EMR)	Monitoring Practice	Investigating or Performing a Root Cause Analysis
• Examples of types of information needed	Procedures: • Lines, drains, airways • Blood administration • Restraints Assessments: • Delirium assessments • Fall risk • Vital signs • Weight • Nursing assessments • Central line assessments Tasks: • Ambulation • Bundle compliance for infection interventions • CAUTI interventions • Medication administration Regulatory: • Tobacco use • Critical lab values • Advance directives Observation: • Documentation rounds	Electronic reports for quality bundles: • CLABSI interventions • CAUTI rounds • Ambulation rounds • Venous thromboembolism rounds Verbal feedback: • Staff • Debriefings • Staff feedback • Unit rounds • Patient rounds Infection prevention: • Hand washing rounds Procedures: • Sedation rounds • Bar code scanning reports EMR: • Quality dashboard	Electronic reports: • Infection report • Incident reports • Fall report • Pneumonia report • Urinary tract infection report • Pressure ulcer report • Pharmacy report EMR: • Nursing assessments • Vital signs • Physician notes • Medication information • Radiologic information • Lab information Verbal information: • Talking to staff Paper forms: • Patient complaints

SUMMARY AND ISSUES

Moving the focus of competencies a layer beyond the frontline healthcare leader, healthcare systems must evolve to be learning organizations; and develop robust and consistent information seeking, and processing behaviors to leverage growing sources of electronic data and information; and operationalize national quality initiatives such as the Triple Aim.

The Triple Aim is focused on the following dimensions:

- Improving the patient experience of care (including quality and satisfaction)
- Improving the health of populations
- Reducing the per capita cost of health care (Berwick, Nolan, & Whittington, 2008)

As a foundation for improving and sustaining high-quality care, there is an increasing movement by hospitals toward becoming high-reliability organizations through investments in leadership, development of a safety culture, and utilization of robust process improvement tools. As an essential factor for achieving high reliability, organizations must invest in information technology to monitor and sustain quality improvement, consistently measure the safety culture, and utilize improvement tools throughout the organization to synthesize and act upon information for quality improvement (Chassin & Loeb, 2011).

Leaders must invest time and effort into understanding data and the sources of data to innovate quality care. Frontline care providers can gather evidence from new technologies, such as wearables, devices, and EMRs, to improve care. Frontline managers and leaders can gather data from reports, systems, and people to facilitate and monitor improvement and quality efforts. Finally, system-level leaders can look for patterns in the data to identify areas, to focus resources for innovation and EBP implementation.

Finally, new technologies are providing data at a rapid rate. The collection of vital signs, continuous alerts, and massive data sets are changing the way healthcare workers manage patient health and care. It is imperative that healthcare leaders of the future continue to assess the relevancy of data using the foundations of EBP. This means that leaders should be open to new sources of data that can inform evidence and also keep a critical eye toward validity, reliability, and application of these new data sources. It will require an innovation mindset to sift through the plethora of technology and data to create new ways of caring for patients, changing the healthcare system, and building EBP.

REFERENCES

Agno, C. F., & Guo, K. L. (2013). Electronic health systems: Challenges faced by hospital-based providers. *Health Care Management (Frederick), 32*(3), 246–252. doi:10.1097/HCM.0b013e31829d76a4

Aitken, M., & Gauntlett, C. (2013). *Patient apps for improved healthcare: From novelty to mainstream.* Parsippany, NJ: IMS Institute for Healthcare Informatics.

Alexander, J. W., & Kroposki, M. (2001). Using a management perspective to define and measure changes in nursing technology. *Journal of Advanced Nursing, 35*(5), 776–783.

American Nurses Association. (2009). *Nursing administration: Scope and standards of practice.* Silver Spring, MD: Nursesbooks.

American Nurses Association. (2014). NDNQI. Retrieved from http://www.nursingquality.org/

Armstrong, K. J., & Laschinger, H. (2006). Structural empowerment, Magnet hospital characteristics, and patient safety culture: Making the link. *Journal of Nursing Care Quality, 21*(2), 124–132.

Ash, J. S., & Bates, D. W. (2005). Factors and forces affecting EHR system adoption: Report of a 2004 ACMI discussion. *Journal of the American Medical Informatics Association, 12*(1), 8–12. doi:10.1197/jamia. M1684

Azaare, J., & Gross, J. (2011). The nature of leadership style in nursing management. *British Journal of Nursing, 20*(11), 672–676, 678–680.

Baker, S., Marshburn, D. M., Crickmore, K. D., Rose, S. B., Dutton, K., & Hudson, P. C. (2012). What do you do? Perceptions of nurse manager responsibilities. *Nursing Management, 43*(12), 24–29. doi:10.1097/01. NUMA.0000422890.99334.21

Banaee, H., Ahmed, M. U., & Loutfi, A. (2013). Data mining for wearable sensors in health monitoring systems: a review of recent trends and challenges. *Sensors, 13*(12), 17472–17500.

Bates, D. W., Saria, S., Ohno-Machado, L., Shah, A., & Escobar, G. (2014). Big data in health care: using analytics to identify and manage high-risk and high-cost patients. *Health Affairs, 33*(7), 1123–1131.

Berner, E. S., & Moss, J. (2005). Informatics challenges for the impending patient information explosion. *Journal of the American Medical Informatics Association, 12*(6), 614–617. doi:10.1197/jamia.M1873

Berwick, D. M., Nolan, T. W., & Whittington, J. (2008). The triple aim: care, health, and cost. *Health Affairs, 27*(3), 759–769.

Berwick, D. M., & Hackbarth, A. D. (2012). Eliminating waste in U.S. health care. *JAMA, 307*(14), 1513–1516. doi:10.1001/jama.2012.362

Bradley, E. H., Holmboe, E. S., Mattera, J. A., Roumanis, S. A., Radford, M. J., & Krumholz, H. M. (2003). The roles of senior management in quality improvement efforts: What are the key components? *Journal of Healthcare Management, 48*(1), 15–28.

Casida, J., & Parker, J. (2011). Staff nurse perceptions of nurse manager leadership styles and outcomes. *Journal of Nursing Management, 19*(4), 478–486. doi:10.1111/j.1365-2834.2011.01252.x

Centers for Medicare and Medicaid Services. (2013). Meaningful use. Retrieved from http://www.cms.gov/ Regulations-and-Guidance/Legislation/EHRIncentivePrograms.html

Centers for Medicare and Medicaid Services. (2014). CMS.gov. Retrieved from http://www.cms.gov/

Chan, M., Estève, D., Fourniols, J. Y., Escriba, C., & Campo, E. (2012). Smart wearable systems: Current status and future challenges. *Artificial intelligence in medicine, 56*(3), 137-156.

Chassin, M. R., & Loeb, J. M. (2011). The ongoing quality improvement journey: Next stop, high reliability. *Health Affairs (Millwood), 30*(4), 559–568. doi:10.1377/hlthaff.2011.0076

Chassin, M. R., Loeb, J. M., Schmaltz, S. P., & Wachter, R. M. (2010). Accountability measures—using measurement to promote quality improvement. *New England Journal of Medicine, 363*(7), 683–688. doi:10.1056/NEJMsb1002320

Chiauzzi, E., Rodarte, C., & DasMahapatra, P. (2015). Patient-centered activity monitoring in the self-management of chronic health conditions. *BMC medicine, 13*(1), 77.

Collaborative Alliance for Nursing Outcomes. (2014). CALNOC. Retrieved from http://www.calnoc.org/

DesRoches, C., Donelan, K., Buerhaus, P., & Zhonghe, L. (2008). Registered nurses' use of electronic health records: Findings from a national survey. *Medscape Journal of Medicine, 10*(7), 164.

Dobkin, B. H., & Carmichael, S. T. (2015). The Specific Requirements of Neural Repair Trials for Stroke. *Neurorehabilitation and Neural Repair*, 1545968315604400.

Effken, J. A., Brewer, B. B., Logue, M. D., Gephart, S. M., & Verran, J. A. (2011). Using cognitive work analysis to fit decision support tools to nurse managers' work flow. *International Journal of Medical Informatics, 80*(10), 698–707. doi:10.1016/j.ijmedinf.2011.07.003

Failla, K. R., & Stichler, J. F. (2008). Manager and staff perceptions of the manager's leadership style. *Journal of Nursing Administration, 38*(11), 480–487. doi:10.1097/01.nna.0000339472.19725.31

Flanagan, M. E., Saleem, J. J., Millitello, L. G., Russ, A. L., & Doebbeling, B. N. (2013). Paper- and computer-based workarounds to electronic health record use at three benchmark institutions. *Journal of the American Medical Informatics Association, 20*(e1), e59–e66. doi:10.1136/amiajnl-2012-000982

Fox, S., & Duggan, M. (2013). Tracking for health. Washington, D.C.: Pew Research Center's Internet & American Life Project. Retrieved from http://www.pewinternet.org/2013/01/15/health-online-2013/

Ganz, D. A., Huang, C., Saliba, D., Miake-Lye, I. M., Hempel, S., Ganz, D. A., . . . & Detsky, A. S. (2013). Preventing falls in hospitals: a toolkit for improving quality of care. *Ann Intern Med, 158*(5 Pt 2), 390–396.

Gartner Hype Cycle. (2015). Hype Cycle Research Methodology. Retrieved from http://www.gartner.com/technology/research/methodologies/hype-cycle.jsp

Grabenbauer, L., Skinner, A., & Windle, J. (2011). Electronic health record adoption—maybe it's not about the money: Physician super-users, electronic health records and patient care. *Applied Clinical Informatics, 2*(4), 460–471. doi:10.4338/aci-2011-05-ra-0033

Hart, M. D. (2010). A Delphi study to determine baseline informatics competencies for nurse managers. *CIN: Computers, Informatics, Nursing, 28*(6), 364–370. doi:10.1097/NCN.0b013e3181f69d89

Institute of Medicine. (2000). *To err is human: Building a safer health system.* Washington, D.C.: The National Academies Press.

Institute of Medicine. (2010). *Clinical data as the basic staple of health learning: Creating and protecting a public good: Workshop summary.* Washington, D.C.: The National Academies Press.

Institute of Medicine. (2012). *Health IT and patient safety: Building safer systems for better care.* Washington, D.C.: The National Academies Press.

Jeskey, M., Card, E., Nelson, D., Mercaldo, N. D., Sanders, N., Higgins, M. S., . . . Miller, A. (2011). Nurse adoption of continuous patient monitoring on acute post-surgical units: Managing technology implementation. *Journal of Nursing Management, 19*(7), 863–875. doi:10.1111/j.1365-2834.2011.01295.x

Kang, C. M., Chiu, H. T., Hu, Y. C., Chen, H. L., Lee, P. H., & Chang, W. Y. (2012). Comparisons of self-ratings on managerial competencies, research capability, time management, executive power, workload and work stress among nurse administrators. *Journal of Nursing Management, 20*(7), 938–947. doi:10.1111/j.1365-2834.2012.01383.x

Keenan, G., Yakel, E., Dunn Lopez, K., Tschannen, D., & Ford, Y. B. (2013). Challenges to nurses' efforts of retrieving, documenting, and communicating patient care information. *Journal of the American Medical Informatics Association, 20*(2), 245–251. doi:10.1136/amiajnl-2012-000894

Kleinman, C. S. (2003). Leadership roles, competencies, and education: How prepared are our nurse managers? *Journal of Nursing Administration, 33*(9), 451–455.

Kossman, S. P. (2006). Perceptions of impact of electronic health records on nurses' work. *Studies in Health Technology and Informatics, 122*, 337–341.

Kossman, S. P., & Scheidenhelm, S. L. (2008). Nurses' perceptions of the impact of electronic health records on work and patient outcomes. *Computers, Informatics, Nursing, 26*(2), 69–77. doi:10.1097/01.NCN.0000304775.40531.67

Lammintakanen, J., Kivinen, T., Saranto, K., & Kinnunen, J. (2009). Strategic management of health care information systems: Nurse managers' perceptions. *Studies in Health Technology and Informatics, 146*, 86–90.

Lammintakanen, J., Saranto, K., & Kivinen, T. (2010). Use of electronic information systems in nursing management. *International Journal of Medical Informatics, 79*(5), 324–331. doi:10.1016/j.ijmedinf.2010.01.015

Lin, L. M., Wu, J. H., Huang, I. C., Tseng, K. H., & Lawler, J. J. (2007). Management development: A study of nurse managerial activities and skills. *Journal of Healthcare Management, 52*(3), 156–168.

Macphee, M., & Suryaprakash, N. (2012). First-line nurse leaders' health-care change management initiatives. *Journal of Nursing Management, 20*(2), 249–259. doi:10.1111/j.1365-2834.2011.01338.x

Mayer-Schonberger, V., & Cukier, K. (2013). *Big data.* New York, NY: Houghton-Mifflin Harcourt.

McCallin, A. M., & Frankson, C. (2010). The role of the charge nurse manager: A descriptive exploratory study. *Journal of Nursing Management, 18*(3), 319–325. doi:10.1111/j.1365-2834.2010.01067.x

Melnyk, B. M., & Fineout-Overholt, E. (Eds.). (2011). *Evidence-based practice in nursing & healthcare: A guide to best practice.* Philadelphia, PA: Lippincott Williams & Wilkins.

Moody, L. E., Slocumb, E., Berg, B., & Jackson, D. (2004). Electronic health records documentation in nursing: Nurses' perceptions, attitudes, and preferences. *Computers, Informatics, Nursing, 22*(6), 337–344.

National Quality Forum. (2004). National voluntary consensus standards for nursing-sensitive care: An initial performance measure set. Washington, D.C.: Author.

National Quality Forum. (2014). National Quality Forum. Retrieved from http://www.qualityforum.org/Home.aspx

Najafi, B., Armstrong, D. G., & Mohler, J. (2013). Novel wearable technology for assessing spontaneous daily physical activity and risk of falling in older adults with diabetes. *Journal of diabetes science and technology, 7*(5), 1147–1160.

Ostrovsky, A., Deen, N., Simon, A., & Mate, K. (2014). A Framework for Selecting Digital Health Technology. *IHI Innovation Report. Cambridge, MA: Institute for Healthcare Improvement.*

Pillay, R. (2010). The skills gap in nursing management in South Africa: A sectoral analysis: A research paper. *Journal of Nursing Management, 18*(2), 134–144. doi:10.1111/j.1365-2834.2010.01063.x

Raghupathi, W., & Raghupathi, V. (2014). Big data analytics in healthcare: Promise and potential. *Health Information Science and Systems, 2*, 3. doi:10.1186/2047-2501-2-3

Raup, G. H. (2008). The impact of ED nurse manager leadership style on staff nurse turnover and patient satisfaction in academic health center hospitals. *Journal of Emergency Nursing, 34*(5), 403–409. doi:10.1016/j.jen.2007.08.020

Robert Wood Johnson Foundation. (2008). High and rising health care costs: Demystifying U.S. health care spending. In *The Synthesis Project* (p. 32). Princeton, NJ: Author.

Rogers, M. L., Sockolow, P. S., Bowles, K. H., Hand, K. E., & George, J. (2013). Use of a human factors approach to uncover informatics needs of nurses in documentation of care. *International Journal of Medical Informatics.* doi:10.1016/j.ijmedinf.2013.08.007

Rouse, R. A. (2009). Ineffective participation: Reactions to absentee and incompetent nurse leadership in an intensive care unit. *Journal of Nursing Management, 17*(4), 463–473. doi:10.1111/j.1365-2834.2009.00981.x

Saleem, J. J., Russ, A. L., Justice, C. F., Hagg, H., Ebright, P. R., Woodbridge, P. A., & Doebbeling, B. N. (2009). Exploring the persistence of paper with the electronic health record. *International Journal of Medical Informatics, 78*(9), 618–628. doi:10.1016/j.ijmedinf.2009.04.001

Shantz, J. A. S., & Veillette, C. J. (2014). The application of wearable technology in surgery: ensuring the positive impact of the wearable revolution on surgical patients. *Frontiers in surgery, 1.*

Soriano, R. M. (2015). *An Examination of How Nurse Managers Access Information for Nurse-Sensitive Quality Measures* (Unpublished doctoral dissertation). University of California, Davis.

Squires, D. A. (2012). Explaining high health care spending in the United States: An international comparison of supply, utilization, prices, and quality. *Issues in International Health Policy* (Vol. 10). New York, NY: Commonwealth Fund.

Staggers, N., Gassert, C. A., & Curran, C. (2002). A Delphi study to determine informatics competencies for nurses at four levels of practice. *Nursing Research, 51*(6), 383–390.

Steinhubl, S. R., Muse, E. D., & Topol, E. J. (2015). The emerging field of mobile health. *Science translational medicine, 7*(283), 1–6.

Swan, M. (2013). The quantified self: Fundamental disruption in big data science and biological discovery. *Big Data, 1*(2), 85-99.

Syoubuzawa, S., Yamanouchi, K., & Takeda, T. (2006). Nursing information processing abilities: A comparison of nursing managers and staff nurses. *Studies in Health Technology and Informatics, 122*, 819.

The Joint Commission. (2014). The Joint Commission. Retrieved from http://www.jointcommission.org/

Thorpe, K., & Loo, R. (2003). Balancing professional and personal satisfaction of nurse managers: Current and future perspectives in a changing health care system. *Journal of Nursing Management, 11*(5), 321–330.

U.S. Department of Health and Human Services. (2013). Benefits of EHRs. Retrieved from http://www.healthit.gov/providers-professionals/electronic-medical-records-emr

Van Den Bos, J., Rustagi, K., Gray, T., Halford, M., Ziemkiewicz, E., & Shreve, J. (2011). The $17.1 billion problem: The annual cost of measurable medical errors. *Health Affairs (Millwood), 30*(4), 596–603. doi:10.1377/hlthaff.2011.0084

Vesterinen, S., Isola, A., & Paasivaara, L. (2009). Leadership styles of Finnish nurse managers and factors influencing IT. *Journal of Nursing Management, 17*(4), 503–509. doi:10.1111/j.1365-2834.2009.00989.x

Wang, T. (2015, January 15). Digital health funding: 2014 year in review [Web log post]. Retrieved from http://rockhealth.com/2015/01/digital-health-funding-tops-4-1b-2014-year-review/

Weberg, D. R. (2013). *Complexity leadership theory and innovation: A new framework for innovation leadership* (Doctoral dissertation, Arizona State University).

Westra, B. L., & Delaney, C. W. (2008). Informatics competencies for nursing and healthcare leaders. *AMIA Annual Symposium Proceedings*, 804–808.

Whittaker, A. A., Aufdenkamp, M., & Tinley, S. (2009). Barriers and facilitators to electronic documentation in a rural hospital. *Journal of Nursing Scholarship, 41*(3), 293–300. doi:10.1111/j.1547-5069.2009.01278.x

Wong, C. A., Recktenwald, A. J., Jones, M. L., Waterman, B. M., Bollini, M. L., & Dunagan, W. C. (2011). The cost of serious fall-related injuries at three Midwestern hospitals. *The Joint Commission Journal on Quality and Patient Safety, 37*(2), 81–87.

Creating a Business Case for Innovation

Cheryl Hoying

CHAPTER OBJECTIVES

Upon completion of this chapter, the reader will be able to:

1. Describe the infrastructure of a patient services department that allows for continuity of care across the organization's healthcare system.
2. Understand the importance of reliability in a healthcare organization and the importance of a resilient staff in achieving reliability.
3. Discuss the role that healthcare systems play in fostering community health and decreasing utilization of the emergency department and hospital services.
4. Recognize the move toward interdisciplinary practice and the benefits to consumers.

INTRODUCTION

In 2001, Cincinnati Children's became one of seven healthcare centers to join Robert Wood Johnson Foundation's Pursuing Perfection initiative. The purpose of the initiative was not just to improve the performance of the seven participating healthcare institutions, but also to demonstrate to the broader provider community that ideal care is attainable (Kabcenell, Nolan, Martin, & Gill, 2010).

That step became a pivotal point in Cincinnati Children's innovative pursuits, spurring leaders to set the strategic objective of transforming health care through organization-wide quality improvement. It was a commitment that quickly spread across the many departments and programs. Subsequent innovative efforts were designed to support the medical center's clinical, teaching, research, and advocacy mission.

Four years later I became Cincinnati Children's new senior vice president of the Patient Services Division. I had come from the Ohio State University Medical Center, where I was responsible for nursing. In my new role at Cincinnati Children's, I also was accountable for nursing and the allied health professions. The added span is now becoming more commonplace—the scope of authority for 60% of chief nursing officers includes areas outside of nursing (Boston-Fleischhauer, 2014b). With this broader role came a new perspective. Not only did I want to determine how we could improve processes, I also wanted to launch the medical center into a new way of thinking interprofessionally.

Discussion

The role of chief nursing officer is expanding to include oversight for allied health and other disciplines. In the future, do you also see the role of nurse manager or director expanding? How? What are the advantages? How might other disciplines react if asked to report to a nurse manager or director? Would a matrix reporting structure be better? Why or why not?

In his book *Leading the Life You Want*, Stewart Friedman states, "Being innovative is to act with creativity and courage in continually experimenting with how things get done, bringing others along with you as you progress toward goals that matter" (2014, p. 14). With this sentiment in mind, we will explore and discuss some of the innovative thoughts and changes that have taken place at Cincinnati Children's over the past 10 years.

A leader's role is to inspire others not just for today but for an extended period of time.

Grow Leaders, Not Managers

Managers are an integral part of organizations. They make sure everyone is doing as they should and that tasks are accomplished as planned. An effective leader, however, should focus on finding and developing more leaders, not managers. Leaders are visionaries. They seek to make changes based on cutting-edge research. Leaders help an organization move forward.

In his book *Joy, Inc.*, Richard Sheridan encourages the elimination of hierarchy: "It's not easy, and some team members grapple with the freedom and responsibility of this leadership style . . . look at every moment, whether difficult or important, as an opportunity see whether a new leader is ready to step up and exercise his or her leadership skills" (2013, p. 144). Sheridan's overarching advice for growing leaders, not bosses, is this:

- "Let your team lead without you" (2013, p. 144). When meetings are unproductive, it may be best to exit, express your confidence, and give your team the authority to make the needed decisions.

- "Be vulnerable" (2013, p. 146). Admit that you are not perfect and do not have all the answers, but say that you will keep trying until you get where you want to be.
- "Encourage new leaders" (2013, p. 148). Do this by being supportive and encouraging your team to develop its own ideas.

The best way to support leadership development in your staff, Sheridan suggests, is to "feed their dream and encourage them as they pursue it" (2013, p. 149).

Innovative leaders rely on both art and science to guide their decision making.

Leaders must be action oriented. Leaders cannot theorize on an idea forever. Instead, effective leaders must push forward, remembering that change is good! At Cincinnati Children's, the effectiveness of new approaches is verified with small tests of change. Implementation takes place in test mode. If it works, roll with it. If it does not work, tweak it and try again. The point is to continue pushing forward for new and better outcomes. Impress this upon staff and shared governance councils. Ask yourself, How can I encourage staff to always be thinking of the next great idea?

Encourage Breakthrough Thinking

Breakthrough thinking is necessary to move forward, but it does not happen without a culture of openness to new ideas and willingness to take risks. Leaders are wise to encourage staff to engage in renewal activities as often as possible. Alison-Napolitano and Pesut, authors of *Bounce Forward: The Extraordinary Resilience of Nurse Leadership*, state that "personal renewal is important for your health and well-being—it allows you to show up for your life, and it gives you energy to do meaningful work . . . Renewal provides you with the interludes you need to solve complex problems with creativity" (2015, p. 42).

Interludes that lead to breakthrough thinking are built into work advances at Cincinnati Children's. During quarterly advances for assistant vice presidents and vice presidents of the Patient Services Division, fun activities pull thinking away from the task of creating strategy or budgets. Cooking healthy meals and repairing a playground for developmentally disabled children provide mental breaks and the opportunity to develop camaraderie and forge personal relationships.

Unlearning May Be Needed

A report published in *Lancet* reviews strategies for transforming education to strengthen health systems in an interdependent world. The authors indicate that competencies to be developed include patient-centered care, interdisciplinary teams, evidence-based practice (EBP), continuous quality improvement, use of new informatics, and integration of public health. In short, undergraduate education needs to provide students with a foundation for lifelong learning (Frenk et al., 2010).

Part of the learning process is unlearning, which is necessary to enhance quality and safety. Unlearning is letting go of old knowledge or old ways of doing business. As difficult as unlearning may be, it is a skill that prepares one for a better way of doing something (Uldrich, 2011). The inability to unlearn can be detrimental to moving forward. As leaders, we can become victims of our own insights and past successes. This can cause us to cling to outdated recipes for success (Porter-O'Grady & Malloch, 2011). They add that "moving into a new age does not mean leaving everything behind. It does mean thinking about what needs to be left behind and reflecting on what does go with us as we move into an age with a different set of parameters" (Porter-O'Grady & Malloch, 2011, p. 10).

Every mile you go in the wrong direction is really a two-mile error. Unlearning is twice as hard as learning.

—ANONYMOUS

Unlearning and breakthrough thinking can be supported by how our workplace and work flow is organized. Often, new structures and processes can help us to see different, more innovative possibilities that can be implemented.

INNOVATIVE ORGANIZATIONAL STRUCTURE

An innovative change in the way the Cincinnati Children's Patient Services Division is organized is making an important impact in patient care and in staff practice. The reorganization gives leaders responsibility for both inpatient and outpatient areas of the medical center. The concept was implemented first with a restructuring of responsibilities for vice presidents in the Patient Services Division. After a year, the division's assistant vice president roles were realigned to include inpatient and outpatient oversight in the patient care areas they managed. Later, the realignment cascaded to directors and managers. This departure from the silo structure of limiting patient care to strictly inpatient or outpatient broadened their perspective while also giving patients the opportunity to see the same caregivers in various healthcare settings.

Most hospital-based staff nursing roles are traditionally designated as either inpatient or outpatient, limiting the nurse's view of practice in other phases of the healthcare continuum. To expand that view, Cincinnati Children's nurse directors are collaborating to design caregiver roles that include work in both inpatient and outpatient settings. It is a major shift in how one thinks about staffing and in how staff think about their work. The newly designed roles place nursing and allied health staff in rotations between inpatient and outpatient settings. The anticipated aim is to do the following:

- Observe the patients' progress along the care continuum.
- Decrease burnout by providing nurses with a break from a highly intense or acute area (such as cardiac intensive care unit) to a lesser acute area (such as cardiology clinic).
- Increase job satisfaction (fewer weekend, holiday, and night shifts in the outpatient setting).
- Maintain skills and technical competence with frequent practice.

After piloting the research study with six nurses in three specialties, which was approved by the institutional review board (Mason & Fiorini, 2013), the study was expanded to 21 nurses in 10 specialties. The end goal is for the nurses to permanently rotate between settings within the same service line and spend half of their work week in each setting. The aim is to determine the impact of the cross-setting role on the nurses' perspective of practice and on job satisfaction and engagement. Preliminary findings show promise in achieving the established aim of the research study.

Preliminary Findings

One nurse who had worked 6 years on the inpatient units found her knowledge broadened in numerous ways when she transitioned to working in the outpatient orthopedic clinics. In the outpatient setting, she learned a patient's entire history, she explained. She saw patients before they had surgery and understood why it was needed. Because of her inpatient experience, she was able to explain to patients and parents exactly what they could expect at the hospital. Then she would see them in the clinic for follow-up visits after surgery. She reported significant learning from being able to observe the entire continuum of care. The experience of interacting with a higher volume of patients and families each day, and the diverse ways of working with families (such as via telephone follow-up calls), has improved her communication skills. The outpatient setting nursing role has an enhanced focus on building relationships, which does not always happen in the hospital where nurses may see patients with short lengths of stay. For nurses who primarily worked in outpatient settings, the foray back into inpatient settings helped them to sharpen their skills, such as using IV pumps, and experience more invasive procedures that are not typically seen in outpatient settings. Another nurse said that rotating helped her understand what happens after the inpatient stay so she can better prepare patients for care beyond the hospital.

Challenges

Rotating nurses through both settings comes with challenges that leaders are working to overcome:

- Scheduling is done differently in inpatient and outpatient settings. If rotating nurses are working a schedule that includes both inpatient and outpatient, the schedules need to accommodate both.
- Inpatient shifts are typically routine hours in the same location. Outpatient shifts often involve different locations and hours in the course of a week. This means that nurses who cannot travel to different locations or work different hours each day due to family obligations may not be suited to rotating schedules.

The best way to fill these blended roles is to have two inpatient nurses from the same service line jointly fill an outpatient job opening. After orientation to the outpatient setting, one nurse works inpatient while the other works outpatient, then they switch.

To further broaden the staff's perspective and to maintain staff competencies, a new organizational model is being implemented at Cincinnati Children's newly expanded Liberty campus, which is located 20 miles north of the hospital's main campus. Many of the operating room staff members at Liberty are the same care providers who work at the base hospital, giving them the experience of urban and suburban settings. As new inpatient staff are hired for the Liberty campus, they are asked to rotate to the main hospital location to enrich their perspective. The pediatric intensive care unit, oncology, and medical–surgical staff also rotate between locations. Doing so allows staff to provide care for two different populations—Liberty is more of a community facility, and the hospital is quaternary (highly specialized care). With the cross-trained staff, greater coverage is enabled because the nurses can provide care where the patient need dictates.

Learning from Diverse Settings: Home Visits

Other organizational changes at Cincinnati Children's are having a positive impact on population health. One significant change resulted from a 2012 visit to Cuba. As an educational endeavor, 11 nurse leaders from across the United States visited the country; the visit included an overview of the Cuban health system. In Cuba, the space and cost of hospitalization is problematic, and home visits to patients are prevalent. These home visits are so effective in Cuba that they were pilot tested and subsequently implemented at Cincinnati Children's with a goal to reduce readmissions for at-risk postacute populations. The program is designed to meet the transition of care needs for patients and families who are not eligible for traditional home health. Families receive a nurse home visit within 48 hours of discharge with this new home visit program.

After 2 years of the Cincinnati Children's home care program, which was funded with a grant from Patient-Centered Outcomes Research Institute (2013), nearly 375 patients were visited in their homes. Within 30 days of each visit, only 6.4% of patients were readmitted. At the same time, an additional 365 patients were referred for home visits, but the patients either refused the visit or the caregiver deemed that a visit was not necessary. Of this second group, 12.3% were readmitted or visited the emergency department. These results demonstrate a significant statistical difference and evidence that in-home assessments provide a valuable service that may reduce readmission for at-risk patient populations. Assessments show multiple examples of patient harm that was averted, improved coordination of care, and an overwhelmingly positive family experience.

Cincinnati Children's decided to initiate a home visit program because it was deemed the right thing to do, regardless of reimbursement. The administrators believed that if patient care could be streamlined with home visits, the finances would follow. The same line of thinking resulted in Cincinnati Children's leadership developing a home visit program for psychiatric patients; nurses provide patients with once-a-month injections to ensure compliance with medication regimes.

Increasing Role of Advanced-Practice Registered Nurses

In 4 years, the number of advanced-practice registered nurses (APRNs) at Cincinnati Children's has increased by 58% to 348. The number is projected to increase to more than 420 by 2017. Their value to the organization and to population health is evident in the number of requests and hires each year. The literature also supports their value. A systematic review (Newhouse et al., 2011) supports a high level of evidence that APRNs provide safe, effective, quality care to a number of specific populations in a variety of settings. Researchers concluded that "APRNs, in partnership with physicians and other providers, have a significant role in the promotion of health" (2011, p. 19). At Cincinnati Children's, APRNs currently work in inpatient and outpatient settings, including the following

- Outpatient clinics in more than 30 subspecialties
- School-based health centers
- Emergency rooms and urgent care settings
- Psychiatry
- Telehealth (pilot program for bariatric surgery patients)

APRNs also provide around-the-clock coverage in numerous inpatient units, including neonatal intensive care, cardiac intensive care, cardiology, neurosurgery, and general/colorectal surgery.

Playing the Role of Disruptor

Innovative organizational structures are designed and led by innovative leaders. One of the roles of an innovative leader is to be a disruptor. If there is an idea that is worth trying, disruptors push to test the implementation of the idea, even if it means treading into new territories. The view that we have never done it that way before is not a reason to shelve a new idea. One former Cincinnati Children's chief executive officer (CEO) instilled this thinking in his leadership staff: it is possible to move in two directions simultaneously.

As Ralph Nader so aptly stated, "I start with the premise that the function of leadership is to produce more leaders, not more followers" (Nader, n.d.). Being a disruptive leader may not be easy, and sometimes it can be uncomfortable, but many believe it is necessary to innovation.

INNOVATIVE PRACTICE MODEL

Health systems have renewed their focus on strengthening interdisciplinary collaboration for at least three reasons (Virkstis, 2012): "First, as the level of collaboration rises, the likelihood of negative outcomes diminishes" (2012, p. 2). Second, "interdisciplinary collaboration enhances the patient experience" (2012, p. 3). Third, "interdisciplinary communication can improve efficiency and reduce costs of patient care" (2012, p. 3).

In its report titled *The Future of Nursing: Leading Change, Advancing Health*, the Institute of Medicine (2011) states that "those involved in the healthcare system—nurses, physicians, patients, and others—play increasingly interdependent roles. Problems arise every day that do not have easy or singular solutions . . . What is needed is a style of leadership that involves working with others as full partners in a context of mutual respect and collaboration" (2011, pp. 222–223). The authors indicated that leadership should flow in all directions at all levels.

In 2002, Cincinnati Children's move to adopt a new multidisciplinary approach to patient care prompted leaders to rethink its practice model and to begin to develop a new model based on interprofessional collaboration. In 2011, the medical center sought to transform the way the organization cares for its patients by building a model that focused on accountable care across the continuum (Hoying et al., 2014). As an academic medical center, Cincinnati Children's already had a history of embracing staff empowerment and shared decision making (Hoying & Allen, 2011). Shared governance for nursing was implemented at Cincinnati Children's in 1989, and a separate allied health structure was created in 1999. However, the two bodies operated in parallel with few occasions to interact and with little collaboration.

By 2005, this increase in collaborative practice precipitated discussions that questioned the purpose and efficiency of two separate structures (one for nursing, the other for allied health). The Patient Care Governance Council (PCGC) was formed in 2006, bringing professional staff together in a patient services shared governance structure. Organized around initiatives, the PCGC's goal was, and continues to be, to deliver better patient care through interprofessional collaboration.

To further enhance collaboration, the immediate past chairs of the Nursing Profession Coordinating Council (NPCC) and the PCGC began attending the Patient Care Committee meetings of the medical center's board of trustees. Also added to the meeting's list of attendees were representatives from pastoral care, physicians, and patients and their families. By 2012, council chairs were named to the medical center's Safety Operations Committee; the chairs of the Interprofessional Management Council and the Nursing Professional Practice Council (NPPC) joined leadership meetings as well. This structure ensures that all voices are heard by senior leadership.

Development of Interprofessional Practice Model

"The articulation of a professional practice model provides a framework for . . . the achievement of exemplary clinical outcomes" (Erickson, 2011, p. 35). Until 2006, the Patient Services Division at Cincinnati Children's had two separate practice models: one for nursing and one for allied health professionals. The two practice models ran parallel to each other and duplicated efforts, yet leaders agreed that achieving exemplary clinical outcomes requires input from all professions. It required new intra- and interprofessional practice behaviors for working together in new ways. To remedy the situation, leaders sought to develop a new practice model that would support the new vision of exemplary interprofessional care.

To allow true collaboration, leadership did not rush the process to develop, adopt, and implement a new practice model. Instead, because the medical center works within a shared governance structure, developing an interprofessional practice model could take shape only after careful analysis, consideration, and feedback from nursing and allied health staff. Development of the new model began in September 2012 when the NPPC initiated the process of reviewing and recommending changes to the nursing practice model. A review group was formed. In November 2012, the group recommended increased nursing participation in developing a revised practice model. Thirteen interdisciplinary focus groups were held to provide feedback and recommendations.

Next, the PCGC reviewed the focus group feedback and revised the practice model. In February 2013, the review group confidently agreed that the new Interprofessional Practice Model (IPM) provided a more succinct yet comprehensive representation of the expectations for nursing practice; the review group recommended that NPPC adopt the IPM as the only practice model for the nursing profession at Cincinnati Children's.

The NPPC agreed. The consensus was that the IPM was considered easier to understand than the current nursing practice model, and the opportunities for the broader interdisciplinary partnership through shared values and expectations outweighed the risks associated with maintaining a discipline-specific model.

Today, the resultant model (**Figure 6-1**) is the overarching conceptual framework for nursing and interdisciplinary patient care at Cincinnati Children's. The figure depicts how all parties collaborate, communicate, and develop professionally to provide patients the highest quality of care. It incorporates these six facets:

- Safety
- Professionalism

Figure 6-1   Working together for optimal outcomes

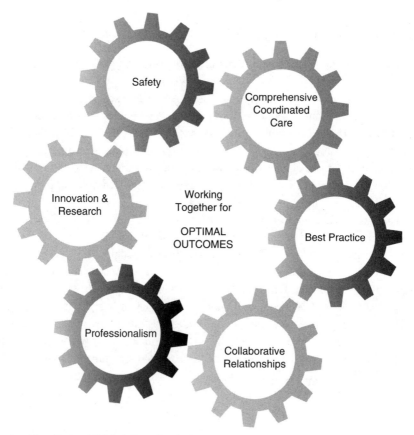

- Best practice
- Collaborative relationships
- Comprehensive coordinated care
- Innovation and research

Since implementation, feedback from frontline nurses about the impact of this new practice model has included the following:

- "It requires mutual respect from the entire care team . . . it is getting us to a new way of practice for the future."
- "It truly is a team-based approach to patient care with the patient's optimal outcome in the center."

The timeline of the IPM's formation, which included allied health, is outlined in **Figure 6-2**.

Figure 6-2 Timeline

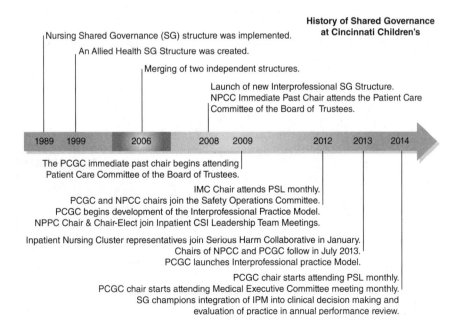

Property of Cincinnati Children's Hospital Medical Center.

The implementation of the new practice model was not without challenges. More than 2 years after the practice model was launched, the level of understanding and implementation varies across the organization. To improve recognition and promote day-to-day usage of the IPM, practice councils continually discuss and review the benefits of using it in problem solving and decision making. For example, clinicians were unable to reach a decision about chlorhexidine baths for patients, so they looked to the gears of the IPM to determine the sticking point. The gears in the model clarify how it works, unlike the former model, which had a lot of words but was not easy to digest.

To help staff effectively use the practice model for decision making and problem solving, a worksheet (**Figure 6-3**) is available on the Cincinnati Children's intranet in the shared governance pages. Staff members are encouraged to use the worksheet to help make decisions and find solutions.

All patient services staff members can submit a problem or idea to the NPCC. This is indicative of the highly collaborative nature of Cincinnati Children's shared governance structure. Accessed online via the shared governance webpage, the submission process gives everyone a voice. After submissions are received, they are reviewed by the NPCC, who then assigns them to the appropriate council for review.

Figure 6-3 Decision-making worksheet

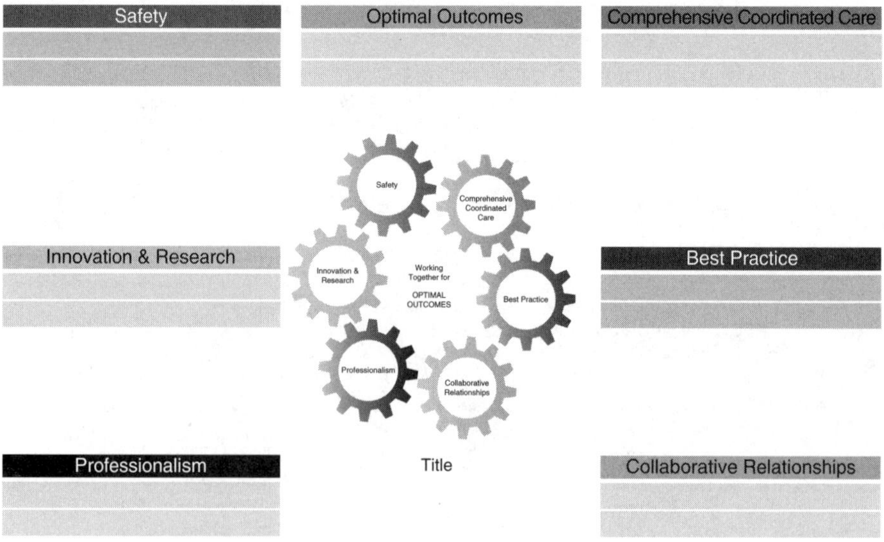

Property of Cincinnati Children's Hospital Medical Center.

An online database charts the progress of each submission; 70 to 80 submissions are received each year.

. . . innovation excellence is often built in a multiyear effort that touches most, if not all, parts of the organization. (de Jong, Marston, Roth, 2015, p. 47)

Since 1989, this staff-driven structure of governance has been at the core of Cincinnati Children's Patient Services Division. Additionally, the inpatient hospital-wide, management-driven Operational Excellence initiative was implemented in 2014. The focus of Operational Excellence is to improve safety, the patient and family experience, and the flow in inpatient areas through empowered and accountable unit leaders. Each unit's clinical director and medical director manage the operations of their units and work together to improve the unit culture and clinical results. These leaders are responsible for a partnered approach to unit-level strategic thinking and planning, communication, and improvement, all with the goal to create focus, define priorities, and build a culture of engagement and ownership. Across the unit leadership, teams apply safety, leadership, and staffing principles, processes, advanced situation awareness, and risk prediction tools.

Shared governance and Operational Excellence share the same passionate intent: to dramatically improve patient care and safety while delivering better outcomes and patient and employee experiences. This intent is also prominent in the medical center's strategic plan.

The challenge for the future at Cincinnati Children's is to develop a model where all staff, in every division and profession, work within the same model and by the same agreed-upon tenets. A step in that direction is still in development.

Interprofessional Education

To fully ingrain the idea of interprofessional practice into the minds of clinicians, one should look upstream to the educational process. This is where clinicians can first learn about the value of an interdisciplinary approach to patient care. The work of the Institute of Medicine (2011) and others has clearly shown that healthcare professionals who understand each others' roles and are able to communicate and work effectively as a team are more likely to provide safe and effective patient care.

> *Continuing to function in the educational silos of current*
> *educational institutions limits formalized exposure to*
> *interdisciplinary opportunities, compromises the ability*
> *to function in future team based practice and research*
> *environments, and contributes to the lack of skill portability*
> *required by students and faculty in diverse and constantly*
> *changing facility and community-based service environments.*
> *(Jansen, 2008, p. 222)*

Jansen believes that multiple barriers exist in the development and teaching of teamwork in healthcare students: "Thus, the emphasis on business values of cost-effective operations means that resources are not readily directed to support the education and development of interdisciplinary teams, a factor that may affect the ability of health professionals to participate in a team context" (Jansen, 2008, p. 220).

Additional barriers include reluctance to alter curricula to include interprofessional education and logistics of scheduling common times for students to engage in interdisciplinary education.

In an unpublished study of the effectiveness of interprofessional teamwork at Cincinnati Children's, 26 nursing and medical students worked together in three pediatric simulation training exercises over an 8-month period. The results indicated that their learned scores were higher than control groups who did not train in an interprofessional setting. Nursing students demonstrated a higher score on teamwork, collaboration, and positive professional identification compared to medical students in both groups. Plans to continue simulation training in an interprofessional environment are underway, with a goal to boost teamwork among all hospital professions.

When representatives from the Robert Wood Johnson Foundation visited Cincinnati Children's in preparation for writing a white paper about interprofessional collaboration, they witnessed the simulation training previously described and the importance of training people in the manner in which they work. "At Cincinnati Children's we were able to see the powerful effects of reflection on a simulation, and how the realizations that occur during reflection can translate to improving interprofessional collaboration and patient care" (Robert Wood Johnson Foundation, 2015, p. 44). Instead of nurses practicing with nurses and doctors practicing with doctors, they witnessed the benefit of training in multidisciplinary teams—physicians, nurses, respiratory therapists—just as in the clinical environment. "At the end of the day, interprofessional collaboration is more than a philosophy—it is about getting real work done through teams" (Robert Wood Johnson Foundation, 2015 p. 45).

> ## Discussion
>
> If you were in a healthcare system, what would be an ideal organizational structure to blend both inpatient and outpatient care delivery? What changes would you make to ensure that caregivers provide services where the need exists instead of expecting patients to come to caregivers? As you contemplate settings, consider community centers, homes, schools.

INNOVATIVE EMPLOYEE ENGAGEMENT

Employees are the cornerstone of a successful organization. They are often the "face" of a healthcare system, and can be the best resource for ideas that improve processes. Employees who feel empowered and appreciated will contribute in immeasurable ways. The topics described below can result in an engaged workforce, satisfied patients, and a safer environment.

You Cannot Be Innovative Unless You Have an Engaged Staff

Effective organizations should have a culture that encourages employee satisfaction. "When employees believe in and trust their management it motivates and encourages employees' participation in decision making which improves employees' efforts, benefits their job satisfaction and commitment to work" (Appelbaum et al., 2013, p. 222).

Yet, as indicated by General Electric in their report *Strategies for Success: Managing Complexity in Health Care* (2015), in the United States less than 43% of the healthcare workforce is happy. That is down from 61% in 1983 and 55% in 2005. It is an even worse situation in Europe, where only 11–23% of the workforce feels engaged. As the authors point out, the constant decline in satisfaction at work is "despite all of the leadership development programs and other initiatives to help managers engage and motivate their teams" (2015, p. 13).

Worse, according to a Gallup report, "30% of U.S. workers are engaged" (2013, p. 8), "52% are not engaged" (2013, p. 12), and "18% are actively disengaged" (2013, p. 13). In a separate study of one hospital system, Gallup found that engagement translates to revenue (Kamins, 2015). The study results indicated that fully engaged physicians were 26% more productive than their less-engaged counterparts, which amounts to an additional $460,000 on average in patient revenue per physician per year.

The authors of the General Electric report (2015) attribute disengagement trends to overcomplicated workplaces. Managers spend about 40% of their time writing reports (matrices, scorecards, etc.) and 30% of their time in meetings, which does not leave much time to work with their teams. As a result, teams do not get the support they need, and consequently they become overworked and disengaged.

The answer, the report states (General Electric, 2015), is not to bring in psychologists to create soft initiatives (a common response). Rather, it suggests the following:

- Simplifying
- Making sure management adds value
- Cooperating
- Giving staff the power to take risks
- Creating feedback loops that expose staff to the consequences of their actions
- Removing layers that do not add value
- Rewarding those who cooperate

The American College of Healthcare Executives (2015) indicates that the most engaged employees are those who are able to make daily progress on meaningful work. They recognize meaningful work as that which helps the organization move forward and achieve its goals. This can be achieved only if the organization's goals are clear, attainable, and broadly communicated.

Discussion Questions

Imagine you are assigned the role of chief nursing officer in a system with poor employee engagement. What ideas would you implement to boost engagement? How would you ensure that long-term engagement remained?

Positioning Nurses to Lead Change

The Institute of Medicine (2011), in response to objectives set forth in the Patient Protection and Affordable Care Act of 2010, states that nurses should be well positioned to lead change and advance health in an evolving healthcare system. The institute's recommendations include the following:

- Remove the scope of practice barriers; nurses should be able to practice to the full extent of their education and training.
- Nurses should achieve higher levels of education and training through an improved education system that promotes seamless academic progression.
- Nurses should be full partners, with physicians and other healthcare professionals, in redesigning health care.

- Effective workforce planning and policy-making requires better data collection and an improved information infrastructure.
- Ensure that nurses engage in lifelong learning. (2011, pp. 29–34)

Shared governance and empowerment go hand in hand; in one study, researchers found that in a hospital setting there was a statistically significant positive relationship between perceptions of shared governance and empowerment (Barden, Griffin, Donahue, & Fitzpatrick, 2011).

Popular author and speaker Matthew Kelly (2011) states, "One of the major issues plaguing human potential in the corporate world today is work-life balance . . . The future of an organization and the potential of its employees are intertwined; their destinies are linked? . . . An organization can only become the-best-version-of-itself to the extent that the people who drive that organization are becoming better-versions-of-themselves" (p. vii).

Broadening the Scope

An innovative way to encourage staff to think beyond their own care setting is being implemented by Intermountain Health System based in Salt Lake City (Boston-Fleischhauer, 2014a). Leaders there have begun a nurse shadowing program, enabling nurses to spend 24 hours over the course of 3 months shadowing a nurse in another care setting within the health system.

For example, a nurse in the pediatric intensive care unit can shadow a nurse in the emergency department. Or a nurse working in an inpatient setting can shadow a nurse in an outpatient clinic, and vice versa. To ensure nurses participating in the program have a meaningful shadowing experience, leaders set clear learning objectives and ask shadowing nurses to write clinical narratives about their experience. **Box 6-1** summarizes the objectives and focus of the shadowing experience.

At Cincinnati Children's, nurses are offered a different shadowing opportunity. For 7 years the Nurse Exchange Program has provided the opportunity for nurses to share their expertise with colleagues from eight pediatric hospitals around the nation. The goal is for experienced nurses to seek, learn, and share best nursing practices. This can be accomplished by adoption of a best practice, improvement science project, or further investigation of research at the unit or organizational level. At Cincinnati Children's, participation is open to RNII-level nurses with a minimum of 2 years of employment.

Employee Engagement and Patient Satisfaction

When their accreditation agency served Midland Memorial Hospital in Midland, Texas, with a leadership deficiency notice, they were faced with an urgent need to boost patient satisfaction scores. The low scores were caused, in part, by low levels

---

Box 6-1 Summary of Shadow Experience

The objectives and focus of the shadowing experience are as follows:

- To understand:
  - The role of the RN
  - The care process
  - Challenges in the setting
  - The patient care operation
  - Clinical goals
  - Compliance and regulatory issues pertaining to nursing practice
  - Role of the patient and family in the care process
  - Patient access to the setting and movement through the setting
- To hear about satisfiers in the setting
- To dialogue:
  - Related to what is important to know about learning to practice here
  - Ideas for nursing practice evolution to meet future patient care needs

---

of employee engagement. Although leaders had assumed that employee engagement and patient satisfaction would improve substantially with the opening of a new tower in late 2012, in reality the reverse occurred. After a year they found that their beautiful new facility raised patient expectations but did not alter the care experience.

Leaders committed to change, and, with assistance from consulting firm Values Coach Inc., they spent 2014 implementing new ideas. Information gleaned from a culture assessment survey of employees confirmed low employee engagement and a perception of an overly negative workplace environment. The results were shared with staff, who were asked to pledge that they would no longer participate in complaining, gossiping, and other negative attitudes. Staff also were asked to recite a daily self-empowerment pledge. Ultimately, the hospital's values statement was rewritten, and all staff were enrolled in a series of courses on personal values.

In a case study on values and cultural initiative (Tye, 2014), Midland Memorial President and CEO Russell Meyers reported, "As a result of our commitment to a culture of ownership, we have documented record-high patient satisfaction and clinical quality indicators and have calculated a cultural productivity benefit of more than $7 million annually" (2014, p. 2).

To create and maintain a healthy work environment, three structures must be in place: leadership, design, and staffing (Dent, Armstead & Evans, 2014). Evidence and scientific data can build a road map to ideal nurse staffing. This road map could lead to higher quality and efficiency in the delivery of care, according to Baggett and colleagues (2014). With these findings in mind, Midland Memorial incorporated evidence and scientific data into the complex process of nurse staffing. Midland Memorial's Robert Dent said the following

Each unit is unique particular to patient populations, acuities of the patients, skill mix of nurses, education and competency of the nurses among other variables to consider in making assignments. Understanding these variables, the clinical managers, staffed mostly 24-hours per day, seven days per week, have the power and autonomy to make appropriate nurse staffing assignments. Nursing leaders must understand data-driven nurse staffing plans to clearly communicate and budget appropriately for nursing resources. (Midland Memorial's Robert Dent, 2015, p. 44)

Empowered Employees Reduce Injury Rate

Cincinnati Children's robust psychiatric program includes 125 beds (acute and long-term care) at three facilities and offers daytime hospitalization for an additional 30-plus patients. Many patients have behavioral challenges. Injuries to mental health specialists and other caregivers unfortunately did occur. In fact, periodic injuries to staff were thought to be part of the job. Asked to make recommendations regarding ways to reduce (ideally to eliminate) staff injuries, the team took a situation awareness approach. Situation awareness is recognized as a way to reduce serious safety breaches in patients, according to a Cincinnati Children's study (Brady et al., 2013).

Empowered with a different mindset (injuries will no longer be considered a routine consequence of the job), the staff developed a situation awareness planning tool (**Figure 6-4**) and an algorithm (**Figure 6-5**) that includes steps for predicting patients at risk, mitigation planning, communication, and next steps if aggression results in staff injury or patient restraint. In the 2 years since the tool was implemented, the baseline days between OSHA injuries more than doubled; and the baseline days between patient injuries that required treatment beyond first aid increased more than six-fold.

Discussion

Although much focus has been placed on patient injury rates, how much focus should be placed on staff injury rates? What are your ideas for boosting resiliency and decreasing stress and injuries among staff? How often should employee injury rates be conveyed? Should employee injury rates be as readily available as patient injury rates? Should they be made public or kept internally?

Figure 6-4   Situation awareness planning tool

Unit: Date: Shift: Outgoing Staff Name: Incoming Staff Name:
  SA Triggers: FR=Flight Risk   WH=Watch Hot   WC=Watch Cold   A=Aggressor   ST=Self Threat   MC = Medical Concern   FC = Family Visitor
                                             Concern

Name, Rm #			
SA Trigger			
S/R High Risk			
Aggression/ Escalation Signs			
Plan			
PRN Medication			
Expected Outcome Must be Yes/No Criteria			
Outcome Deadline (specific time)			
Escalation/ Contingency Plan			

Property of Cincinnati Children's Hospital Medical Center.

Empowerment, Engagement, and Recognition

Staff should be encouraged to suggest new ideas to improve outcomes then be willing to test their implementation. They will not always be successful, but improvement comes only with the willingness to try. It is important to applaud the efforts of staff who are eager to test new ideas. Recognizing and celebrating achievements can go a long way in boosting engagement, even if those achievements are small. Harvard Business School researchers found that when it comes to change, recognizing small wins serve to regularly confirm for staff that they are making progress on meaningful work (Amabile & Kramer, 2011).

INNOVATIVE THINKING

Empowering employees not only results in engagement, it also can generate innovative ideas. The following are examples of innovating thinking that are impacting patients at Cincinnati Children's. Ideas can originate from expected (and sometimes unexpected) sources, such as leaders, staff, patients, and families.

Figure 6-5 Situational awareness algorithm

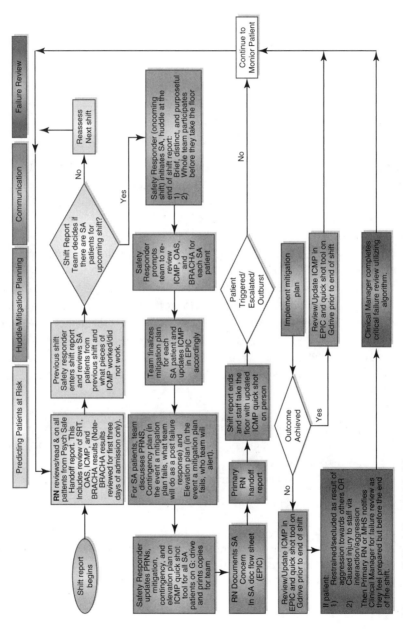

Predicting Patients at Risk | Huddle/Mitigation Planning | Communication | Failure Review

Property of Cincinnati Children's Hospital Medical Center.

Collaborating for Patient Safety

. . . there's no proven formula for success, particularly when it comes to innovation. (de Jong, Marston, Roth 2015, p. 37)

Sometimes a good idea evolves into a great idea. Children's Hospitals Solutions for Patient Safety (www.solutionsforpatientsafety.org) is one such example. Here is how the idea got its start.

In the 1980s, pediatric hospitals in Ohio formed the Ohio Children's Hospital Association (OCHA) to advocate for legislative and regulatory issues that affect children's health. Over time the group's aim broadened to emphasize quality and safety. As Ohio state officials became more aware of OCHA and their success in improving quality and safety, they asked for OCHA's involvement on quality improvement projects. The results were impressive and included reducing surgical site infections, adverse drug events, and serious harm events.

After achieving significant results in the state, Ohio's children's hospitals were asked in 2011 to lead a national effort to implement their strategies in children's hospitals throughout the country. In 2012, 25 hospitals from across the nation joined the Ohio hospitals, forming the Children's Hospital's Solutions for Patient Safety (SPS) network.

By 2015 the SPS network—funded in part by the Cardinal Health Foundation— had grown to more than 80 children's hospitals nationwide. Their shared visions are as follows:

- No child will ever experience serious harm while we are trying to heal them.
- By putting aside competition and sharing our safety successes and failures, we can achieve our goals faster.
- We all learn from and all teach each other to ensure every child is safe in our care, every day.

The network members support each other on their journey toward zero harm by providing frequent training and learning opportunities, tools, data collection and analysis, and opportunities to collaborate. Together they have committed to these shared network goals of harm reduction for 2015–2016:

- 40% reduction in hospital-acquired conditions
- 10% reduction in readmissions
- 25% reduction in serious safety events

To achieve these goals, CEOs, hospital boards of trustees, and clinical leaders are aligning their organizational goals with the network harm reduction goals in a way that is transforming the safety and quality of care delivered in children's hospitals in the United States.

Discussion

How can hospitals be more transparent with patients on their quality scores? What role can partnerships among hospitals play in boosting quality and safety? Using SPS as an example, how would you initiate such a partnership?

Daily Briefs Focus on Quality and Safety

Huddles can lead to improved efficiencies and quality of information sharing, as well as increased levels of accountability, empowerment, and sense of community, according to researchers Goldenhar, Brady, Sutcliffe and Muething (2013). Together these create a culture of collaboration and collegiality that increases the staff's quality of collective awareness and enhanced capacity for eliminating patient harm.

With true collaboration, everyone's voice is heard.

Although small huddles take place frequently throughout all Cincinnati Children's locations, a house-wide daily safety brief, held each morning at 8:35, recaps the previous day and plans for the current day. Key leaders from the following areas attend in person or via phone:

- Employee safety
- Family relations
- Emergency department
- Inpatient services
- Perioperative area
- Outpatient services
- Psychiatry
- Home health

- Pharmacy
- Radiology
- Laboratory
- Infection prevention and control
- Supply chain
- Information services
- Protective services
- Facilities

The briefing puts real-time knowledge into the hands of those who can predict and solve problems. The following occurs at each daily safety brief:

1. A review of safety and quality issues from the past 24 hours
2. Discussion of quality and safety issues that may occur in the next 24 hours so they can be anticipated, predicted, and planned for
3. Follow-up report on issues identified today or on previous days and what is being done to resolve them (e.g., repair plan for malfunctioning equipment, update on manufacturer backorder on equipment, update on pharmaceutical shortage)

These morning gatherings have plenty of benefits, including the following: (1) help the journey to high reliability by making sure staff are preoccupied with quality and safety; (2) keep staff at all sites on the same page; (3) identify and fix problems while they are small; and (4) provide a distinct determination of who is responsible for an issue and when the fix will occur.

Each day, units and departments have their own safety briefs. The information that is compiled and shared at these smaller briefs are fed to the house-wide brief.

Three Daily Huddles for Perioperative Safety

As previously mentioned, huddles can create a culture of collaboration and collegiality that increases the staff's quality of collective awareness and enhances the capacity for eliminating patient harm. Cincinnati Children's perioperative team is aiming to accomplish each of these objectives with three daily huddles (**Table 6-1**).

At each huddle, the patient status (**Table 6-2**) is recorded and tracked throughout the patient's stay. This status is reported at Cincinnati Children's daily operations brief, previously mentioned.

At any time, any staff member is eligible to throw in the red card. Doing so stops activity until the concern is resolved. Convincing nurses to feel comfortable stopping a procedure can be challenging, yet nurses have an important voice that must be heard.

Table 6-1   Huddle Summary

Time of Huddle	Who Attends	Reason for Huddle
6:45 a.m.	• Charge nurse for same-day surgery, OR, and PACU • Anesthesiologist • Perioperative coordinators • SPD manager • VAT, MRI	• Review the status of every patient • Change a patient's risk level if appropriate
2:15 p.m.	• Charge nurse for same-day surgery, OR, and PACU • Anesthesiologist • Perioperative coordinators • SPD manager • VAT, MRI	The charge nurse runs the huddle • Every patient's risk level is determined based on health condition, procedure, or both • Patients arriving the next day are reviewed
9:00 p.m.	• OR and PACU charge nurse • Anesthesia board runner	Patient status is reviewed with input from staff and perioperative coordinators, who have been updated by surgeon and anesthesia

Table 6-2   Patient Status Color Tracking

Color	Description
Green	All clear, patient prepared and verified that there are no threats to patient safety through the perioperative area.
Yellow	Keep close watch; elevated risk factors for patient safety identified (e.g., another patient has same last name, patient has behavioral issues or comorbidities). Proceed with caution. Communicate additional needs to charge nurse.
Orange	High alert risk for patient vulnerability during the perioperative process (e.g., transplant patient). Requires additional resources and/or support from perioperative expert.
Red	The highest indicator, which requires stopping the line until the perioperative safety communication system has resolved the identified threat (e.g., equipment is malfunctioning).

The following excerpt from an article published by the Robert Wood Johnson Foundation speaks to the need for all voices to be heard:[1]

> Mary Jean Schumann DNP, MBA, RN, CPNP, executive director of the Nursing Alliance for Quality Care, a Foundation-funded partnership among the nation's leading nursing organizations and consumer groups touts shared decision-making and better communication as effective strategies, and says it "comes down to the culture. Everyone needs to be heard." Too often, she notes, nurses are not in the room when solutions are devised and are brought in only when it's time to talk about implementation. Even when nurses are included in problem-solving, "a single nursing voice is not enough," she cautions.
>
> Aline Holmes MSN, RN, director of the New Jersey Hospital Association's Institute for Quality and Patient Safety says nurses need to push themselves as well. "We need to get out there, develop more leadership skills—but top leadership needs to support that too. They need to focus on quality and safety, and bring nurses into those conversations." (Robert Wood Johnson Foundation, 2011, para. 13–14)

The Robert Wood Johnson Foundation (2010) commissioned a poll that found that large majorities of opinion leaders would like to see nurses exert more influence in a number of areas. Reducing medical errors and improving patient safety (90%) and improving quality of care (89%) topped the list.

Reuniting Patients and Their Pets

Oftentimes great ideas come from patients. At Cincinnati Children's, one such idea came from a teenage cancer patient. She spent so much time in the hospital, she knew the pain of not being able to spend time with her beloved dogs, so she set a goal to see that other kids would not feel that pain.

We have known that animal-assisted interventions, which include both animal-assisted activities and therapies, have historically been beneficial to human health. When the animal is the patient's beloved pet, the benefits might be even greater. "Animal-facilitated therapy has shown to decrease pain, change vital signs, provide distraction, decrease fear, increase socialization, increase pleasure and decrease emotional distress in hospitalized pediatric patients" (Urbanski & Lazenby, 2012, p. 272).

In 2013, thanks to efforts by the teenage cancer patient and others, a grant was secured and the Pet Center at Cincinnati Children's opened, enabling reunions between sick children and their beloved pets. Since then, reunions are commonplace, including

---

[1] Robert Wood Johnson Foundation. (2011). Nurses are key to improving patient safety. Retrieved from http://www.rwjf.org/en/library/articles-and-news/2011/04/nurses-are-key-to-improving-patient-safety.html. Copyright 2011. Robert Wood Johnson Foundation. Used with permission from the Robert Wood Johnson Foundation.

patients who, after weeks in isolation due to a bone marrow transplant, are wheeled to the Pet Center for what they describe as the best day they had during their month in the hospital. Since the Pet Center opened, dogs, cats, a guinea pig, and a rabbit have enjoyed visits with their owners. Many families indicate the reunion is the first time things felt normal since their child was admitted.

The Pet Center, believed to be one of the few of its kind in the country, is mostly indoors. Radiant heat makes it comfortable except during Cincinnati's coldest winter days. Pet visits are available to children who have been hospitalized 5 or more days, pending approval of their medical team. Many children have not seen their pet in months. Their emotional reunions are exactly what the teenage cancer patient had in mind, says her mother. Sadly, the patient lost her battle with cancer at age 19, shortly after the Pet Center opened. However, this young woman's dream to reunite patients with their pets has resulted in an enduring legacy.

One-of-a-Kind Program Has Worldwide Impact

A frustrated emergency department nurse manager at Cincinnati Children's came up with an idea that has had worldwide impact (Riehle, Daston, Rutkowski, & Wehman, 2012). Erin Riehle, MSN, RN, had a difficult time keeping the emergency department supply room stocked, and she eventually hired a young woman with Down syndrome for the job. This was the beginning of Project SEARCH, a one-of-a-kind program that helps young people with intellectual and developmental disabilities make successful transitions from school or sheltered workshops to integrated, competitive employment.

Since that day in 1996 when the program began, Project SEARCH has grown to more than 400 sites in a variety of businesses across the United States and in Canada, England, Scotland, Ireland, and Australia. In the near future, programs are likely in Germany, Gibraltar, Holland, India, Israel, and Wales.

Project SEARCH programs serve nearly 3,500 young adults each year, totaling nearly 30,000 young adults with disabilities since its inception. The rate of employment is 69.5%, which means that 20,850 young adults with significant disabilities have found jobs that translate to more fulfilling lives, work in inclusive settings, access to employer-paid benefits, and the potential to live independently.

Project SEARCH is an impressive example of the results that can be attained not only by empowering staff, but by having the willingness to test new ideas.

Partnering to Improve Outcomes

Cincinnati Children's 2015 strategic plan calls all staff to lead, advocate, and collaborate to improve the health of local children with asthma, the most common childhood chronic illness affecting children. Asthma is especially prevalent among Cincinnati's African American children from low socioeconomic and inner-city backgrounds. Within Hamilton County, where Cincinnati resides, one child in every six has been diagnosed with asthma. One of the most common barriers that impedes positive health outcomes for this population is medication adherence (Burgess, Sly & Devadason, 2012).

Obtaining a child's corticosteroid inhaler in a timely manner was often hampered by logistical problems (Crosby, 2012). To alleviate the obstacle and to help prevent visits to the emergency department, Cincinnati Children's formed innovative partnerships with local pharmacies. Tapping into recent advancements in technology for prescription refill automation, affected patients now are provided automated refills and home delivery of medications. Initially the goal was to increase the inhaled corticosteroid refill rate from 20% to 50% through these partnerships. After the intervention, the monthly fill rate now is 80%, and the program has spread to a second county near Cincinnati.

Partnering with school nurses has further improved outcomes for children with asthma, as reported by Kimberly Toole (2013). What began in 2006 in eight schools now has spread to the entire Cincinnati public school district. The partnership provides school nurses with additional training about asthma and access to a student's asthma action plan and medication records via access to the electronic health record. The goal of these interventions, although not yet determined, includes increased school attendance for the students living with asthma and increased work time for parents.

Box 6-2 A Fun Tweak to Discharge Instructions

It is common to send an asthmatic child home from the hospital with written discharge instructions. It can be more effective to demonstrate the proper use of an inhaler with an instructional video starring the patient.

Discussion

Think of a time that you proposed a new idea to a colleague or supervisor and answer the following questions:

- How did you make your case for your suggestion?
- Did it encompass both art and science?
- How was your suggestion received?
- Did it get implemented?
- If it was deployed, what were the results?
- If not acted upon, would your suggestion work today?

Providing a Service: The Right Thing to Do

According to the American Hospital Association (2012), annually one in four Americans experiences a behavioral health-related illness. Nearly half of all Americans will develop a mental illness during their lifetime, and 27% will suffer from a substance abuse disorder. Although chronic behavioral health disorders primarily affect adults, half of all chronic mental illness begins by the age of 14 years, and three-quarters begin by the age of 24 years. Of the adults with mental illness, the majority also have a comorbid physical condition. In fact, one of every four admissions to a general hospital has a behavioral health disorder.

To help address the need for highly specialized hospital-based behavioral health services, Cincinnati Children's has devoted a total of 125 beds (acute and long-term care) at three facilities to patients with behavioral issues. The decision to do so, in spite of a lack of financial reimbursement, was made because it was necessary and important. The medical center's former CEO believed that, when faced with a dilemma, ask yourself three times "Is it the right thing to do?" If the answer is always yes, then it must be done, no matter how hard it is to pursue. Using this thinking, although caring for psychiatric patients is costly and challenging, it is best for the community.

Sam, an adolescent female, is a perfect example of how facing the challenges of caring for psychiatric patients can have far-reaching benefits. "After losing her father, Rob, to suicide in 2008, Sam struggled with depression and post-traumatic stress disorder. More than two years after his death, Sam thought about suicide herself and on two different occasions spent time at [Cincinnati] Children's Hospital" (Salmons, 2014).

Because she does not want children in similar situations to feel as helpless and alone as she once did, Sam founded Rob's Kids, "an organization 'passionately committed to making a difference in the lives of children who struggle with depression or post-traumatic stress disorder'" (Salmons, 2014).

Benefits Patient and Pharmacist

Traditionally, Cincinnati Children's lung transplant clinical pharmacist and cystic fibrosis clinical pharmacist have visited only the hospital's inpatients. By expanding their reach to the hospital clinics, the pharmacists have provided continuity of care for their patients (previously, clinic patients did not see a pharmacist during visits). The change has also provided pharmacists with a broader perspective of their work.

During a trial period, in addition to inpatient visits, the lung transplant clinical pharmacist saw four patients in the clinic for a total of 10 separate encounters. The average time spent during each encounter was 1 hour. Follow-up comments from the pharmacist indicate significant benefits to the patient. The pharmacist's notes include the following:

- Identified inappropriate medication list and updated with the coordinator
- Identified inappropriate dosages of medications due to patient's weight gain
- Numerous recommendations for antibiotics, weaning of sedation medications, immunizations, switching from liquid to tablet form (patient could not tolerate liquid, but care team was not aware of this)
- Patient counseling occurs at every visit; many patients are on more than 15 medications with multiple drug–drug and drug–nutrient interactions

In this same period of time, the cystic fibrosis clinical pharmacist saw 30 individual patients during clinic visits. Learnings from this pharmacist include the following:

- During visits, discrepancies on the patients' medication lists were caught
- Medication education is helping to increase adherence and understanding
- Involvement in two patient admissions from clinic to hospital. They are able to assist the physician with the choice of antibiotics and any medication changes that should be made during hospitalization

Because visiting clinic patients is in addition to the pharmacists' already crowded workload, a challenge moving forward will be to find the time and resources to accommodate the expanded appointment schedule. Pharmacists and staff who go the extra mile and are willing to try innovative new ideas that improve patient care also need to be encouraged to care for themselves. Innovators need resiliency!

INNOVATIVE WAYS TO BUILD RESILIENCY

Resilience is defined as the ability to become strong, healthy, or successful again after something bad happens. In the healthcare arena, resilient staff can more quickly recover from the frequent disruptions, stressful situations, and turbulence of our constantly changing environment. A person with a high level of resilience tends "to be skilled in preparing for emotional emergencies (as can happen frequently in patient care settings) and adept at accepting what comes at them with flexibility rather than rigidity—times are tough but I know they will get better" (Waters, 2013, para. 5).

Authors Zolli and Healy indicate that personal resilience is a habit: "Whether cultivated through wise mentors, vigorous exercise, access to green space, or a particularly rich relationship with faith, the habits of personal resilience are habits of mind—making them habits we can cultivate and change when armed with the right resources" (2012, p. 130).

A 2012 Gallup poll (Bass & McGeeney, 2012) found that nurses, along with the general adult population, are more likely to smoke and less likely to eat healthy and exercise than physicians. Obesity is more prevalent among nurses than physicians. Armed with the knowledge that resilience can be developed over time and that nurses lag behind their physician colleagues in healthy behaviors, Cincinnati Children's has implemented numerous programs aimed at improving staff resilience, health, and wellness.

Walking Desks

Staff members who spend most days sitting at a desk can get a boost of energy and improve their mood with a quick exercise break. To make those breaks easier to take, walking desks were installed in areas of Cincinnati Children's where staff members are less likely to be on their feet at work, including the administrative area in the Specialty Resource Unit. The desks provide the opportunity to walk in place while working on a laptop or taking a break. In an interview in *Nursing Administration Quarterly* (Sanford, 2015), Senior Vice President of Patient Services Cheryl Hoying indicates, "I have a walking desk in my office so I can get 10,000 steps a day in while I work" (2015, p. 100).

Another frequent walker at Cincinnati Children's states, "The desk in my area is a great way to boost my energy level and decrease my stress after long periods sitting. I love that I can be active at work while still completing my job responsibilities." With a walking desk, leaders are able to model good behavior by exercising while answering e-mails and other seated tasks.

Healthy Challenge

Regular exercise can help prevent the impact of stress on the body. There are "substantial and highly statistically significant associations between the frequency of moderate to vigorous physical activity (MVPA) and different indicators of psychological distress. Frequent participation in MVPA reduces psychological distress and decreases the likelihood of falling into a high-risk category" (Perales, Pozo-Cruz, & Pozo-Cruz, 2014, p. 91).

Encouraging a healthier lifestyle through regular exercise, proper nutrition, and healthier habits as a way to improve staff resilience is the goal of a quarterly healthy challenge for the Patient Services Division at Cincinnati Children's. Each challenge enables staff to earn points in the workplace wellness program that supports employees as they adopt and sustain behaviors that reduce health risks and improve quality of life.

More than 1,000 staff routinely accept the challenge each quarter. Some challenges are suggested by staff who are eager to engage their coworkers in the typically fun activities. Challenges have included the following:

- Trying a new vegetable each week for 4 weeks
- Doing one new thing each week for 4 weeks that will result in less stress and a calmer holiday season
- Completing a triathlon over a 4-week period
- Kicking a bad habit

Schwartz Center Rounds

Could the stresses of today's healthcare system threaten the delivery of compassionate care? Schwartz Center Rounds, implemented at Cincinnati Children's in 2014, provides an outlet to openly and honestly discuss the social and emotional issues caregivers face in working with patients and families. Each monthly session begins with panelists from diverse disciplines, including physicians, nurses, social workers, psychologists, and allied health professionals, who share an experience on an identified case or topic. Afterwards, caregivers in the audience are invited to share their own perspectives on the case and broader related issues. The premise is that caregivers are better able to make personal connections with patients and colleagues when they have greater insight into their own responses and feelings.

This national program is now in place at more than 400 healthcare facilities. The Schwartz Center website (www.theschwartzcenter.org) reports these benefits as expressed by participants:[2]

- Increased insight into the social and emotional aspects of patient care, increased feelings of compassion toward patients, and increased readiness to respond to patients' and families' needs.
- Improved teamwork, interdisciplinary communication, and appreciation for the roles and contributions of colleagues from different disciplines.
- Decreased feelings of stress and isolation and more openness to giving and receiving support.

Topics discussed at Cincinnati Children's Schwartz Center Rounds have included experiencing the death of a patient, running on empty, and compassionate care for international patients.

---

[2] The Schwartz Center for Compassionate Healthcare. (2016). Schwartz Center Rounds®. Retrieved from http://www.theschwartzcenter.org/supporting-caregivers/schwartz-center-rounds/

The Schwartz Center was begun by healthcare attorney Ken Schwartz, a nonsmoker and health advocate who was diagnosed with advanced lung cancer at age 40 years. During his 10-month ordeal, Ken came to realize that what matters most during an illness is the human connection between patients and their caregivers. He wrote movingly about his experience in an article for the *Boston Globe Magazine*. At the end of his life, Ken outlined the organization he wanted to create and founded the Schwartz Center in 1995—just days before his death—to ensure that all patients receive compassionate and humane care.

OTHER RESILIENCY BUILDERS AND STRESS RELIEVERS AT CINCINNATI CHILDREN'S

It can be physically and emotionally difficult for healthcare providers to care for fragile patients on a daily basis. Even the most resilient staff struggle when a patient's health suddenly deteriorates or a patient dies. The ideas on the following pages describe stress-relieving processes available to staff in the Patient Services Division of Cincinnati Children's. The staff's ability to effectively deal with the inevitable stress of their job helps them to be more resilient.

Emotional Support Team

When two or more individuals experience a sudden, unanticipated event, such as an employee or patient death, situation, or injury, Cincinnati Children's Emotional Support Team (EST) will establish a confidential support session. The EST is intended to facilitate the processing of emotions. The team helps employees handle the distress, pain, confusion, and fear that can result from crisis situations. The EST also helps employees continue to deliver safe patient care by providing a timely and appropriate outlet for their emotions.

Time to Grieve

Staff in the pediatric intensive care unit experience the death of a patient more often than other areas of the hospital. Should a death occur, the unit's policy is to allow the caregiver to take the rest of the day off to privately deal with the grief.

Assistance from Police Psychologist

The hospital environment is focused on providing the best possible medical and quality of life outcomes. When a serious safety event occurs, the effect on staff can be devastating. To improve resiliency during these difficult times, Cincinnati Children's has enlisted the help of a local police psychologist who routinely assists law enforcement staff in stress management and counsels police officers and families. While the two disciplines are different, both involve stress while providing service to the public.

The path to achieving better outcomes is transparency.

"An important aspect of critical incident is the feeling of helplessness when facing a life or death situation," explains James M. Daum (2015). In his work with police, Daum has learned that after an incident, a police officer typically will try to "recollect and sequence what was experienced, and determine whether there was any alternative to firing shots or taking the action they chose. Emotional reactions can include guilt, anger, depression, anxiety or numbness. Physical symptoms such as nausea, gastro-intestinal disturbance, headaches, fatigue and sleep disturbance are common" (2015).

During a mandatory psychological debriefing, which is strictly confidential, the police officer is given support in his or her efforts to regain a sense of self-control and well-being. Similar debriefings are under consideration for Cincinnati Children's staff who are involved in a serious safety event. The goal is a return to work feeling healthy and emotionally ready.

Gauging Stress

The noise of hospital construction can be difficult for parents of sick children to handle, especially when those children are critically ill. During months of construction in Cincinnati Children's neonatal intensive care unit, leaders wanted to be certain that parents were getting the support they needed. As a gauge, parents were asked to place a yellow, orange, or red fuzzy ball into a fishbowl (**Figure 6-6**) at the unit's reception desk to indicate if they were getting the support they needed. When orange or red balls made their way to the fishbowl, it was time for a staff huddle to determine why.

Construction noise can also adversely affect caregivers, so the neonatal intensive care unit staff has their own fishbowl. Four times each day, team leaders and charge nurses use colored ball to gauge stress. The results are charted. When stress is high, it is time to find out why and make adjustments.

Lowering the Noise

The potentially dangerous effects of noise fatigue have been made apparent by The Joint Commission. In April 2013, The Joint Commission issued a sentinel event alert (2013) warning of the dangers of alarm desensitization and urging hospitals to improve alarm management protocols and alarm-setting guidelines. The Joint Commission followed up by requiring hospitals to demonstrate that they have made alarms an organizational priority and identify the types of alarms they plan to target. By 2016, hospitals will need to develop and implement specific protocols aimed at curbing unnecessary alarms.

Figure 6-6   Fuzzy ball stress gauge

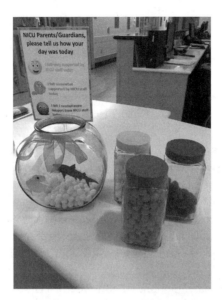

Excessive cardiac monitor alarms lead to desensitization and alarm fatigue. Researchers at Cincinnati Children's created and implemented a standardized cardiac monitor care process (CMCP) on a 24-bed pediatric bone marrow transplant unit. The aim of the project was to decrease monitor alarms through the use of team-based standardized care and processes.

Using small tests of change, researchers developed and implemented a standardized CMCP that included four components:

- A process for initial ordering of monitor parameters based on age-appropriate standards
- Pain-free daily replacement of electrodes
- Daily individualized assessment of cardiac monitor parameters
- A reliable method for appropriate discontinuation of the monitor

By implementing these standardized CMCP, Cincinnati Children's researchers (Dandoy et al., 2014) found that cardiac monitor alarms significantly decreased per patient day from 180 to 40. Overall compliance with the CMCP increased from a median of 38% to 95%.

Alarms are not the only source of disruptive noise in hospitals. After identifying the sources of noise on one unit at Cincinnati Children's, the following changes were made:

- Repaired noisy carts/ice machines
- Hung reminder signs to minimize noise

- Lowered volume on pagers
- Replaced phone ringers with lights
- Closed doors during rounding
- Asked that new trash bags be shaken outside patient rooms

Taking Fun Seriously

Cincinnati Children's Patient Services Division routinely incorporates exercise and fun into the workday to relieve stress. Activities include a monthly dress up day, when staff are invited to do things like celebrate the start of a sports season by wearing a favorite team's jersey or be a twin for the day by dressing exactly like a coworker. The medical center's annual fitness on the field event lets staff and their families participate in fun activities on the turf at the Cincinnati Bengals' stadium. After work neighborhood walks and weekend hikes led by hospital leadership demonstrate a commitment to staff health and wellness.

Ideas for maintaining a healthy mind and body are a regular part of new staff orientation. Maintaining financial stability also is discussed during orientation. It is recognized that personal finances can be a persistent source of stress that affects staff. For example, new graduates may be burdened with student loans. Addressing financial stability in orientation is an important support. Advice on how to systematically reduce debt and save for retirement are examples of topics discussed.

OTHER IDEAS FOR BOOSTING RESILIENCY

Mindfulness

Mindfulness practice holds promise for increasing individual and workplace resilience (Goldstein, 2013). The research team sought to evaluate the effectiveness of a mindfulness-based program for increasing health, a sense of coherence and decreased depression, and anxiety and stress in nurses and midwives. Mindfulness is described as paying attention on purpose, in the present moment, and nonjudgmentally to the unfolding of experience from moment to moment. Learning to become more present frees us to be more flexible and creative—and ultimately, more resilient, enjoying better health and well-being.

In his book *The Equanimous Mind* (2011), Manish Chopra, PhD, recommends one of India's most ancient techniques of meditation to reach the highest happiness. Called vipassana, this meditative practice helps one learn more about one's own thoughts, feelings, and judgments. Vipassana focuses on the deep interconnection between mind and body. "It is this observation-based, self-exploratory journey to the common root of mind and body that dissolves mental impurity, resulting in a balanced mind full of love and compassion" (Chopra, 2011, p. xi).

Modeling Healthy Behavior

Physical activity is a key factor in resilient behavior, suggests molecular biologist John Medina, PhD (2014). "When combined with the health benefits exercise offers, we have as close to a magic bullet as exists in modern medicine" (2014, p. 22). Referring to physical activity as cognitive candy, Medina reports that research has consistently shown that exercisers outperform couch potatoes in tests that measure long-term memory, reasoning, attention, problem solving, and fluid intelligence. Nurse leaders would do well to model physical activity at every opportunity (e.g., walking desks, participating in fundraising walks, and taking the steps instead of the elevator).

Alone Time

Nurses and other care providers should not deny the pressures and stresses they are experiencing in their life—at home and at work (Wicks, 2014). "That is the first piece of what makes a resilient organization and leader: facing the issues directly" (2014, p. 11). To boost resiliency, Wicks encourages people to

find crumbs of alone time in their day and look for places where they can have some kind of silence and solitude for reflection so they can process things . . . Because with the right perspective, it's not the amount of darkness in the healthcare system or in our family or ourselves that matters; it's how we stand in that darkness. And that requires patience, perseverance and courage if we are going to be a leader, which requires a period of debriefing. (2014, p. 14)

Reduce Nurse Workload

Reducing nurse workload may be one way to avoid burnout and boost resiliency. Nurse workload, such as nurse-to-patient staffing ratios, can influence nursing care quality and lead to adverse patient outcomes. A growing body of research in pediatrics demonstrates this relationship. Tubbs-Cooley, Cimiotti, Silber, Sloane, and Aiken (2013) from the University of Pennsylvania demonstrated a significant increase in the odds of pediatric readmission in hospitals with leaner pediatric nurse-to-patient ratios, leading the team to speculate that higher workloads may result in rushed or incomplete discharge preparation. Beginning in 2013, Tubbs-Cooley is leading a team of researchers at Cincinnati Children's Hospital Medical Center to study relationships among nurse workloads, missed nursing care, and patient outcomes to better understand how shift-to-shift variation in bedside nurse workload causally impacts nursing care quality and patient outcomes. This work, focused primarily in neonatal intensive care, has established preliminary linkages among nurse workloads, missed care, and outcomes:

- In a pilot study of 230 certified neonatal intensive care nurses, the nurses reported missing oral care for vented babies, missing discharge preparation, and missing oral feedings on their last shift worked. Nurses cited workload-related factors as the most significant reasons for missed care.
- Missed oral feeding opportunities led to significant prolongation of feeding milestones and neonatal intensive care hospitalization among preterm infants.
- Intubated infants whose nurses report missed adherence to ventilator-associated pneumonia guidelines during a shift are up to four times more likely to experience an unplanned extubation on the same shift.

Prioritizing

Leaders should recognize that they cannot do everything. They should engage in true prioritization to determine what should be done first. Kraemer (2011) describes true prioritization as a list of all items to be accomplished, from most important to least important. This process enables leaders to "commit your time, attention, and resources to what matters most" (2011, p. 18). This may seem simple, but often the most straightforward and effective strategies can be overlooked. Modeling good prioritization practices is a powerful opportunity for leaders that can result in a ripple effect of better prioritization throughout the organization. Simultaneously, another valuable practice is *exnovation*, the purging of non-value-added practices to allow the organization to adopt different and fresh thinking to new activities.

Microsystem Stress Reduction

Remember that if you don't prioritize your life someone else will. (McKeown, G. 2014, p. 235)

Nurse fatigue and information overload can result in patient care error (Sitterding & Broome, 2015). The inability to control attention can result in failure to notice something about the current situation or the failure to notice that something is different. This possibility of patient harm is what has spurred nurse leaders at Cincinnati Children's to investigate.

Believing that unexpected increases in patient volume may be causing stress to staff, and concerned that this stress correlates with levels of patient harm, Cincinnati Children's nurse leaders have initiated a study to validate and mitigate this hypothesis. Nursing hours per patient day and qualitative stress (a four-point scale) are under review on a shift-by-shift basis by microsystem (unit-level) charge nurses and clinical supervisors. They also are being reviewed on a weekly basis, along with other measures, including operational vacancy rate, percentage of float staff used, 13-hour shifts, and shifts that reported high levels of stress. Data is currently being analyzed, and mitigation strategies are being developed.

Short-Termism

Even the most resilient staff today may find themselves lacking in the long run, particularly those who practice short-termism—that is, tuning out everything except the most immediate outcomes. Laurence Fink (2015), chairman and CEO of BlackRock, believes this craving for immediate gratification prevents leaders from "grappl[ing] effectively with complex, long-term challenges . . . There seems to be a great deal more upside to placing a simple bet for quick win than for staying the course through difficult times to create sustainable gains that are more widely shared" (2015, para. 3).

Other Ideas for Building Resiliency

An American Psychological Association webpage called Road to Resilience recommends implementing the following ideas to build resiliency:

1. Make connections. Good relationships with close family members, friends or others are important. Accepting help and support from those who care about you and will listen to you strengthens resilience. Some people find that being active in civic groups, faith-based organizations, or other local groups provides social support and can help with reclaiming hope. Assisting others in their time of need also can benefit the helper.
2. Avoid seeing crises as insurmountable problems. You can't change the fact that highly stressful events happen, but you can change how you interpret and respond to these events. Try looking beyond the present to how future circumstances may be a little better. Note any subtle ways in which you might already feel somewhat better as you deal with difficult situations.
3. Accept that change is a part of living. Certain goals may no longer be attainable as a result of adverse situations. Accepting circumstances that cannot be changed can help you focus on circumstances that you can alter.
4. Move toward your goals. Develop some realistic goals. Do something regularly—even if it seems like a small accomplishment—that enables you to move toward your goals.

Instead of focusing on tasks that seem unachievable, ask yourself, "What's one thing I know I can accomplish today that helps me move in the direction I want to go?"

5. Take decisive actions. Act on adverse situations as much as you can. Take decisive actions, rather than detaching completely from problems and stresses and wishing they would just go away.

6. Look for opportunities for self-discovery. People often learn something about themselves and may find that they have grown in some respect as a result of their struggle with loss. Many people who have experienced tragedies and hardship have reported better relationships, greater sense of strength even while feeling vulnerable, increased sense of self-worth, a more developed spirituality and heightened appreciation for life.

7. Nurture a positive view of yourself. Developing confidence in your ability to solve problems and trusting your instincts helps build resilience.

8. Keep things in perspective. Even when facing very painful events, try to consider the stressful situation in a broader context and keep a long-term perspective. Avoid blowing the event out of proportion.

9. Maintain a hopeful outlook. An optimistic outlook enables you to expect that good things will happen in your life. Try visualizing what you want, rather than worrying about what you fear.

10. Take care of yourself. Pay attention to your own needs and feelings. Engage in activities that you enjoy and find relaxing. Exercise regularly. Taking care of yourself helps to keep your mind and body primed to deal with situations that require resilience. (Comas-Diaz et al., 2015, page 4 of website, para 1-10)

Staff resiliency is vital to healthcare organizations. It enables staff to refresh, move forward, develop new ideas, and implement change.

CONCLUSION

Any conversation about innovation should include the importance of change. Change is constant, and it waits for no one. To keep innovating, one must be open, enthusiastic, and continually asking questions. Without it, stagnancy sets in. By coproducing creative solutions with patients and staff, better health and value will be achieved.

REFERENCES

Advisory Board. (2014). *Intermountain Health System nurse shadowing program.* Washington D.C.

Alison-Napolitano, E., & Pesut, D. (2015). *Bounce forward: The extraordinary resilience of nurse leadership.* Silver Spring, MD: American Nurses Association.

Amabile, T. M., & Kramer, S. J. (2011, May). The power of small wins. *Harvard Business Review, 89*(5). Retrieved from https://hbr.org/2011/05/the-power-of-small-wins

American College of Healthcare Executives. (2015). *Congress on healthcare leadership. COO bootcamp.* Presented by R. Brace & W. Riley. Retrieved from https://www.ache.org/Congress/bootcamps.cfm

American Hospital Association. (2012). *Bringing behavioral health into the care continuum: Opportunities to improve quality, costs and outcomes*, 48(3). Retrieved from http://www.aha.org/research/reports/tw/12jan-tw-behavhealth.pdf

Appelbaum, S., Louis, D., Makarenko, D., Saluja, J., Meleshko, O., & Kulbashian, S. (2013). Participation in decision making: A case study of job satisfaction and commitment. *Industrial and Commercial Training, 45*(4). doi:10.1108/00197851311323510

Baggett, M., Batcheller, J., Blouin, A.S., Behrens, E., Bradley, C., Brown, J.J. . . . Yendro, S. (2014). Excellence and evidence in staffing: A data-driven model for excellence in staffing. *Nursing Economics, 32*(Suppl. 3), 3–35.

Barden, A. M., Griffin, M. T., Donahue, M., & Fitzpatrick, J. J. (2011). Shared governance and empowerment in registered nurses working in a hospital setting. *Nursing Administration Quarterly, 35*(3), 212–218. doi:10.1097/NAQ.0b013e3181ff3845

Bass, K., & McGeeney, K. (2012). U.S. physicians set good health example. Retrieved from www.gallup.com/poll/157859/physicians-set-good-health-example.aspx

Boston-Fleischhauer, C . (2014a). Aiming for care continuity? Help staff see beyond their own care setting. Retrieved from http://www.advisory.com/research/nursing-executive-center/expert-insights/2014/help-staff-see-beyond-their-immediate-care-setting

Boston-Fleischhauer, C. (2014b). The changing CNO role (and how to succeed within it). Retrieved from http://www.advisory.com/research/nursing-executive-center/events/meetings/2014/2014-2015-nursing-executive-center-national-meeting-cno-roundtables/locations/dc/120814/the-changing-cno-role/presentation#slide/2

Brady, P.W., Muething, S., Kotagal, U., Ashby, M., Gallagher, R., Hall, D. . . . Wheeler, D.S. (2013). Improving situation awareness to reduce unrecognized clinical deterioration and serious safety events. *Pediatrics, 131*(1), e298–e308. doi:10.1542/peds.2012-1364

Burgess, S., Sly, P., & Devadason, S. (2012). Adherence with preventive medication in childhood asthma. *Pulmonary Medicine.* doi:10.1155/2011/973849

Chopra, M. (2011). *The equanimous mind.* Singapore: Author.

Comas-Diaz, L., Luthar, S., Maddi, S., O'Neill, H., Saakvitne, K., & Tedeschi, R. (2015). *The road to resilience: 10 ways to build resilience.* Retrieved from http://apa.org/helpcenter/road-resilience.aspx

Crosby, L. K. (2012). *Exploration of Cincinnati Children's Hospital Medical Center* (Unpublished doctoral dissertation). Wright State University, Dayton, OH.

Dandoy, C. E., Davies, S. M., Flesch, L., Hayward, M., Koons, C., Coleman, K., . . . Weiss, B. (2014). A team-based approach to reducing cardiac monitor alarms. *Pediatrics, 134*(5). doi:10.1542/peds.2014-1162

Daum, J. M. (2015). [Biographical information presented at a meeting with Cincinnati Children's]. Copy in possession of Cheryl Hoying.

de Jong, M., Marston, N. & Roth, E. (2015). The eight essentials of innovation, *McKinsey Quarterly, 2015*, No. 2. (p. 37, 47).

Dent, R. L. (2015). Nine principles for improved nurse staffing. *Nursing Economics, 33*(1), 44.

Dent, R. L., Armstead, C., & Evans, B. (2014). Three structures for a healthy work environment. *American Association of Critical-Care Nurses Advanced Critical Care, 25*(2), 94–100.

Erickson, D. (2011). Professional practice model: Strategies for translating models into practice. *Nursing Clinics of North America, 46*(1), 35.

Fink, L. (2015). Our gambling culture. Retrieved from http://www.mckinsey.com/insights/strategy/our_gambling_culture

Frenk, J., Chen, L., Bhutta, Z.A., Cohen, J., Crisp, N., Evans, T. . . . Zurayk, H. (2010). Health professionals for a new century: Transforming education to strengthen health systems in an interdependent world. *Lancet, 376*, 22.

Friedman, S. (2014). *Leading the life you want*. Boston, MA: Harvard Business Review Press.

Gallup. (2013). State of the American workplace. Retrieved from www.gallup.com/services/178514/state-american-workplace.aspx

General Electric. (2015). Strategies for success: Managing complexity in health care, p. 13. Retrieved from http://www3.gehealthcare.com/en/insights/forward_thinking/forward_thinking/strategies_for_success_managing_the_complexity_in_health_care

Goldenhar, L., Brady, P., Sutcliffe, K., & Muething, S. (2013). Huddling for high reliability and situation awareness. *BMJ Quality and Safety, 22*(11), 899–906. doi:10.1136/bmjqs-2012-001467

Goldstein, E. (2013). *The now effect: How a mindful moment can change the rest of your life*. New York, NY: Atria Books.

Hoying, C., Lecher, W. T., Mosko, D. D., Roberto, N., Mason, C., Murphy, S. W., . . . Britto, M. T. (2014). On the scene: Cincinnati. *Nursing Administration Quarterly, 38*(1), 27–54.

Hoying, C., & Allen, S. (2011). Enhancing shared governance for interdisciplinary practice. *Nursing Administration Quarterly, 35*(3), 252–259.

Institute of Medicine. (2011). *The future of nursing: Leading change, advancing health*. Washington, DC: National Academies Press.

Jansen, L. (2008). Collaborative and interdisciplinary health care teams: Ready or not? *Journal of Professional Nursing, 24*(4), 220, 222.

Kabcenell, A., Nolan, T. W., Martin, L. A., & Gill, Y. (2010). The pursuing perfection initiative: Lessons on transforming health care (IHI Innovation Series white paper). Cambridge, MA: Institute for Healthcare Improvement.

Kamins, C. (2015). What too many hospitals are overlooking. Retrieved from www.gallup.com/businessjournal/181658/hospitals-overlooking.aspx

Kelly, M. (2011). *Off balance*. New York, NY: Hudson Street Press.

Kraemer, H. M. J. (2011). *From values to action*. San Francisco, CA: Jossey-Bass.

Mason, C., & Fiorini, P. (2013, September 27). Nurses' practice, experiences, and satisfaction with the inpatient outpatient role at Cincinnati Children's Hospital Medical Center (IRB approved unpublished research). Cincinnati, OH.

McKeown, G. (2014). *Essentialism: The Disciplined Pursuit of Less*. New York, NY: Crown Business.

Medina, J. (2014). *Brain rules*. Seattle, WA: Pear Press.

Nader, R. (n.d.). BrainyQuote.com. Retrieved from http://www.brainyquote.com/quotes/quotes/r/ralphnader110188.html, para 1.

Newhouse, R., Stanik-Hutt, J., White, K. M., Johantgen, M., Bass, E. B., Zangaro, G. . . . Weiner, J. P. (2011). Advanced practice nurse outcomes: A systemic review. *Nursing Economics, 29*(5), 19.

Patient-Centered Outcomes Research Institute. (2013). Improving post-discharge outcomes by facilitating family-centered transitions from hospital to home. Retrieved from http://www.pcori.org/research-results/2013/improving-post-discharge-outcomes-facilitating-family-centered-transitions

Perales, F., Pozo-Cruz, J., & Pozo-Cruz, B. (2014). Impact of physical activity on psychological distress: A prospective analysis of an Australian national sample. *American Journal of Public Health, 104*(12), 91.

Porter-O'Grady, T., & Malloch, K. (2011). *Quantum leadership*. Sudbury, MA: Jones & Bartlett Learning.

Riehle, E., Daston, M., Rutkowski, S., & Wehman, P. (2012). *High school transition that works: Lessons learned from Project SEARCH*. Baltimore, MD: Brookes.

Robert Wood Johnson Foundation. (2010). Groundbreaking new survey finds that diverse opinion leaders say nurses should have more influence on health systems and services. Retrieved from http://www.rwjf.org/en/library/articles-and-news/2010/01/groundbreaking-new-survey-finds-that-diverse-opinion-leaders-say.html

Robert Wood Johnson Foundation. (2011). Nurses are key to improving patient safety. Retrieved from http://www.rwjf.org/en/library/articles-and-news/2011/04/nurses-are-key-to-improving-patient-safety.html

Robert Wood Johnson Foundation. (2015). Lessons from the field: Promising interprofessional collaboration practices. Retrieved from http://www.rwjf.org/en/library/research/2015/03/lessons-from-the-field.html

Salmons, S. (2014). Burlington teen is 'making a difference.' *Cincinnati Enquirer.* Retrieved from http://www.cincinnati.com/story/news/local/burlington/2014/05/03/burlington-teen-making-difference/8682341/

Sanford, K. (2015). The resilient nurse leader. *Nursing Administration Quarterly, 39*(2), 100.

Sheridan, R. (2013). *Joy, Inc.: How we built a workplace people love.* New York, NY: Portfolio/Penguin.

Sitterding, M., & Broome, M. (2015). *Information overload: Framework, tips and tools to manage in complex healthcare environments.* Silver Spring, MD: American Nurses Association.

The Joint Commission. (2013). *Sentinel event alert: Medical device alarm safety in hospitals.* Issue 50, April 8, 2013. Retrieved from http://www.jointcommission.org/assets/1/18/SEA_50_alarms_4_5_13_FINAL1.PDF

Toole, K. (2013). Helping children gain asthma control: Bundled school-based interventions. *Pediatric Nursing, 39*(3). 115–120

Tubbs-Cooley, H., Cimiotti, J., Silber, J., Sloane, D., & Aiken, L. (2013). An observational study of nurse staffing ratios and hospital readmission among children admitted for common conditions. *BMJ Quality Safety, 22*(9), 735–742.

Tye, J. (2014). *Midland Memorial Hospital case study on values and culture initiative.* Solon, IA: Values Coach.

Uldrich, J. (2011). *Higher unlearning: 39 post-requisite lessons for achieving a successful future.* Edina, MN: Beavers Pond Press.

Urbanski, B., & Lazenby, M. (2012). Distress among hospitalized pediatric cancer patients modified by pet-therapy intervention to improve quality of life. *Journal of Pediatric Oncology Nursing, 29*(5), 272–282. doi:10.1177/1043454212455697

Virkstis, K. (2012). Strengthening interdisciplinary collaboration: Best practices for enhancing partnership and communication. Retrieved from http://www.advisory.com/research/nursing-executive-center/studies/2012/strengthening-interdisciplinary-collaboration

Waters, B. (2013). 10 traits of emotionally resilient people. Retrieved from https://www.psychologytoday.com/blog/design-your-path/201305/10-traits-emotionally-resilient-people

Wicks, R. (2014). The resilient leader: Mind, body and soul. *Healthcare Executive, 29*(6), 11.

Zolli, A., & Healy, A. (2012). *Resilience: Why things bounce back.* New York, NY: Simon & Schuster Paperbacks.

CHAPTER 7

Emergence and Disruption: Working on the Edge of Evidence

Cathy Lalley and Kevin Clouthier

CHAPTER OBJECTIVES

Upon completion of this chapter, the reader will be able to:

1. Identify human patterns with a complexity science lens.
2. Compare and contrast characteristics of complex responsive processes and complex adaptive systems.
3. Describe innovation in real time.
4. Define the practice of reflexivity.
5. Outline the effects of relational leadership to advance evidence and emergence in healthcare practices.

MEANING MAKING IN ORGANIZATIONAL LIFE

The goal of this chapter is to share contemporary thinking relevant to the edge of evidence-based patterns. However, when the term *evidence-based* is deconstructed, do we share a common understanding of what we are discussing? Alternatively, might you have a different view than we do? Is the evidence of which we speak based in the cold objective eye of the scientific paradigm of the Newtonian physical world, or might it be grounded in a different paradigm? When speaking of evidence based, are we referencing practice that is grounded in what has been previously determined to be best in prior work, or does it mean what is best in the current situation in which we are working? Finally, does it mean the best that emerges from our practice or best determined through controlled experimentation in a laboratory in some other place, culture, and clinical setting? If we are to communicate, it would be beneficial to determine what we are discussing together.

Before we embark on this journey, it may be important to include the words of Ken Gergen, a prominent voice in social constructionism, who has raised a question of the presumed logic of cause and effect (2009). When regarded from the relational view, it is the effect that is required to be known before the cause can be determined. So, in the case of evidence-based practice, might it be necessary to have practice before we are able to determine the causes of evidence based? It is in the practice of health care where human patterns emerge to determine the causes of best practices.

What began as a simple title to a chapter on evidence-based practice has become a conundrum of muddles, words, and unclear meanings that demand our attention before proceeding. Yet how can this be done when you are reading these words? How will we pattern our interaction to create common meaning as we share our collaborative journey through the remainder of this chapter? That is a tall challenge, indeed.

What we will provide throughout this chapter is grounded in a particular construction of the development of evidence that becomes apparent in the creation of relationships between people in the workplace and the meanings that are co-constructed through their interactions together. Our intention is to provide a glimpse into practices that occur in the living present to inform novelty (innovation) in collaborative work. Just as you, the reader of this chapter, and we, the authors of this work, collaboratively determine the meaning that comes from our interaction through these pages, we will look at how this is accomplished through the creation of relationship. As all living organisms, such as swarm bees and even slime mold, move about and transform in relationship to survive, so do humans in organizations. To begin, we will introduce a foundation for us to continue our journey.

COMPLEXITY SCIENCE FOR COMPLEX ENVIRONMENTS

The practice of health care takes place in the context of human interactions in complex environments. Complexity science gives us a lens to explore and understand human interactions because it is the study of dynamic behaviors of many complexly interacting, interdependent, and adaptive agents responding to internal and external forces in the environment (Marion, 2008). Healthcare organizations come to life through human interactions and can no longer be described or understood solely in terms of linearly organized, predictable, or from a control-based paradigm (Lindberg, Nash, & Lindberg, 2008; Porter-O'Grady & Malloch, 2011; Uhl-Bien & Marion, 2008). Health care is delivered in relationships by clinicians who engage in multidirectional interactions that are not predictable, whereby the power influencing the interaction is from the interaction itself; not an outside force.

ONE UMBRELLA

Fitting within the umbrella of complexity science, two leadership theories have been generated in an attempt to understand and describe organizations: complex adaptive systems (CAS) and complex responsive processes (CRP). Common elements of theories based in complexity science are temporal and relational dynamics. Time in complexity theories is emergent and irreversible. Leadership theories understood from complexity science understand that agents are humans who are interdependent, engage in self-organizing nonlinear interactions, require diversity to survive, embrace uncertainty, and are able to respond rapidly and creatively to environmental changes (**Box 7-1**). Both CAS and CRP leadership theories recognize that change emerges in response to internal and external pressures; change is continuous in living systems (CAS) or in human inter-actions (CRP). For example, clinicians' responses to evidence in clinical practice occurs continuously. Clinicians respond to practice recommendations based in evidence while continuously seeking to improve quality of care. Within complexity-based theories of leadership there is variation in the unit of analysis and power dynamics.

UNIT OF ANALYSIS

CAS leadership theory describes the evolution of complex systems with multiple, di-verse, interconnected elements. When using a CAS model, the investigator must define the system's boundaries, including what is inside the system and what is outside the system (Dooley, 2004), recognizing the primary unit of analysis is the defined CAS itself such that the behaviors of the agents are always understood within the context of the CAS (Uhl-Bien, Marion & McKelvey, 2008). The boundaries of the CAS are per-meable so that agents and other CAS can cross over the boundary (Bennet & Bennet, 2004). When exploring outcomes of a defined system or group, this leadership theory can offer insight. However, when using a CAS perspective, the specific interactions

---

Box 7-1 Common Characteristics Among Leadership Theories Based in Complexity Science

- Time emergent and irreversible
- Agents are interdependent
- Agents participate in self-organizing nonlinear interactions
- Requires diversity to survive
- Thrives in uncertainty
- Agents are able to respond rapidly and creatively to environmental changes

and movement among agents within the CAS are overlooked for the outcome of the whole CAS. Thus, nurses may be diverse interdependent agents participating in self-organizing nonlinear interactions, capable of responding rapidly to environmental changes when evidence is presented to guide their practice although the specific behaviors of the nurses are not explored within the CAS, only the behaviors and outcomes of the entire CAS are measured. To explore how change emerges within an organization at the edge of evidence, behavior of diverse interdependent agents participating in self-organizing nonlinear interactions is needed.

An assumption within CRP is the reason for organization is purposeful joint action required for human living and sustained by individual and group identity with the potential to transform it (Stacey, 2001). CRP provides a view of change where apparently paradoxical perspectives, such as the application of evidence into practice, can be embraced in the living organization, including a healthcare work group, through human interaction. The unit of analysis in CRP is the interaction itself. Human interactions do not have boundaries around them; they include agents within a work group as well as agents in other work groups. CRP is the lens to observe change occurring in the here and now among diverse interdependent agents participating in self-organizing nonlinear interactions (**Figure 7-1**).

POWER DYNAMICS

Power dynamics refers to how change occurs. Traditionally, healthcare leaders have attempted to control change through defined processes, such as planned implementation of evidence-based practice guidelines. Although we have all observed change that

Figure 7-1   Change in CAS compared to CRP

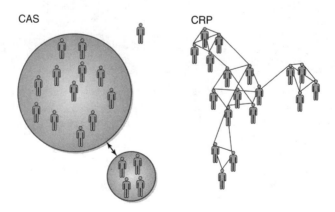

is both planned and unplanned, there have been successful campaigns for planned change that are consciously conceived of and implemented by knowledgeable actors; it was scripted or controlled and left little opportunity for innovation (Poole & Van de Ven, 2004). In planned change, the potential for local response and modification are limited because a normative cast is applied to improve a situation with a stated reference point (Poole & Van de Ven, 2004). Unplanned change implies that change to some degree is a force in its own right and is not susceptible to control or management (Poole & Van de Ven, 2004). Often with planned change, such as implementation of evidence-based practice guidelines, unplanned domestication occurs at the local level (Poole & Van de Ven, 2004). Poole and Van de Ven cautioned managers and change agents, suggesting that they "should realize how difficult change and innovation are to script and manage, as these processes constantly move in unexpected directions and are driven by dynamics that are either too powerful to control or too subtle to understand" (2004, p. 5). The mechanisms for change among CAS and CRP leadership theories are diverse.

Change in CAS

After the boundaries of a CAS are defined, the agents inside and outside the CAS are defined as well, including the leader of the CAS. The administrative leader of a CAS is an outside objective observer of the CAS who creates the conditions for change and observes movement of the CAS. The outside objective observer role of the leader appears much like the traditional leader role from the industrial age. The leader plans, organizes, leads, implements, controls, and evaluates change programs. When the leader attempts to control change, such as with the implementation of evidence-based guidelines, the leader attempts to hold power over workers by defining steps in the change process and identifying the persons involved in the change. To advance the goals of the system, the leader will implement practice patterns based in evidence, while agents or healthcare clinicians within the CAS participate in self-organizing interactions to respond to environment pressures. In this example, the outcome of the CAS is practice based in evidence according to a predefined metric, and the agents that respond to the environmental pressures are found within the boundaries of the system. From the CAS perspective, change in practice is measured by the outcome of the CAS.

After the boundaries are described in a CAS, change is explored at those boundaries. According to Poole and Van de Ven (2004), change is a difference in state, quality, or form measured at two or more points in time in an organizational entity. Change is the outcome of the system where one looks for new patterns or products. In this approach, the micro interactions within the CAS go ignored and change is not identified in the human-to-human interactions. The leader tries to influence the outcome of the system by standing outside of it and directing activities. When the focus is on change of the CAS as a clearly defined system, then the human-to-human interactions are seen as a means to the outcomes but not quantifiable or describable in any outcome metrics. The dynamic power of human interaction can be seen through the lens of CRP.

Change in CRP

CRP is a lens used to explore the conditions for change or the power dynamic within an organization without defined boundaries but with purposeful joint action. With a CRP perspective, power or the force for change occurs in human interactions. It is in micro interactions that variation arises from diversity within the organization (Stacey, Griffin & Shaw, 2000). The power dynamic occurs in the micro interactions where ideology and power relations are negotiated among those in the interaction; power is *with* the interaction rather than a force *over* interactions.

According to Stacey and Griffin (2005), the cooperative social process of self-organization is both enabled and constrained by rules of power relations, including norms, values, and accounting to one another. The organizing principles governing fluid human interactions are formed by and form power relations and ideology. Stacey and Griffin (2005) explain that ideology is composed of norms and values and is the evaluative criterion of choices. Norms are "evaluative criteria taking the form of obligatory restrictions which have emerged as generalizations and become habitual in a history of social interaction" (Stacey & Griffin, 2005, p. 6). Values are "individually felt voluntary compulsions to choose one desire, action or norm over another" (Stacey & Griffin, 2005, p. 6); they arise in social acts.

Power relations are ongoing processes clinicians participate in as they negotiate with each other regarding what they do or do not do. In these processes, clinicians may find that by using language that is persuasive, they are in, or accepted, while others may find themselves out, or not accepted. It is in processes of accounting to one another on the basis of ideology and power relations that clinicians' individual and collective identity is formed, and so are differences. The application of evidence to clinical practice is influenced by power relations in such a manner that those who are most persuasive to implement a specific guideline or those who are most persuasive to customize the evidence-based guideline find themselves in the in group that forms the norms and values of the larger group.

WORKING IN REAL TIME: SENSING THE EMERGENCE OF INNOVATION

The ancient Greek philosopher Heraclitus observed that the only constant in our world is change. Improved outcomes, higher profitability, faster production cycles, and higher quality represent a partial list of the drivers of innovation that motivate leadership in the clusters of human interaction that have been stabilized around specific themes that are continually reproduced—what we more commonly refer to as organizations (Fonseca, 2002). In a seeming contradictory note to Heraclitus's observation, the previous statement (referencing human interactions that are stabilized around themes) suggests that while there is a drive for innovation there is also a need for stability in human interactions in organizations to sustain an identity as an organization. At the same time, there would be a similar requirement for members of an organization to sustain their identity within an organization. Simultaneously there exists both stability and change. The potential for transformational change emerges as people conduct their business through local interactions.

What has hopefully become apparent in what has been described thus far is that through a lens of CRP, the emphasis or focus of observation is not a presence of a superordinate system that extends control of processes. Rather, attention is directed to the interdependent processes that occur among people—in this case, healthcare professionals and their interactions as they simultaneously influence and are influenced by the evolution of the organization. Due to contemporary interprofessional practices that are inherent in healthcare organizations, there is a fundamental degree of complexity present as the various roles interact with each other and alongside ever-increasing technological innovations. While there are actions that support continuation of the identity of individuals and the organization, so too are novel actions introduced in practice or process (Mereth, Aasen, & Johannessen, 2009). Meanings are continuously negotiated as people go about the tasks in their work (Durrant, 2004). As can be anticipated, there is a dynamic tension that exists between what is and what is aspired to be achieved in a desired future. The dynamic nature of this tension is not played out in a sequential, linear manner. Rather, is it evidenced in the paradoxical occurrence of the desire to sustain identity through stability in combination with the desire to effect change simultaneously.

These desires to advance the work of the organization commonly referred to as innovation practices emerge through the patterning of power relations and novelty that is introduced to the interactions among interdependent people (Fonseca, 2002). As members of a clinical team interact, the power relations that emerge are asymmetrical. Elias (1978) has offered that the nonlinear nature of human interaction has the potential to lead change that is disproportionate to the initial condition from which that change has emanated. The introduction of novelty that emerges as people negotiate meaning through their interactions represents the foundation of difference that is potentially amplified through conversational processes leading to change in practice or innovation (Fonseca, 2002).

Imagine a clinical team that has engaged in a familiar practice over an extended period of time. Their experience and interactions are based on known meanings of words and actions that have become well established. Such norms formed as meanings are established through the responses that are provided to gestures that have been expressed (Mead, 1934). Imagine further that this work process is interrupted through the introduction of a novel interaction that represents a difference in the usual process. In this circumstance, the previously held meaning associated with the interaction no longer holds true. In effect, there emerges various degrees of misunderstanding about what the meaning now entails (Fonseca, 2002). As the team members grapple with this potential transformation through social interactions of gesture and response, the misunderstanding that has been generated through the dissolution of the previously held norm is dissipated and new meanings are negotiated that become associated with the introduction of new practices. As the conversations ensue, additional ideas are introduced as diversity and the process of co-creating meaning of the new process expands. Should there be a successful negotiation of new meaning through conversation and actions among participants, the newly formed norm signals a successful innovation to the previous way of accomplishing the task. The process that has been described may be regarded as a counterintuitive perspective of innovation in that the introduction of novel ways of interacting creates a new pattern of behavior. This is contrasted with a more traditional view of innovation process that proposes that people coalesce around a common cultural attribute designed to transform the organization (Fonseca, 2002).

THE ITERATIVE INNOVATION PROCESS

In this CRP way of understanding innovation, what cannot be overlooked is simultaneous potential of both change and stability. A shift in power relations through the introduction of novelty leading to increased levels of diversity can prompt the experience of a risk to identity. This dynamic tension may be experienced in the form of the potential of discovering that one is excluded through persistent association with a preference to sustain known processes associated with previously held narrative themes and meanings (Stacey, 2001). The dynamic tension can be seen when a clinician is reluctant to implement a new evidence-based practice guideline because the practice is outside his or her comfort level. This person is commonly understood by others as a laggard. These sorts of experiences inherently possess the potential to a rise in lived anxiety (Fonseca, 2002). When the level of experienced anxiety is overwhelming, the transformational power of the proposed novelty is likely to be squelched by the desire to reduce anxiety by maintaining the status quo. Unlike the generative conversations that promote transformation, conversations occurring under this kind of threat are dominated by repetitious meaning associated with the usual way of conducting business. The result of this pattern of interaction is the victory of stability over change.

How is it that a proposed diversity of practice can overcome the retreat from anxiety to fulfill its transformational potential? Sproedt (2012) has proposed that innovation is largely achieved through the creation of social interaction grounded in trust and identity that emerges through the process of interactions that encourage and promote common meaning. Stated otherwise, the presence of positive relationships among interdependent members of an organization is a necessary precondition for innovation success.

USING OUR WORDS TO LEVERAGE RELATIONAL PRACTICES

Before proceeding, allow us to refine some earlier points as we return once again to this notion of relationship. We proposed in the introduction that there were three separate elements involved in sharing our work: you the reader, we the authors, and this chapter as the vehicle for communication. Our hope is that our words have assisted in identifying these three objects that together forge our emerging relationship. We premise this notion on the assumption that the authors and readers have a shared understanding of our chosen words. If the words that we were using to write this story were uniquely our own, it would be likely that you would not recognize them. If this were so, we could hardly expect that the publisher would print them. In actuality, as you are no doubt aware, the words that we have chosen are ones that we have encountered innumerable times, and these words form meaning through our communal understanding. In an effort to be completely transparent, we also acknowledge that many of the words that we have chosen to make up this chapter are words that have come to us from others who, in turn, had borrowed them from still others. In effect, who do these words belong to as you read them? Gergen (2009) raised this very issue and proposed that through these words, we share a relationship.

Yet it is a frequently held view that the sole purpose of words is to identify objects within our reality. If this were the only purpose of words, we would discover that we were living an experience in which we would be separated from the reality that words describe (Shotter, 2012). In truth, the flexibility with which we use words, according to Lock and Strong (2012), accomplishes far more to contribute to our reality other than merely naming objects in the world. Lock and Strong suggest that words do accomplish additional achievements, such as performing acts as demonstrated in the statement "I pronounce thee husband and wife." While reading the words "I pronounce thee husband and wife," you may well experience an image of a wedding in a house of worship, at city hall, or perhaps in a meadow or on a seashore. In effect, what you accomplish through such visualization is the creation of a social context in which the words have relevance (Shotter, 2012). Absent a context, words cannot convey a story that is comprehensible. Thus, the context that serves as the backdrop in the service of words offers opportunity for another important capacity of language: to provide meaning.

A shared network that is based in common context is necessary for meaning to emerge. Through these networks, people do not merely utter words to each other but instead engage in a responsive interactional process (Lock & Strong, 2012; Shotter, 2012). Reaching back to Foucault for support, Lock and Strong identify that as we engage each other in this form of social interaction, we find that we are in a journey of sharing ideas, thoughts, beliefs, and ways of understanding that all coalesce into a discourse that constructs our world.

By way of example, suppose we declare that stealing is a good action. You may be confused and perhaps incredulous that we would utter such a statement. However, when we set the context for this statement to be in reference to the game of baseball, we may be more readily greeted with understanding of our meaning by some readers. In such a situation, the baseball discourse constructs meaning. Others, even with this additional information, may be less inclined to agree and remain confused because they do not share this discourse that permits understanding of the game of baseball. These people might be immersed in a discourse pertaining to social justice that provides a negative evaluation of stealing. These people may remain confused because they would not include themselves in the group that shares in the meaning attributable to this baseball discourse. In effect, these people remain excluded from the meaning system that has emerged and thereby cannot claim to share in this construction of stealing.

What becomes available to us in this example is that there are at least two meanings of the word *stealing*. Neither of these meanings is reflective of an external reality. It is rather the co-created meaning that is shared. The conceptualization of stealing is made possible through a shared discourse premised upon the presence of a relationship among members. All that remains is for members of the group with knowledge to share their knowledge with those who are excluded so they can be in a relationship with others who are knowledgeable of the nuances of baseball.

This is relevant to the discussion of CRP. Remaining momentarily with our baseball stealing metaphor, those people who did not comprehend the unique meaning of stealing in baseball find themselves excluded from the conversation. The transformation of their membership group occurred through the transfer of knowledge via communication (Stacey, 2001). Through a process of being in a relationship and sharing conversation, knowledge or the meaning of stealing in baseball emerged.

From a more generic frame of reference, what can be claimed through this metaphorical example is that change can and is achieved through a process of shared knowledge that has been organized through relationships and that organizes the relationships themselves. More specifically, change occurs through communication. The transformational power resides in the interaction that occurs among participants. Gergen (2009), who has proposed that process informs evidence in a similarly counterintuitive perspective, has proposed that individuals do not create relationship. Rather, individuals emerge from relationship.

Such a frame of reference holds huge potential for healthcare organizations and those who work within them. The reductionist metaphor of an organization that is compartmentalized through boundaries that define roles, divisions, and functions recedes as human interaction gains prominence (Wheatley, 2006). By implication, Wheatley highlights that when operating from a framework that honors human interaction, leaders will organize their practices to engage the energy inherent in power that is generated through high-quality relationships. Plowman and colleagues (2007) note that rather than seeking stability through control and planning, leaders might instead become enablers of the emergence of the future by engaging in dialogues that create meaning of events. They continue to encourage leaders to promote dialogical practices, noting that unlike a traditional organization, one that is based in emergent dialogue leads to the realization of work contexts in which workers do not wait for direction from managers. Instead, their experience indicates that workers demonstrate ownership of their performance.

Inherent in the adoption of these practices is a concomitant shift from seeing events as isolated incidents. Pronouncing a couple husband and wife is an experience that will endure through time, although the words are uttered in mere moments. Enabling emergence within the workplace through dialogue similarly occurs through ongoing processes. Splicing these experiences together into a tapestry of continuing processes further expresses the emerging stories of our relationships in the world (Shotter, 2012).

RELATIONSHIP AS THE VEHICLE FOR CHANGE

Meanings of words and actions emerge through social interaction. Purposeful change in health care that utilizes evidence-based practice is facilitated through human relationships. The human relationships that influence practice patterns include the researcher or author of the evidence, clinicians, patients or clients for whom the evidence supports improved care, professional practice communities, and other individuals in the organization who also must make sense of the evidence to create implementation methods.

As described in the discussion of CRP, organizations are understood as processes of conversations through which power relations and ideology emerge in the living present. One of these power relations that has the potential to be overlooked is the relationship between evidence-based practice and practice-based evidence. Swisher (2010) pointed to the inseparability of the two forms of research. They are in relationship with each other. Swisher, who is a practitioner, observed the necessity to decipher the findings of empirical research in combination with evidence based in practice. For a practitioner to fully participate in an individual relational practice with another, it is necessary for the practitioner to engage in the reflexive practice with both forms of evidence. How does a clinician engage in such a reflexive practice? To develop a relationally grounded practice with individual clients that is based in evidence, the practice of reflexivity is needed.

REFLEXIVITY

Reflexivity is the activity of paying attention to one's experience. These experiences are simultaneously individual and social processes of making sense of one's interactions with others in the here and now (Stacey & Griffin, 2005). Clinicians practicing reflexivity reflect upon their own experience of simultaneously being formed by and informing the collective identity of the work group when applying evidence to clinical practice. In this process of forming and being formed by identity, the clinician is influenced by power relations, such as norms and values of those in their work group and their client or patient, as well as the authors of evidence-based practice guidelines, for example. A clinical practice utilizing reflexivity means that the clinician is conscious in the present moment of the power dynamic that is enacted when he or she is presented with evidence to guide practice. In the power dynamic, identity is both formed by and forms the local interactions where practice emerges on the edge of evidence.

By paying attention in the here and now to emergent processes of individual and group formation in the interactions around them, clinicians are practicing reflexivity. It is what occurs in the local situation, at the point of service, where the clinician's identity forms and is formed by interactions. A clinician responding to evidence to guide his or her practice is necessarily making explicit his or her way of thinking that is both formed by and forming the evolving relationship with patients or clients, other clinicians, and the authors of the presented evidence.

With a CRP lens, there are many opportunities to explore change in organizations using reflexivity. The opportunities for change lie in the dynamics of human interaction. Power relations are ongoing processes that nurses participate in as they negotiate with each other regarding what they do or do not do. In these processes, some nurses may find that by using language that is persuasive that they are in, or accepted, and others may find themselves out, or not accepted. Reflexivity is practiced in the processes of accounting to one another on the basis of power relations that includes norms and values. In the process of accounting to one another nurses' individual and collective identity is formed, so is difference. Change occurs in human interaction. Organizational change may be noticed in one single human-to-human interaction, or the change may emerge after many iterations of interacting together. In the end, the emergence of new patterns based on evidence occur in human interaction.

When new evidence is presented to improve clinical practice in an organization, implementation is simultaneously a social and an individual process. It is an individual and social process as the clinician's identity is formed by and forms interactions with others in response to the evidence-based practice guideline. The clinician may value the evidence and change his or her practice according to the guidelines; the clinician may also feel the voluntary compulsion to follow the practice guideline to contribute to the formed collective identity with other practitioners of having an evidence-based practice.

Influenced by power relations, including norms and values, the clinician is formed by and forming identity in the here and now. Quite possibly, clinicians may find that the evidence-based practice guideline needs to be adapted to the local situation, and patient needs and preferences. Thus, the clinicians may also form and be formed by patterns of relating that are patient centered. The clinician's response to evidence in clinical practice occurs through this dynamic of the clinician being formed by and forming identity with others by paying attention to identity (individual and collective) in the here and now.

NEW LENS, NEW OPPORTUNITIES FOR CHANGE

A case study is presented to demonstrate nurses paying attention in the here and now processes of formation for individual and collective identities in their clinical practice that was influenced by evidence-based guidelines. In this case study, nurses demonstrated interdependence and identity as they worked together on a medical–surgical–telemetry unit. These nurses were engaged in self-organizing nonlinear interactions. They embraced uncertainty and diversity in work flow solutions, and as a result they were able to respond rapidly and creatively to environmental changes. Ultimately this led to the nurses being able to safely administer ordered medication to patients.

This case study describes nurses formed by and forming identity while endeavoring to improve patient outcomes with a medication administration process. Nurses administer medications after verifying the five rights: right patient, right drug, right route, right dose, and right time (Federico, 2011). According to the evidence, bar code medication administration (BCMA) improves patient outcomes with medication administration thus it has been recommended to be implemented in hospitals to enhance the quality and safety of patient care (Institute of Medicine, 2001; Koppel, Wetterneck, Telles, & Karsh, 2008; Poon et al., 2010).

Case Example: Improving patient outcomes with BCMA

To improve the medication administration process, a Magnet hospital in the southwest United States implemented BCMA technology. On one medical–surgical–telemetry unit of the hospital, the nurses found that the BCMA technology did not function as they had been shown 2 months prior to the technology going live in their training sessions. Several of the nurses said the way they were shown to use the technology was to take the medication into the patient's room, scan their employee identification badge, and look at the top bar of the computer screen to ensure they were in the correct clinical application. Then they were to use the handheld scanner to pick up the bar code on the patient's wristband to confirm the right patient to receive the medication. Next, the nurse was to review the medication administration screen on the computer to ensure the correct screen was displayed because there are two different computer modules: one for documenting medications and another for intravenous fluids. If tablets were to be administered, the nurse would then look at the screen to confirm that the correct medication module of the electronic medication record was displayed. Then the nurse would scan the bar code on the medication package, look at the computer screen for alerts (such as not on medication list or administering too early), then the medication would be automatically highlighted in yellow on the screen to indicate that the five rights were aligned. The nurse would then give the tablets to the patient and select OK on the screen to save the information.

However, the nurses found that the technology did not operate as they expected. The nurses scanned the bar code on their employee identification badge to record who was administering the medication. Then they scanned the bar code on the patient's identification band, but the patient's electronic medication record did not appear on the computer screen. When the nurse first experienced this obstacle, she stopped the medication process and located a coworker to ask for help. In the interaction between the two nurses, they found that they experienced the same problem in the BCMA process. One nurse called the in-house help desk while the other nurse asked a more experienced nurse about his experience with BCMA. The help desk technician was unable to guide the nurse through the BCMA process because he did not understand the designed process from a clinician's point of view. From the interaction among the three nurses at the patient's bedside, they found that they could use the computer keyboard and mouse to highlight the patient's name. Then, instead of scanning the bar code on the patient's identification band, the nurses used the keyboard and mouse to highlight the patient's name and scanned the bar code on the medication package. The nurses looked at the computer screen for any alerts before administering the medication to the patient.

The nurses agreed that the technology was not bringing up the patient's electronic medication record as expected. It was a norm on this unit for nurses to place patients' needs at the center of their activities, including administering ordered medication to patients at the scheduled time. Each nurse in this interaction valued efficient and safe medication administration. The nurses consulted with another nurse and tried again to follow the designed process for BCMA.

In the interaction, the nurses found that if they responded to the designed process in their local situation, they could highlight the patient's name in the electronic medical record using the keyboard and mouse, then highlight the patient's electronic medication record. After the patient's electronic medication record was on the computer screen, they could scan the bar code on the medication package and look for alerts on the computer screen, such as a violation of the five rights. If no alert was on the screen, the nurse would administer the medication and press the Enter key three times to record the medication administration. A new practice pattern emerged in the current situation as the nurses were forming and formed by individual and collective identity. As other nurses experienced this same problem with the BCMA, they asked their coworkers for a solution, and the use of the keyboard and mouse became the standard of practice within this unit.

The emerging medication process came out of the nurses' interactions that were influenced by norms, values, and power relations. The nurses worked on a unit where efficient and safe care was a norm. Each nurse in this medical–surgical–telemetry unit had an individual compulsion to find a way to administer the medication using BCMA in what they believed was an efficient and safe manner. The work-around to pull up the patient's electronic medication list using the keyboard and mouse became the standard process because their actions were influenced by power relations, including norms and values. The nurses, who were respected by their peers and who used persuasive language to respond to the evidence to improve medication administration safety with the designed process in their local situation, were forming the in group with the revised way to use BCMA. In these interactions, the nurses were formed by and forming identity while working on the edge of evidence.

Questions

1. How did evidence stimulate a practice change?
2. Described a situation in which you participated in a discussion with coworkers to find a better way to achieve the desired outcome.
3. Was a better way to achieve the outcome met? How was the outcome received by those outside the discussion? Who else do you think should have been involved in the discussion?
4. How many times a week do you think you participate in such discussions?

Case Example: Patient therapeutic process

The previous case study demonstrates the process of change within a work team in a healthcare organization. In the following case study, novelty is introduced through a 1:1 therapeutic conversation that took place between a psychotherapist and a client, Gary, who was a healthcare worker when he experienced a transition to a new team at work. This conversational process is influential in the transformational change that Gary experienced in his workplace relationships that, in turn, positively impacted his personal familial relationships.

Gary had been introduced to a new work team and was tasked with responsibility to effect changes in practice on a health team. From a CRP perspective, without the benefit of positive relationships with colleagues and the mandate to effect change, Gary was thrust into a situation fraught with potential for anxiety through exclusion. Indeed, as he described his experience to the therapist, his story suggested that he was coping with tremendous anxiety associated with an experience of rejection by the work team as he introduced new practices in the workplace. In turn, Gary noticed that he was managing his anxiety by experiencing escalating bouts of despondency and withdrawal that produced a pattern dislocating him from his partner, who did not know how to support or resolve his behavior.

As he related his story, my experience, as the psychotherapist, was that of tremendous misunderstanding of the purpose of our conversation. Although there was a clear description of being unhappy, I had yet to understand, make sense as it were, of any purpose in our coming together. When people come together to work in a therapeutic engagement and begin to have a conversation, assuming one therapist and one client, both participate from a position that honors the traditions or norms that each hold and have evolved through their lived experience (McNamee & Hosking, 2012). To develop a shared purpose and process, both have a need to resolve the misunderstandings that exist when they begin. For instance, I could not presume to know what Gary meant when he spoke about his unhappiness. Our challenge is to begin our conversational journey to better understand each other. Through this process, the relative misunderstandings that dominated early conversations begin to dissolve. Said otherwise, as meaning emerges, so too does potential for movement (McNamee & Hosking, 2012).

However, when this process is viewed through the CRP lens, if the story sustains its focus upon only the description of how the experience is unpleasant, nothing else happens and the conversation will stagnate in a state of equilibrium or stability (Fonseca, 2002). As the psychotherapist, my role then is to continually introduce additional novelty to the conversation that spurs the necessity for additional meaning-making processes that move the system toward transformation. This is an iterative process that is the necessary energy required to spark change.

This would be a simple enough process to pursue in the psychotherapeutic conversation and coconstruct conditions that are associated with the preferred future if the process was a linear one organized toward resolution of the presenting problem. However, CRP highlights the simultaneous tension that exists between stability and transformation (Stacey, 2010; Stacey et al., 2000; Stacey & Griffin, 2005). When this tension is contained adequately, transformation is possible. Alternatively, should the tension overwhelm the people involved in the conversation, transformation is seen as being a threat and there is a retreat toward stability.

Returning to the story of the psychotherapeutic conversation, Gary had commented in a nonchalant manner, about 30 minutes into our discussion, that the administrator and others had complimented him for his excellence in the work that he had accomplished. With that said, the conversation returned to the earlier oppressive story of sadness and hurt. Just before the end of the conversation I commented that he had been acknowledged by his colleagues and supervisor for the excellent work he has accomplished. I also mentioned that it must be comforting to be surrounded by people who show appreciation for him at work and at home in the way that they do. I asked what had been helpful for him in the conversation that we had shared. Gary noted that it was good to have an independent party listen to him because he had been carrying the story quietly within himself. He asked to return in a week.

In the second conversation, I began by exploring what was significant from the first conversation. Gary noted that my acknowledgement of his contribution to the workplace was something that really stood out for him. He had heard my comments that echoed those from others but that had not impacted him when the words had originally been expressed. Gary expressed his curiosity that the comments had not registered as being news to him when he had first heard them. Reflexively, I wondered whether he heard it from me because he identified me as an independent third party. It occurred to me that these comments offered within the safety of the therapeutic conversation had introduced diversity (Fonseca, 2002). I followed up this conversational highlight by inquiring whether this revelation had made any other difference for him. Gary noted that he had taken this revelation to heart, and in turn it prompted him to have good days at work with colleagues, which he had previously reported as not being possible. Continuing our conversation, he spoke about seeking relief from profound sadness. We explored his values, what he wants, and the norms that he understood to be getting in the way of him achieving his preferred experience. I saw that my role in the process was to continually ask him common questions about reframing his experience, such as "What would be different when . . . ," "Who will notice if . . .," and "How he and others will notice and make other inquiries to provoke consideration of living life beyond the problem." Although this is a collaborative process, from the perspective of CRP in this segment, our power relationship was organized through continuous curiosity that introduced diversity into the conversation. In turn, Gary's responses prompted additional inquiries and curiosity.

Returning to the exploration of the sadness, we discussed how his previous pattern of behavior had served him well, but that it was perhaps now time to do something different. He commented that he wondered why now was the time. Then, unexpectedly, he interrupted himself and said it was less important to learn about why by looking at the past. Instead, it would be better to focus on the future and make things better. I made sense of this as being an invitation to address the anxiety associated with transformation (Stacey, 2010; Stacey et al., 2000; Stacey & Griffin, 2005). I checked with Gary to learn what we needed to do to create safety for him to pursue his goal. He said that he was feeling comfortable and nothing further was needed. He trusted the process.

The preferred future emerged when he noted that he will feel at peace and respect the decision of others rather than encourage them to meet his needs. I asked how much detail of the preferred future he believed he required to discuss his view of the transformation. Gary thoughtfully responded that minimum detail was necessary. As Fonseca (2002) has proposed, his declaration suggested that only a minimal description is needed for a sense of the future to emerge.

What is fascinating is that we informed each other about what direction the conversation would take. In this coaction (Gergen, 2009), his comments invited my contribution, which, in turn, invited his contributions. A method of introducing degrees of difference in the therapeutic process is to question people on a scale of 0 to 10, with 10 representing the best possible outcome that they can imagine and 0 representing the problem when it was at its worst. I asked Gary how he understood things on that scale to be different as we spoke as opposed to when we first began our encounter. He said he experienced an improvement of 5 points in the two conversations. He saw potential for change and expressed his experience that he knew he could feel the freedom to go slow and be deliberate in his actions.

Questions

1. Think back to a time when you had a conversation with a colleague and you experienced confusion. How did you manage that experience? In light of this chapter, what might you have done differently to alleviate your confusion?
2. How might you manage stressful work relationships in the future with knowledge of the process of creating innovative workplace relationships?
3. When you next engage a new work team, what might you do to foster a sense of well-being and collective purpose?
4. What is one thing that you can do tomorrow in your workplace to help foster a sense of relational practice?

In the long history of humankind (and animal kind, too) those who learned to collaborate and improvise most effectively have prevailed.

—CHARLES DARWIN

ORGANIZATIONAL AND HUMAN PATTERNS ADVANCE INNOVATION

Organizational patterns made up of human interactions advance evidence into practice. Leaders who hold the CRP perspective to organizational change recognize the practice patterns response to evidence occurs in human interactions in the present moment and that these interactions are influenced by norms, values, and power relations. To be part of the practice pattern response to the evidence, leaders will put themselves in relationships—in interactions with other members of the organization at the point of service. The leader understands the power relations dynamic that is influenced by norms and values of the work group. This leader will have a practice based in reflexivity because he or she knows to pay attention to interactions including evidence, the patient or client, clinicians, professional practice communities, researchers or authors, and other members of the organization. Conversations with those who are most persuasive will influence when and how evidence advances practice that forms and is forming identity.

Figure 7-2 schematically depicts the processes involved in emergent meaning (innovation) creation and implementation of innovation from the lens of CRP. This depiction of a Venn diagram demonstrates that the processes associated with innovation in the moment, relational conversations, knowledge, evidence, and negotiation of

Figure 7-2 Four elements in the innovation process

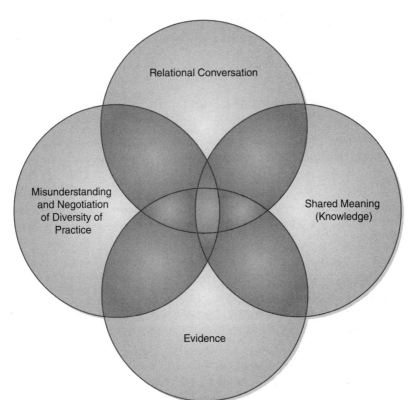

diversity interact with one another in a pattern that has no definitive direction or order. Indeed, the processes are iterative as the experience of energy and anxiety ebb and flow as the conversational processes progress. The diagram also depicts meaning emerging with the confluence of these practices, also calming anxieties that are associated with such transformation. Alternatively, should any of the four processes be underdeveloped so that anxiety prevails, the core of the process, emergent meaning, will remain an elusive target and the previous process will persist. The best hope that there will be sufficient awareness of the potential for innovation in the moment is presence of reflexive processes by the members of the team. Through such action, sensitivity to the identity of each member as a team and of the team itself will pave a pathway grounded in the trust built in relationships to implement new practices.

A leader who practices reflexivity is conscious and pays attention to the present moment knowing innovation in the form of local response will emerge in human interaction. Emergence of new patterns and disruption of ineffective patterns occurs in local interactions of clinical practice. As clinicians, patient or clients, professional practice communities, researchers or authors, and other members of the organization interact to respond to the evidence, the human patterns emerge by each individual and the collective by paying attention to their experience in the here and now.

EMERGENCE IN THE MOMENT

Such attentiveness to the micro-level processes that are occurring in the living present give rise to the potential for innovation in practice to become known. Through interactional processes that honor the presence of divergent perspectives, potential new practices are emerging. There is no necessity for there to be a coordinated overseer to direct the process. As conversations are undertaken, people's identities are being formed as they are forming the identity of others and the organization overall. Such generative interactions capture the energy that flows from power relations that emerge, shift, and churn as possibilities present themselves from thematic conversations that transpire. Should expressions of anxiety become pronounced through repetitive commentaries extolling the benefit to sustain old practices, slowing of the speed of change to ensure integrity of identity through conversation can calm mounting fears and will ultimately lead to successful change. This is aptly described in the work-around case presentation in which nurses remained tethered to the value and identity of providers of safe and efficient patient care as they collaboratively responded with novelty to a technological process that did not provide the promised process. The safety extended by the presence of a secure identity created a social context through which ingenuity transformed a potentially dangerous situation into a successful innovation to practice. Alternatively, the counseling case highlighted the emergence of a powerful identity through transformation of meanings that had been attributed to an anxiety-filled work experience. In this situation, novelty resolved misunderstanding that potentiated a different view of the workplace transformation.

To be highlighted is the acknowledgement that through conversation, meaning occurs only in and through the interactions of people. The patterns of interaction organize us as we conduct our business. When the diversity is sufficient and anxiety (although present) is contained, it becomes possible to transform meaning, knowledge, and practice.

LEVERAGING RELATIONAL PRACTICES TO CREATE CHANGE

For any reader who has engaged in a process similar to those that have been described in the case examples, you are familiar with the activity that is occurring during these interactions. Just as we have suggested in the previous discussion, you are no doubt aware of the multiple relationships that you are engaged in during the moments of interactions with the patient or client. In addition to the relationship with the evidence-based practice that has formed and is forming your identity and practice, you are processing information from your professional body, your disciplinary college, codes of conduct, and policies and procedures in your organization while simultaneously engaging with the person or people with whom you are interacting. No doubt there are numerous other relationships that are influencing you at the same instant. The interactions we all participate in every day influence our identity, individual and collective, and our response to evidence. Oftentimes we are not aware of how interactions form and are forming our identity. The interactions are not merely a conduit for an evidence-based practice that is formed by and informing identity, but in this collaborative process meaning is created, which is practice-based evidence.

Recall that in an earlier section of this chapter, we referenced Gergen (2009), who spoke of the need to appreciate that the effect be known before the cause can be identified. Extrapolating from this logic, it can be stated that the challenge that is being confronted is the source of innovation, which is found in interactions where meaning is created. Through reflexivity, as a practitioner you incorporate views and perspectives that are formed by and forming with others. What becomes abundantly clear through such a process is the necessity for the development of a sense of trust within the variety of relationships. It is trust that is the basis of the relationship informing your practice. With trust there is a foundation from which the possibility to engage in conversation that disturbs the status quo is established. Through a process of describing and amplifying new meaning, a credible innovative process with participants of the conversation emerges. Without the development of such trust, anxiety associated with the disruption of the power relationships that have persisted (Sarra, 2005) will threaten the cohesion that can thwart the change. Relationship becomes the vehicle by which power relations transition from an experience of *power over* to provide a pathway to experience *power to promote* new meaning and ultimately innovation (McNamee & Hosking, 2012). Our ability to relationally engage with each other provides opportunity for multiple perspectives of meaning, perhaps one perspective for each participant, to be shared in a context of trust and openness. During such conversations, fresh understanding that is shared with colleagues introduces new frames that were previously unknown. Misunderstanding may result. Through this conversational sharing, the possibility is present for the introduction of novelty that potentiates fresh meaning and, ultimately, innovation. This collaborative meaning-making through conversation creates the space for fresh ideas to emerge and provides opportunities to innovate in the present moment. This, in turn, creates space for collaboratively developing meaning through conversational processes on the edge of evidence.

REFERENCES

Bennet, A., & Bennet, D. (2004). *Organizational survival in the new world.* Boston, MA: Elsevier.

Dooley, K. J. (2004). Complexity science models of organizational change and innovation. In M. S. Poole & A. H. Van de Ven (Eds.), *Handbook of organizational change and innovation* (pp. 354–373). Oxford, UK: Oxford University Press.

Durrant, T. (2004). The strategic management of technology and innovation. In T. Durrant, O. Grandstrand, C. Herstatt, A. Nagel, D. Probert, B. Tomlin & H. Tschirky (Eds.), *Bring technology and innovation into the boardroom* (pp. 19–46). London, UK: Palgrave McMillian.

Elias, N. (1978). *What is sociology?* New York, NY: Columbia University Press.

Federico, F. (2011). The five rights of medication administration. Retrieved from www.ihi.org/knowledge /Pages/ImprovementStories/

Fonseca, J. (2002). *Complexity and innovation in organizations.* New York, NY: Routledge.

Gergen, K. J. (2009). *Relational being: Beyond self and community.* New York, NY: Oxford University Press.

Institute of Medicine. (2001). *Crossing the quality chasm: A new health system for the twenty-first century.* Washington, DC: National Academies Press.

Koppel, R., Wetterneck, T., Telles, J. L., & Karsh, B. (2008). Workaround to barcode medication administration systems: Their occurrences, causes, and threats to patient safety. *Journal of the American Medical Informatics Association, 15,* 428–423. doi:10.1197/jamia.M2616

Lindberg, C., Nash, S., & Lindberg, C. (2008). *On the edge: Nursing in the age of complexity.* Bordentown, NJ: Plexus Press.

Lock, A., & Strong, T. (2012). Discursive therapy: What language, and how we use it in therapeutic dialogues, matters. In A. Lock & T. Strong (Eds.), *Discursive perspectives in therapeutic practice* (pp. 1–22). Oxford, UK: Oxford University Press.

Marion, R. (2008). Complexity theory for organizations and organizational leadership. In M. Uhl-Bien & R. Marion (Eds.), *Complexity leadership* (pp. 1–15). Charlotte, NC: Information Age.

McNamee, S., & Hosking, D. M. (2012). *Research and social change: A relational constructionist approach.* New York, NY: Routledge.

Mead, H. G. M. (1934). *Mind, self and society.* Chicago, IL: University of Chicago Press.

Mereth, T., Aasen, B., & Johannessen, S. (2009). Managing innovation as communicative processes: A case of subsea technology R&D. *International Journal of Business Science and Applied Management, 4*(3), 22–33.

Plowman, D. A., Solansky, S., Beck, T. E., Baker, L., Kulkarni, M., & Travis, D. V. (2007). The role of leadership in emergent self-organization. *Leadership Quarterly, 18*, 341–356.

Poole, M. S., & Van de Ven, A. H. (2004). *Handbook of organizational change and innovation.* Oxford, UK: Oxford University Press.

Poon, E. G., Keohane, C. A., Yoon, C. S., Ditmore, M., Bane, A., Levtzion-Korach, O., . . . Gandhi, T. K. (2010). Effect of bar-code technology on the safety of medication administration. *The New England Journal of Medicine, 362*, 1698.

Porter-O'Grady, T., & Malloch, K. (2011). *Quantum leadership: Advancing innovation, transforming health care.* Sudbury, MA: Jones & Bartlett Learning.

Sarra, N. (2005). Organizational development in the national health service. In R. D. Stacey & D. Griffin (Eds.), *A complexity perspective on researching organizations: Taking experience seriously* (pp. 173–200). New York, NY: Routledge.

Shotter, J. (2012). Ontological social constructionism in the context of a social ecology: The importance of our living bodies. In A. Lock & T. Strong (Eds.), *Discursive perspectives in therapeutic practice* (pp. 83–105). Oxford, UK: Oxford University Press.

Sproedt, H. (2012). *Play, learn, innovate: Grasping the social dynamics of participatory innovation.* SØnderborg, Denmark: Books on Demand.

Stacey, R. (2001). *Complex responsive processes in organizations: Learning and knowledge creation.* London, UK: Routledge.

Stacey, R. (2010). *Complexity and organizational reality: Uncertainty and the need to rethink management after the collapse of investment capital* (2nd ed.). New York, NY: Routledge.

Stacey, R., & Griffin, D. (2005). *A complexity perspective on researching organizations.* London, UK: Routledge.

Stacey, R. D., Griffin, D., & Shaw, P. (2000). *Complexity and management: Fad or radical challenge to systems thinking?* London, UK: Routledge.

Swisher, A. K. (2010). Practice-based evidence. *Cardiopulmonary Physical Therapy Journal, 21*(2), 4.

Uhl-Bien, M., & Marion, R. (2008). Introduction: Complexity leadership—a framework for leadership in the twenty-first century. In M. Uhl-Bien & R. Marion (Eds.), *Complexity leadership* (pp. xi–xxiv). Charlotte, NC: Information Age.

Uhl-Bien, M., Marion, R., & McKelvey, B. (2008). Complexity leadership theory. In M. Uhl-Bien & R. Marion (Eds.), *Complexity leadership* (pp. 185–224). Charlotte, NC: Information Age.

Wheatley, M. J. (2006). *Leadership in the new science.* San Francisco, CA: Berret-Koehler.

CHAPTER 8

The Information Revolution: Using Data and Technology to Support Patient Care

Robert C. Geibert

CHAPTER OBJECTIVES

Upon completion of this chapter, the reader will be able to:

1. Name four online resources that provide reliable health-related information.
2. Define peer-to-peer health care.
3. Define big data and small data and provide examples of how each is used in health care.
4. Define mHealth and describe five ways that mobile communication devices have been useful in seeking and providing health-related information.
5. Define Virtual Nursing Grand Rounds and explain how they have been used to support evidence-based practice.

The diffusion of technology into every aspect of the healthcare system and the power of the Internet are perhaps the most significant factors that have supported the integration of evidence-based practice (EBP) into the provision of patient care. With 24/7 access to clinical data, clinicians can search for information from a growing number of online resources sponsored by organizations worldwide and incorporate their findings into their clinical decision-making process at a faster rate. Some resource examples are the Agency for Healthcare Research and Quality (http://www.ahrq.gov), the Joanna Briggs Institute (http://www.joannabriggs.org), and the Cochrane Library (http://www.cochranelibrary.com), to name a few.

The availability of electronic networks provides access to data at the point of care, whether that location is the clinic exam room, the hospital bedside, a patient's home, or a clinic in rural India. It is no longer necessary to visit a medical library during its limited hours of operation to find answers to clinical questions. This chapter discusses how innovations in technology and access to vast amounts of health-related information can support EBP and improve patient outcomes.

THE EXPANDING ROLE OF TECHNOLOGY

Healthcare practitioners are not the only beneficiaries of this wealth of information. Healthcare consumers can also access a significant amount of fact-based health-related data via the Internet at sites such as those operated by WebMD (http://www.webmd .com), the Mayo Clinic (http://www.mayoclinic.com), and PubMed (http://www.ncbi .nlm.nih.gov/pubmed). PubMed is a service sponsored by the U.S. National Library of Medicine that includes more than 22 million publication citations from MEDLINE, some of which are available in full-text versions. In fiscal year 2014, MEDLINE added 765,860 new citations (U.S. National Library of Medicine, 2015a).

The National Institute of Health's website MedlinePlus (http://www.medlineplus .gov) has information on more than 950 health topics in English and Spanish and is designed for use by anyone. It includes a medical encyclopedia, a medical diction-ary, drug information, videos, and links to thousands of clinical trials, and it does not contain advertising or endorsements. In 2014, MedlinePlus webpages were viewed 986 million times! Nearly 108 million unique visitors accessed the site in the first quarter of 2014 (U.S. National Library of Medicine, 2015b). The term *unique visitor* refers to the number of different people who have accessed a site within a specific period of time, such as the first quarter of a year. Although a user may visit the site multiple times, the visitor is counted only once. With this enormous availability of online health-related information, consumers have an opportunity to be better informed about their care. It is unknown, however, if those who have accessed information made changes in their behavior to improve their health.

The Internet has made access to this vast amount of health-related information possible. According to Internet Live Stats (2015), there are now more than 3 billion Internet users in the world. The Internet Live Stats data indicate that about 40% of the world's population has an Internet connection and that the United States follows China as the leader in Internet usage. The United States has approximately 280 million users, which equals 86.75% of the country's population, a finding that was validated by the Pew Research Center in a 2014 survey (Pew Research Center, 2014).

A 2012 Pew Research Center survey found that 72% of Internet users said they had looked online for health information within the past year. Search engines were used as the starting point by 77% of the respondents, and another 13% began at a site that specialized in health information, such as WebMD. The most commonly researched topics were specific diseases or conditions, procedures or treatments, and doctors or other health professionals. Half of the searches were conducted on behalf of someone else (Pew Research Center, 2013).

The researchers inquired about the source of information that the respondents ac-cessed for help when they had a serious health issue. They found that 70% of U.S. adults got information, care, or support from a doctor or other health professional; 60% received information or support from friends and family; and 24% turned to others who had the same health condition.

Discussion

In the past 6 months, how have you used online resources to locate health-related information? Did your searches focus on your needs, or were you researching on the behalf of others? How easy was it to find reliable information? How did you determine if the information was reliable? How often have you had to help a patient or family member interpret healthcare data?

Online social networking is playing an important part in connecting those with similar health conditions. The Pew Research Center refers to these connections as peer-to-peer health care (Fox, 2011). Some online users may live in small communities where access to others who are living with the same issues are limited or not available. Others may have a rare condition, which is defined in the United States as affecting fewer than 200,000 Americans at the same time (Rare Disease Day, 2015). One can find many touching stories about life-changing online connections that have been made, often because a person no longer feels like he or she is the only one who is living with a certain condition. Numerous lifelong friendships have been formed, and some users have met face to face.

Caregivers were another group that the Pew Research Center studied to examine their information-seeking behaviors (**Figure 8-1**). They discovered that 39% of adults in the United States care for an adult or multiple adults. They also learned that caregivers are heavy users of technology and differ from noncaregivers in their information-seeking activities (Pew Research Center, 2013).

During the survey, researchers identified that 45% of U.S. adults were dealing with at least one chronic condition. Of those with two or more conditions, 78% had high blood pressure and 45% had diabetes. Researchers examined information-seeking behaviors of those with chronic conditions and found that those with one or more chronic conditions were no more likely to track their weight, diet, or exercise routine than other adults. However, 19% of those reporting tracked health indicators or symptoms. Tracking rates increased with the number of conditions; for example, 40% of adults with one condition and 62% with two or more conditions.

In summary, the number of consumers who use technology as a tool to seek health-related information is growing rapidly. The use of innovative technologies is clearly

Figure 8-1 Caregivers and health activities

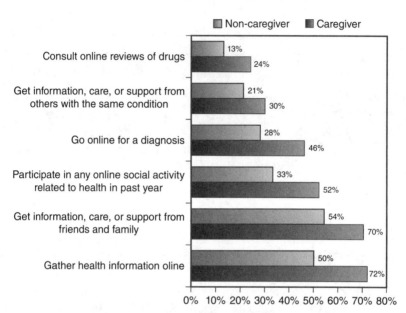

Reproduced from "Family Caregivers are Wired for Health," Pew Research Center, Washington, DC (June, 2013). Retrieved from http://www.pewinternet.org/files/old-media/Files/Reports/2013/PewResearch_FamilyCaregivers.pdf

providing useful tools that enable them to become better informed and to be collaborative contributors as decisions are made about their health care. The work of healthcare organizations is to help consumers turn information into action because accessing information and not using it is the same as not accessing it. A tool is useless unless it is used. Nurses are in a unique position to assist patients and their families in accessing both useful and reliable online health information as a part of their self-care strategies.

BIG DATA

The online healthcare information that is provided by reputable organizations is based on enormous amounts of data that are drawn from many sources. Healthcare organizations also collect and analyze millions of pieces of data. These data are commonly referred to as *big data*.

Big data is a "buzzword, or catch-phrase, used to describe a massive volume of both structured and unstructured data that is so large it is difficult to process using traditional database and software techniques" (Beal, 2014, para. 1). Big data generally comes from multiple sources and has value when the data sets are integrated and analyzed.

IBM (2015) informs us that we create 2.5 quintillion bytes of data every day. We have generated so much data that 90% of the data in the world today has been created in the past 2 years. Those data come from everywhere: sensors used to gather climate information, posts to social media sites, digital pictures and videos, purchase transaction records, cell phone GPS signals, and more.

Big data tells us *what* is happening but generally fails to tell us *why* it is happening. However, uncovering "what" can be the first step to uncovering "why". Henly (2014) informs us that the dimensionality of big data is huge, that data types are diverse, and that there are innumerable interconnections among the data. Henly states that instead of using data for explanation, the three goals of big data use are to describe, integrate, and predict. Healthcare organizations can use data science to analyze these large amounts of data to inform decision making.

The complexities of big data are often characterized as three Vs: volume, velocity, and variety (Thorpe & Gray, 2015):

- Volume represents enormous repositories of data; for example, millions of data pieces collected from millions of patient electronic health records and other data sources. The low cost of data storage and the increasing use of electronic health records are factors that are encouraging massive data collections.
- Velocity refers to the increasing rate at which data flows into an organization (Dumbill, 2012), which is often a near real-time stream of data. Dumbill informs us that data must be analyzed quickly so that appropriate feedback can occur. In some cases, so much data may arrive that useless data must be filtered out and discarded to provide sufficient space for data that are useful.
- Variety refers to the many forms of structured and unstructured data that are collected from numerous sources. Thorpe and Gray (2015) tell us that structured data includes quantitative information that is always entered in the same format across systems, such as a patient's name, address, medical record number, and vital signs. Unstructured data represents qualitative information that is often generated as narrative notations; some identify this as storytelling.

Nursing frequently uses this type of documentation to describe situations and environmental factors that affect outcomes because flow sheets are generally not designed to accommodate narrative data. Therefore, these types of data are difficult to capture and analyze in a meaningful way. However, artificial intelligence is being used to explore ways to code these textual entries to produce structured data.

Marcus (2014), in a document from the National Institute of Standards and Technology Big Data Working Group, suggests that three other Vs should be considered in relationship to healthcare data: veracity, variability, and value:

- Veracity refers to the accuracy of the data. Unfortunately, data may be inaccurate when it is generated, or it may lose meaning when it is translated. Therefore, veracity is extremely important when making clinical decisions.
- Variability must be considered when the same information can have different meanings; for example, listing Oxford as a patient's location may refer to Oxford in 23 states or 4 countries. Therefore, it is important to resolve these ambiguities to enhance the accuracy of data analysis.
- Value is enhanced when the aggregation of information into a data set, such as big data, enables analysis to reveal correlations, trends, and patterns across populations that may not be possible when analyzing smaller data sets.

Marcus (2014) informs us that big data analysis is not only useful in answering research questions, but it has been used to develop and test models for predicting outcomes for interventions, costs, and readmissions. The availability of big data and its analysis is an important tool that can be used to identify evidence-based best practices.

The use and analysis of big data in the healthcare industry lags behind industries such as finance, insurance, and pharma. Dan LeSuer of the HealthCatalyst group suggests that there are five reasons that healthcare data are unique and difficult to measure (LeSuer, 2014):

1. Much of the data are in multiple places, and the sources are not interconnected. In healthcare organizations, data may come from electronic medical records, pharmacy, laboratory and radiology systems, membership databases, and others. It also comes in different formats, such as text, numeric, paper, digital, pictures, and so forth. More sources of data from patient-generated tracking devices, like fitness monitors and blood pressure sensors, will soon be integrated.
2. The data are structured and unstructured. LeSuer (2014) notes that although electronic medical records provide a platform for consistent data capture, clinicians are used to documenting in ways that are most efficient for them without regard for how the data could eventually be aggregated and analyzed. For example, there are times when documenting in fields of a flow sheet cannot adequately describe a situation. It is easier to write a narrative, even though it is likely that the data will not be captured or useful during data analysis.
3. Definitions are inconsistent and variable. EBP guidelines and new research are coming out every day. The amount of available healthcare data continuously changes, and interpretation is often variable. Reaching consensus on definitions

or conditions may be difficult, if not impossible. Therefore, identifying ways to structure the data are challenging.

4. The data are complex and are often derived from multiple sources that are not connected. LeSuer (2014) notes that developing standard processes to improve quality outcomes is one healthcare goal; however, the number of variables makes it challenging. The human body is much more complex, and the variety of data collected from multiple information systems is much more difficult to analyze than in other industries, such as manufacturing.

5. Regulatory requirements are increasing and evolving. LeSuer (2014) posits that traditional approaches to data management do not work in health care because of the complexities previously listed. He writes that health care is unlike industries in which business rules and definitions remain unchanged for long periods of time. LeSuer suggests that "the volatility of healthcare data means a rule set today may not be a best practice tomorrow" (2014, p. 5).

Learning Activity

1. Contact your organization's nurse researcher or the information technology and marketing departments and ask them how big data collection and interpretation has contributed to the organization's plan of action.
2. Knowing that big data tells you the what but not the why (cause), how do you determine cause?

SMALL DATA

As you become more aware of the value big data can bring to healthcare outcomes, it is important to understand the role that small pieces of data play in the journey to big data. Small data refers to data that are in a "volume and format that makes it accessible, informative and actionable" (TechTarget, 2013, para. 1). Small data generally provide information that answers a specific question, or it may address a specific problem. General examples include inventory reports or weather forecasts. The data are often displayed visually to enhance understanding (TechTarget, 2013).

In health care, small data are generated each time a patient interacts with a clinician and the findings are documented in an electronic health record. That data then becomes part of big data. McCartney (2015) suggests that when nurses are documenting their nursing assessments, nursing care, and outcomes in an electronic health record, they are doing more than charting. In fact, they are creating small data which then becomes a part of big data. McCartney (2015) notes that contributing to big data may have the potential to create new knowledge and advancements in patient care.

Sacristán and Dilla posit that "there are no big data without small data" (2015, p. 3). They suggest that big data should be analyzed and translated into information. However, it is easy to drown in data and yet be starved for information. Because the amounts of big data are generally enormous, it is possible for analysts to identify megatrends that cannot be extracted from small data. For example, big data can tell a healthcare system how many patients fill, or do not fill, a particular prescription, such as a statin. What big data cannot tell us is why patients are deciding to fill, or not fill, that prescription.

Sacristán and Dilla believe that "information is only useful if it is translated into knowledge and knowledge is only useful if it is used to improve the health of individual patients" (2015, p. 2). Therefore, it is critical to standardize ways in which high-quality small data are collected. In addition, they inform us that each medical act is the intersection between small data and big data (**Figure 8-2**).

I routinely use an electronic health record during my work in an oncology infusion center. Multiple pieces of small data are captured and documented during each patient visit. For example, it is necessary to document a nursing assessment, vital signs, the patient's readiness for receiving treatment, IV insertion and discontinuation, medication administration safety and nursing double checks, medication start and stop times, the patient's response to treatment, chemotherapy plan completion of days and/or cycles, the creation of orders that are used to bill for nursing assessment and time, narrative descriptions of qualitative observations and/or patient interactions, verification that subsequent appointments have been scheduled, and more. It is difficult to remember if

Figure 8-2   Learning healthcare system

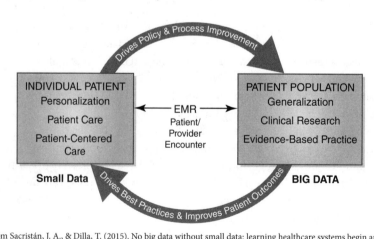

Data from Sacristán, J. A., & Dilla, T. (2015). No big data without small data: learning healthcare systems begin and end with the individual patient. *Journal of Evaluation in Clinical Practice*. Advance online publication. doi: 10.1111/jep.12350.

all these pieces of data have been documented before closing an encounter, especially when working with multiple patients throughout a hectic day.

I receive a pop-up message when attempting to close an encounter if a chief complaint is not documented or if orders have not been signed. However, I question why a sophisticated electronic health record system does not notify me when the multitude of nursing documentation requirements are unmet. Even when completing many simple online forms as part of a routine Internet visit or registration, a user will generally receive a pop-up message that identifies the missing data that must be entered before the form can be submitted successfully.

SMALL DATA FEEDS ELECTRONIC HEALTH RECORD BIG DATA

In recent years, a rapidly increasing number of healthcare organizations have created electronic portals that are enhancing communication opportunities among consumers, their healthcare providers, and other health-related services. For example, e-mail your doctor capabilities are providing patients with 24/7 opportunities to communicate with their healthcare providers from any Internet-connected computer in the world. Making appointments, viewing lab results, renewing prescriptions, viewing immunization records, and accessing a portion of their electronic health record are frequently provided features. In addition, many organizations are using, or exploring, the use of videoconferencing appointments, frequently via smartphone, and/or telephone appointments.

APPOINTMENT VIA VIDEOCONFERENCE

I have a colleague who travels frequently. He was on a flight from Atlanta to San Francisco when he noticed that his right eye was irritated and had a thick discharge. He was concerned that he might have an eye infection. Because he was leaving very early the following morning for an international trip to a country where healthcare services are below U.S. standards, he decided to seek medical care before departing. Unfortunately, it was after hours, and his physician's office was closed. However, he called the office 24-hour advice nurse help line and requested advice and a same-day appointment.

He was informed that an appointment by videoconference was available 2 hours later. Because my colleague was very familiar with this form of communication, he accepted the appointment without hesitation. At the appointment time, my colleague connected to the call via his iPad that he had connected to an external high-definition camera. He reported that the visual and audio qualities were excellent and that the physician asked him to bring his eye close to the camera to facilitate an assessment. A diagnosis was made, and an antibiotic was ordered that my colleague could pick up at his pharmacy that evening.

This example demonstrates how innovations in technology are being used to improve access to care, to provide opportunities for effective patient and clinician interactions, and to successfully diagnose and treat a condition that resulted in a high level of patient satisfaction.

DIRECT TRANSFER OF SMARTPHONE DATA TO A PATIENT'S ELECTRONIC HEALTH RECORD

The ability to transfer a patient's personal health data directly from his or her smartphone to the healthcare organization's electronic health record is receiving substantial media attention. Apple is a leader in developing this innovative technology and has been working with numerous healthcare organizations and application developers to apply this new technology.

The release of the Apple iOS 9 operating system contained many new features. The included Health iPhone app is attracting a significant amount of attention in the healthcare industry. This very user-friendly app can track and display health-related information, including the following: Body measurements, Fitness, Me, Nutrition, Results, Sleep, Vitals, and Reproductive Health (**Figure 8-3**).

Figure 8-3 iPhone health application

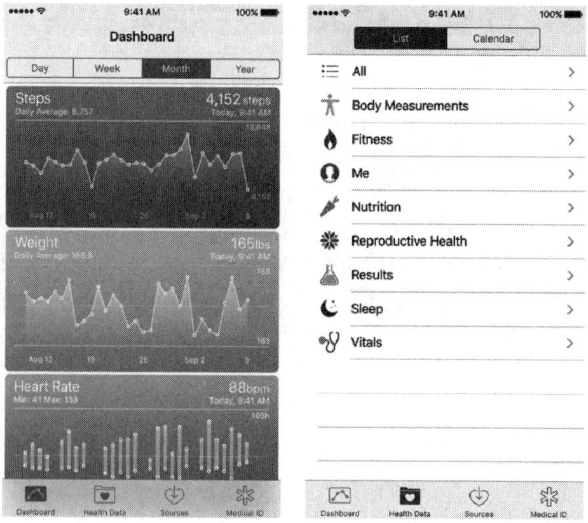

Screen shots reprinted with permission from Apple Inc.

Some data is automatically tracked by the app without user intervention. For example, steps are tracked on iPhone 5s, iPhone 6, iPhone 6 Plus, iPhone 6s, or iPhone 6s Plus, and flights of stairs climbed are tracked on iPhone 6, iPhone 6 Plus, iPhone 6s, or iPhone 6s Plus (Keirn Swanson, 2015). The Health app easily interacts with many other free and paid compatible health and fitness apps. For example, Keirn Swanson suggests the ARGUS Motion and Fitness Tracker that can be downloaded from the iTunes store (2015). It can track steps, and it uses GPS data to track running and cycling activities. It can also track fluid intake and numerous other items. Some of the tracking data is automated, and other data must be entered manually.

To enable third-party apps to integrate with the Health app, Apple has created a HealthKit tool that it distributes to app developers. This tool, coupled with Epic Systems (http://www.epic.com) electronic healthcare records, is enabling the integration of personal health data into an electronic health record, as described later.

The Cedars-Sinai Medical Center in Los Angeles recently announced that more than 87,000 of the patients who are already using their online patient portal would be able to use the HealthKit technology on their smartphones to transfer data from their devices directly into their electronic health record (Comstock, 2015). Patients can choose which information to transfer, including weight, blood pressure, steps, pulse, glucose, and SpO2 data.

With regard to collecting data, it is interesting to note that Darren Dworkin, the organization's chief information officer, stated, "To be perfectly candid, we're not sure what we're going to do with that information" (Comstock, 2015, para. 2). He indicated that there is interest in discovering what information their patients will decide to share.

Learning Activity

1. In relation to the prior activity, ask the departments you contacted to describe what small data was collected and how it contributed to the big data that was analyzed and used to change practice.
2. What type of small data feedback do you receive where you work?

MHEALTH

The term *mHealth* refers to "the delivery of healthcare services via mobile communication devices" (Torgan, 2009, para. 6). The Pew Research Center recently reported that nearly two thirds of Americans now own a smartphone and that more than half of smartphone owners have used their phone to get health information (Pew Research Center, 2015b) (**Figure 8-4**).

The Apple and Android app stores are full of fitness and health-related apps. It is difficult to determine how many of these apps are available for download. I have seen estimates that range from "a bucket full" to tens of thousands. Determining the quality

Figure 8-4   Smartphone activity summary

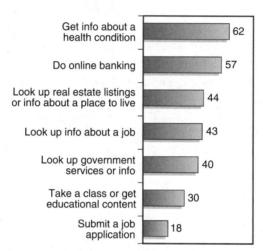

of an app's content is challenging. Although numerous websites advertise lists of the best apps or must-have apps, a *Harvard Men's Health Watch* journalist offered the best advice: be skeptical ("Better health with smartphone apps," 2015).

It is important to stop and consider the following questions: What makes us sure that information from the Internet will be used more frequently, or better than, information gained during a human encounter? Does access to, and information obtained from, electronic healthcare resources change behavior, especially in relationship to our personal health? If so, what are the effective motivating factors? Is a human component necessary, or can bots play that role? Does a combination of technology and human interaction make a difference? Are responses different among various age groups?

In an attempt to answer some of these questions, I performed multiple, comprehensive searches using Internet search engines, consumer reference databases, and databases used by healthcare professionals. I found a small number of studies that explored the veracity of the healthcare information that the app provided, in comparison to the marketing blurbs. Some studies reported behavioral changes; however, the sample sizes were frequently small and the changes were not sustained, or they required frequent human follow up and support. Although some apps provided individualized computer-generated support, that was generally not an effective approach.

Quite surprisingly, no information was found that identified apps that used successful behavioral change theories to enhance user responses. In fact, the vast majority of apps acted as data trackers, such as documenting weight loss or the number of steps taken in a day. It was the user's responsibility to view and analyze the data collected by the app, to make an action plan, and to carry it out. I believe that most users will soon begin to suffer from app fatigue. After the novelty wears off, will the thrill of learning new things or the excitement about tracking user-selected health-related items wane? Or will healthcare apps become the new treadmill in the bedroom that receives a lot of use when it is new then gradually becomes an electronic clothing rack?

BE SKEPTICAL

When we look at and use apps with a bit of skepticism, we will discover that not all apps are good. In 2013, the Reuters news agency reported a study that reviewed the accuracy of several apps that were designed to screen for skin cancer (Pittman, 2013). Because the apps were marketed as educational, the U.S. Food and Drug Administration (FDA) did not regulate them. Researchers used photos of 188 prediagnosed lesions that included melanomas and benign lesions, and they checked the accuracy of three algorithm-based apps. The most accurate app missed 18 of the 60 melanomas and mistakenly classified them as lower risk. As healthcare providers, we know that it is wise for consumers to have any areas of concern evaluated by a dermatologist; however, some app users may not have financial or other resources to seek professional care and will rely on the app's findings. This can prove to be deadly.

Dr. Orrin Franko of the American Academy of Orthopedic Surgeons informs us that developers of health-related apps do not need to be medical professionals, nor do they need to seek medical input to ensure accuracy (Franko, 2013). He says that although some apps may include a legal statement, the app developers are not required to disclose their sources of information or their limitations.

This author suggests that the vast majority of consumers accept an app's content to be factual, especially if they have paid for it. Marketing departments are very creative in describing the value that their app will bring to the consumer who uses or buys it, even though the claims may not be supported by evidence.

Discussion Questions

What criteria would you use to assess the veracity of a particular app? How would one be able to confirm that the content of a healthcare app is reliable? What apps have you seen patients and families use?

SMARTPHONES USED TO ACCESS MEDICAL ADVICE DURING A DISASTER

Nepal experienced a serious 7.9 magnitude earthquake on April 25, 2015, that caused thousands of deaths and extensive damage. A World Health Organization press release on May 1 reported that hospitals in four of the most-affected districts were completely destroyed or too badly damaged to function (2015).

A Web-based organization named AskTheDoctor (http://www.askthedoctor.com) offered their services free of charge for 2 months to patients and medical officials in Nepal who needed medical advice. According to the organization's website, one can receive immediate advice from a doctor, or access a database of more than 200,000 questions and answers. Access is available via smartphones, text messaging, e-mail, and video chats.

According to the company's CEO, Prakash Chand, by May 1 more than 3,000 people in Kathmandu had used their services (Wicklund, 2015). He reported that the most commonly asked questions were about fractures and dislocations, amputations, wounds and infections, and head and facial injuries. He continued by saying that roughly 85% of the requests from Nepal were made from smartphones.

USING MOBILE TECHNOLOGY TO SUPPORT ASTHMATICS

Asthma is a chronic condition in which the airways narrow, swell, and produce extra mucus. These actions can make breathing difficult and may trigger coughing, wheezing, and shortness of breath (Mayo Clinic, 2015). An oral inhaled medication like albuterol is commonly used as a rescue treatment.

A company called Propeller Health (http://www.propellerhealth.com) has created an FDA-approved tracking and monitoring system for metered-dose inhaler use that is helpful in asthma and chronic obstructive pulmonary disease management. A small device called a sensor attaches to the top of an inhaler and sends wireless signals to a user's smartphone via Bluetooth technology whenever that inhaler is used. The sensor can be used with rescue and controller medications.

A user's Propeller iOS or Android smartphone app tracks the time and date of use and, with the user's permission, can use the phone's geolocation services to identify where the inhaler was used. The app can display trends of use that may help the user identify usage patterns. In addition, the app will also provide personalized feedback and education regarding ways to improve asthma control (**Figure 8-5**).

The Propeller technology also makes it possible for healthcare providers to collaborate with their patients who are using the system. The provider can use the technology

Figure 8-5   Propeller app for iOS

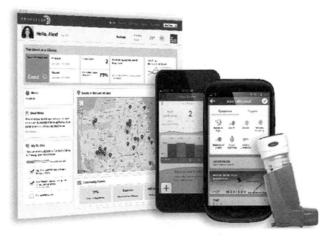

Used with permission. Propellerhealth.com; http://propellerhealth.com/solutions/.

to monitor the patients' inhaler use, identify compliance with a treatment plan, and advise when medication or other changes may be needed.

Although an individual user can benefit greatly from the sensor technology, researchers are also using the system to track large numbers of asthmatic residents within a community. For example, Kentucky has the fourth highest adult asthma prevalence in the United States, and Louisville consistently ranks among the top 20 cities where asthmatics find it challenging to live (Naber, 2015). On March 20, 2015, a project named AIR Louisville was launched. According to the press release, it marks the "first-of-a-kind data-driven collaboration among public, private and philanthropic organizations to use digital health technology to improve asthma" (Naber, 2015. para. 1). A goal of the project is to use the data about when and where residents are having asthma attacks to help determine what actions might improve air quality in the community. It is also the aim of AIR Louisville to help asthmatic residents become better informed about asthma, improve their asthma management, and avoid locations that may lead to asthma attacks.

A grant from the Robert Wood Johnson Foundation and participation from local employers and healthcare organizations are funding the project. AIR Louisville will provide more than 2,000 sensors to residents who will collect data during the 2-year program. This is yet another innovative use of mobile technology that has the potential to improve health.

VIRTUAL NURSING GRAND ROUNDS

The Vietnam Nurse Project (VNP) is an international nursing education practice among the University of San Francisco School of Nursing and Health Professions, four medical centers (Thanh Nhan Hospital, National Hospital for Tropical Diseases, Bach Mai Hospital, and Viet Duc Hospital), and Thanh Nhan Hospital Intensive Care Unit (TNH/ICU) in Hanoi, Vietnam. Virtual nursing grand rounds (VNGR) are an important component of the project, with the goal of improving nursing practice in TNH/ICU. VNGR is the first program of its kind for nurses in Hanoi (Crow, Nguyen, & DeBourgh, 2014).

VNGR is a fully interactive, real-time computer technology assisted point-to-point program that uses low-cost technology to provide ongoing evidence-based staff development and consultative services (Crow et al., 2014). Videoconferencing broadcast sites are at the University of San Francisco and TNH/ICU and are enabled by the following technologies: iPads; laptop computers; LCD monitors; a wireless network with Internet access; a cloud-based digital drop box; and Zoom (http://www.zoom.us), a video conferencing application.

Broadcast topics are based on educational needs assessments and requests from the TNH/ICU nursing staff and its medical director. Each 90-minute broadcast is based on patient cases and generally focuses on a body system and related nursing care priorities. Broadcast topics have included the following: care of patients with acute pneumonia (either community- or hospital-acquired); oral care in mechanically ventilated patients; chest physiotherapy; urinary catheter care; care of patients before and after hemodialysis; and proper patient hygiene (Nakhongsri & Crow, 2015). All broadcast content is translated into Vietnamese in real time, and PowerPoint slides are translated prior to the presentations.

The broadcast content is based on the nursing process and includes nursing solutions and approaches. Examples include pathophysiology, primary diagnosis, priority assessment, specific measurable patient goals, specific nursing interventions to meet the patient care goals, and appropriate documentation of the nursing interventions (Nakhongsri & Crow, 2015).

Another successful VNGR focused on wound care assessment and management. The TNH/ICU nurses took an iPad to patients' bedsides and photographed their wounds. These photographs were transmitted to U.S. wound care nurse experts for assessments and recommended plans for nursing interventions. The experts prepared a response and presented it to the TNH/ICU nurses via a VNGR.

In another case, the TNH/ICU nursing and medical staff requested a consultation regarding a patient in their unit who was suffering with necrotizing fasciitis. According to the Centers for Disease Control and Prevention (2015), necrotizing fasciitis is a rare and serious bacterial infection that spreads rapidly and kills soft tissue. The media commonly refers to it as a flesh-eating infection.

In this situation, after the patient gave consent, photographs were taken and sent to the VNP director. He distributed the information to certified wound care nurses who assessed the situation and offered recommendations for treatment and care. This information was then presented to the ICU staff. It is important to note that this was accomplished within 6 hours of receiving the consultation request. It is also important to note that, because of collaborative teamwork between nurses and physicians and because the recommendations of the wound care nurse experts were put into action, the patient's status improved dramatically and he was eventually discharged from the hospital.

VNGR Broadcasts Support EBP

Two doctor of nursing practice (DNP) students at the University of San Francisco collaborated with the VNP to improve nursing practice in the TNH/ICU and the TNH outpatient endocrinology department. They worked with nurses in these two departments to introduce and integrate an evidence-based protocol into their nursing practices.

Both nurses went to Vietnam for an on-site visit to meet department leaders and nurses who worked in those units. They then developed their projects with support and guidance from their DNP nursing faculty project chairperson and director of the VNP.

The titles of their projects were as follows:

- *Implementing an Evidence-Based Oral Hygiene Protocol for Mechanically Ventilated Patients in the Intensive Care Unit, Thanh Nhan Hospital, Ha Noi, Vietnam: A Practice Improvement Project*
- *Implementing an Evidence-Based Foot Assessment Protocol for Use by Nurses Caring for Adult Diabetic Patients Seeking Care in the Thanh Nhan Hospital Endocrinology Department, Ha Noi, Vietnam*

The success of both projects depended on the creative use of technology to bridge the 7,340 miles and 14-hour time difference that separate the University of San Francisco and TNH. Examples include the following:

- VNGRs were a useful tool to inform and support the Vietnamese nurses throughout the projects.
- E-mail was frequently used to communicate with project participants, such as the ICU head nurse, who completed chart audits to collect compliance data. After removing patient identifiers, the audit documents were scanned and e-mailed to the University of San Francisco.
- Audiovisual conferencing with Apple FaceTime was frequently used, often via smartphones.

Successful implementation and outcomes of the two evidence-based protocols have positively impacted and improved nursing practice. The oral care protocol was the first evidence-based nursing protocol in the Hanoi public health department facilities. Because of its success, the protocol has been shared and implemented in four other hospital ICUs in Hanoi. Prior to the implementation of the foot care protocol, nurses were not allowed to do foot assessments or document in a patient's medical record. However, they now routinely perform assessments and document their findings in the medical record. In addition, the foot care protocol is now a part of the entire Hanoi Department of Health's 37 facilities. This is an example of how technology is helping to elevate the practice of nursing in Hanoi by expanding practice.

Learning Activity

1. Think of ways that you or your colleagues could use a VNGR to support the desired outcomes of your job.
2. How could a VNGR be used to create a nursing EBP consortium, and how would that benefit practice and patient outcomes?

THE FUTURE

The innovation and development of new technologies, and the diffusion of those technologies into healthcare environments, will be useful in supporting nurses as they incorporate evidence into their practices. When evidence-based care is provided, patients will experience better outcomes. Wireless and mobile technologies will increasingly enhance data access and will be useful tools in decision making.

Patients will also have opportunities to become better informed, often from their smartphones, wearable devices, or equipment in their homes. They will become more active participants in their health care as the small data that has been generated from their smart devices becomes integrated into their electronic health records and becomes big data.

An increasing number of medical apps will be developed that will integrate with medical devices used at home. For example, a smartphone user will be able to collect a small sample of blood for a complete blood count, or many other diagnostic tests, which will then be analyzed by a smartphone app that may be interconnected with other devices. This data will be transmitted directly into the user's electronic health record and become immediately available to the user's healthcare team.

Clothing will be designed to collect and transmit data. For example, Sensilk is a company that has developed a comfortable and fashionable bra that contains a SOAR biometric soft sensor (http://www.sensilk.com). The sensor can track heart rate, heart rate variability, heart rate recovery rate, respiratory rate, calories burned, and distance traveled, and it assigns each workout a fitness score. According to Hap Klopp, founder of the North Face outdoor clothing company, "a lot of wearable tech is oriented around the engineering associated with those product [sic] . . . But to reach women, you have to be equally attentive to fashion: fit, design, appropriateness, and current looks" (Taraska, 2015, para. 11). Sensilk designed their bra with that in mind.

Videoconferencing appointments via smartphones or other mobile devices will increasingly become the norm as more diagnostic workup data is collected and compiled at home and becomes available and integrated into an electronic health record. Users will be able to access this care 24/7 from any Internet-connected computer in the world. Patients will be relieved that they can avoid spending time driving to and from an appointment and waiting for long periods of time while surrounded by sick patients in a clinic waiting room. The costs for these appointments will continue to decrease as the technology becomes ubiquitous.

It will be possible for a small group of friends, or even online pals, to support each other in achieving fitness goals, such as walking 10,000 steps per day. The team members can be anywhere in the world; however, it is important to coordinate meeting times with various time zones in mind. Using audiovisual technology via their smartphones, each person in the group will be able to see and hear each other during a walk. This, most likely, will encourage motivation. Each team member will be able to see a graphic representation of each other's step history at any time. This feature is another motivational tool as team members support each other.

The development of healthcare apps will require clinician involvement to ensure that the content is accurate. Apps will be reviewed and rated for their content and effectiveness, and they will be certified by well-known healthcare organizations. Healthcare apps that are designed to change behavior will be developed with the use of evidence-based protocols that have been proven to be effective change agents. Children of all ages will be able to access a variety of healthcare-related apps that have been specifically designed for their levels of interest and comprehension.

Teleconsultation opportunities between professional nurses and other healthcare clinicians will be facilitated with the availability of wearable high-definition devices. These devices will enhance communication and will be available to transmit and receive data from specially equipped clinic exam rooms, hospital rooms, bedrooms and living rooms, and the field.

Healthcare clinicians who are interested in information technology and improving health care through innovative uses of technology will experience an increasing number of opportunities to become certified in healthcare analytics. In addition, the number of nurse informaticists will grow, and the infusion of their knowledge and skills will become increasingly apparent in healthcare organizations.

As our ability to collect data and turn it into meaningful information continues to grow at an exponential rate, and as healthcare providers and patients develop stronger collaborative partnerships, we can anticipate better patient care outcomes—one of the main goals for infusing innovative technology into health care.

Learning Activity

Read current literature and/or search online to identify ways that innovations in technology are being used to improve health care. Share your findings with colleagues. Would these methods be useful in your organization?

Learning Activity: Technology Project Scenario

1. Your organization is aware of your interest in using technology to improve care. A high-level executive has requested your assistance in helping to brainstorm innovative ways that technology could be used to enhance patient care in your department. Although the organization has not identified specific goals, they are looking for ideas regarding the state-of-the-art mobile technology to support health care. You are asked to make a presentation to organization leaders in 2 weeks.
2. Create an outline that describes the content of your presentation.

REFERENCES

Beal, V. (2014). Big data. Retrieved from: http://www.webopedia.com/TERM/B/big_data.html

Better health with smartphone apps. (2015). *Harvard Men's Health Watch*. Retrieved from http://www.health.harvard.edu/staying-healthy/better-health-with-smartphone-apps

Centers for Disease Control and Prevention. (2015). Necrotizing fasciitis: A rare disease, especially for the healthy. Retrieved from: http://www.cdc.gov/features/necrotizingfasciitis/

Comstock, J. (2015). Cedars-Sinai CIO: Let the patients decide what data to share via Apple HealthKit. Retrieved from: http://mobihealthnews.com/42966/cedars-sinai-cio-let-the-patients-decide-what-data-to-share-via-apple-healthkit/

Crow, G. L., Nguyen, T., & DeBourgh, G. A. (2014). Virtual nursing grand rounds and shared governance. *Nursing Administration Quarterly, 38*(1), 55–61.

Dumbill, E. (2012). What is big data? Retrieved from https://beta.oreilly.com/ideas/what-is-big-data

Fox, S. (2011). Peer-to-peer health care. Retrieved from http://www.pewinternet.org/2011/02/28/peer-to-peer-health-care-2/

Fox, S., Duggan, M., & Purcell, K. (2013). Family caregivers are wired for health. Retrieved from http://pewinternet.org/Reports/2013/Family-Caregivers.aspx

Franko, O. J. (2013). How helpful are mobile healthcare apps?: Without clinician input and validation, healthcare apps could be a liability. Retrieved from http://www.aaos.org/news/aaosnow/mar13/managing5.asp

Henly, S. J. (2014). Mother lode and mining tools: Big data for nursing science. *Nursing Research, 63*(3), 155.

IBM. (2015). What is big data? Retrieved from http://www-01.ibm.com/software/data/bigdata/what-is-big-data.html

Internet Live Stats. (2015). Internet users. Retrieved from http://www.internetlivestats.com/internet-users

Keirn Swanson, J. (2015). How to use Apple's Health app. Retrieved from http://www.maclife.com/article/howtos/how-to-use-apple-health-app-iphone—slide-0

LeSuer, D. (2014). 5 reasons healthcare data is unique and difficult to measure. Retrieved from https://www.healthcatalyst.com/5-reasons-healthcare-data-is-difficult-to-measure

Marcus, B. (2014). Brainstorming outline: Combining subgroup deliverables. (M0092). Retrieved from http://bigdatawg.nist.gov/show_InputDoc.php

Mayo Clinic. (2015). Asthma definition. Retrieved from http://www.mayoclinic.org/diseases-conditions/asthma/basics/definition/con-20026992

McCartney, P. R. (2015). Big data science. *MCN: The American Journal of Maternal/Child Nursing, 40*(2), 130.

Naber, A. (2015). Louisville to use technology and innovation to reduce burden of asthma [Press release]. Retrieved from http://propellerhealth.com/2015/03/louisville-to-use-technology-and-innovation-to-reduce-burden-of-asthma/

Nakhongsri, A., & Crow, G. (2015). Virtual nursing grand rounds: Improving practice overseas. *Nursing 2015, 45*(5), 18–21.

Pew Research Center. (2013). Health fact sheet. Retrieved from http://www.pewinternet.org/fact-sheets/health-fact-sheet

Pew Research Center. (2014). Internet user demographics. Retrieved from http://www.pewinternet.org/data-trend/internet-use/latest-stats/

Pew Research Center. (2015a). More than half of smartphone owners have used their phone to get health information, do online banking. Retrieved from http://www.pewinternet.org/2015/04/01/us-smartphone-use-in-2015/pi_2015-04-01_smartphones_03/

Pew Research Center. (2015b). U.S. smartphone use in 2015. Retrieved from http://www.pewinternet.org/2015/04/01/us-smartphone-use-in-2015/

Pittman, G. (2013). Skin cancer phone apps aren't very accurate: Study. Retrieved from http://www.reuters.com/article/2013/01/16/us-skin-cancer-idUSBRE90F1H920130116

Rare Disease Day. (2015). What is a rare disease? Retrieved from http://www.rarediseaseday.org/article/what-is-a-rare-disease

Sacristán, J. A., & Dilla, T. (2015). No big data without small data: Learning health care systems begin and end with the individual patient. *Journal of Evaluation in Clinical Practice*. Advance online publication. Retrieved from http://onlinelibrary.wiley.com/doi/10.1111/jep.12350/abstract

Taraska, J. (2015). Smart bras aren't as stupid as they sound. Retrieved from http://www.fastcodesign.com/3046580/wears/smart-bras-arent-as-stupid-as-they-sound

TechTarget. (2013). Small data. Retrieved from http://whatis.techtarget.com/definition/small-data

Thorpe, J. H., & Gray, E. A. (2015). Big data and ambulatory care: Breaking down legal barriers to support effective use. *The Journal of Ambulatory Care Management, 38*(1), 29–38.

Torgan, C. E. (2009). The mHealth summit: Local and global converge. Retrieved from http://caroltorgan.com/mhealth-summit/

U.S. National Library of Medicine. (2015a). Citations added to MEDLINE by fiscal year. Retrieved from http://www.nlm.nih.gov/bsd/stats/cit_added.html

U.S. National Library of Medicine. (2015b). MedlinePlus statistics. Retrieved from http://www.nlm.nih.gov/medlineplus/usestatistics.html

Wicklund, E. (2015). mHealth comes to the rescue in Nepal. Retrieved from http://www.mhealthnews.com/blog/mhealth-comes-rescue-nepal

World Health Organization. (2015). WHO issues rapid health assessment on Impact of Nepal earthquake. Retrieved from http://www.who.int/mediacentre/news/releases/2015/health-assessment-nepal/en/

Measuring Innovation

Setting the Stage for an Evidence-Based Practice Culture and Emergence of Innovation

Dolora Sanares-Carreon and Diane Heliker

CHAPTER OBJECTIVES

Upon completion of this chapter, the reader will be able to:

1. Describe cultures of evidence and innovation.
2. Apply Disciplined Clinical Inquiry (DCI) methodology for evidence and innovation practices.
3. Discuss four qualities of an evidence and innovation culture.

Cultures are comprised of many features including social and organizational practices, understandings about the world, beliefs concerning what is good, what is important, rituals, language, and technology (Polkinghorne, 2004, p. 12).

Practices are always situated within a cultural context . . . Practices are human interventions that make things in the world different from what they were . . . alter the status quo and produce change . . . Once knowledge about how to do things (e.g., evidence-based practice [EBP]) is developed, it can be shared with others. Thus it can become the possession of a whole society [e.g., the nursing profession], spreading among its members through various modes of communication [e.g.. the DCI pathways] and social institutions [e.g., healthcare complexes]." (Polkinghorne, 2004, p. 9)

Continuous inquiry is a key attribute in setting the stage for an EBP culture. For this type of culture to persist, a transparent process for a disciplined clinical inquiry has to be created. Another attribute is an inquiry that is cyclical. If continuous cyclical inquiry is not present, the culture withers away because of the changing nature of the evidence supporting the practice. Change is driven by the complexity of the context, the people, and the other elements interacting within and beyond the fringes of the ecosystem.

The purpose of this chapter is to invite discussions to initiate further exploration of our understanding and recognition surrounding the creation of a culture of EBP and the emergence of innovation embedded in the DCI model. More specifically, this chapter will discuss DCI as a cornerstone of an EBP culture; describe how engagement in EBP through DCI sparks new insights and refines creative ideas; probe strategies for setting the stage toward innovation; and explore pathways for mapping the transformation of creative ideas and adapting a new practice in complex adaptive systems.

EBP: THE PRACTICE OF THE 21st CENTURY

The practice of the 21st century evolved from growing cynicism over the prominence of expert opinion toward a shift to research-based practice that subsequently primed the revolution toward EBP. Over the past 5 decades EBP has spawned highly polarized discourses among scholars, leaders, and practitioners. Some envisaged promising possibilities, and some voiced skepticism about the true value of EBP in reforming the healthcare delivery system. Streams of change occurred at organizational, national, and global levels. Eventually, evidence of efficacy and effectiveness has been conscientiously melded with what matters most to the recipients of care. The following discussion is a brief account of the waves of EBP as it cascaded across the micro, macro, and mega healthcare delivery systems.

The Global Movement to EBP

The exponential growth of biomedical research that occurred during the second half of the 20th century opened the floodgates for discourses over the eminence of expert-based medical practice. The tsunami of new knowledge further heightened the variations in practice. The medical community contended that the culprit was inaccessibility to high-quality evidence for those who make everyday patient care decisions. In 1972, Archie Cochrane, a British epidemiologist, published "Effectiveness and Efficiency:

Random Reflections on Health Services," a paper that strongly criticized the lack of reliable evidence behind many of the commonly accepted healthcare interventions. After 2 decades, the Cochrane Collaboration was founded in his honor. It formed an accessible international database of systematic reviews (Claridge & Fabian, 2005; Goodman, 2002).

In 1991, Canadian cardiologist Gordon Guyatt brought to the fore an approach to teach bedside medicine that added more certainty to clinical decision making. Dr. Guyatt presented his idea to the faculty of McMaster University and called the reframed approach for medical residency training program, evidence-based medicine. An oral history of evidence-based medicine from the proponents' personal account of the past, present, and future is accessible at http://ebm.jamanetwork.com/ (Smith & Rennie, 2014). In 1996, Guyatt's mentor, David Sackett, an American-born and Canadian-naturalized epidemiologist, formally defined evidence-based medicine as the "conscientious, explicit, and judicious use of current evidence in making decisions about the care of individual patient" (Sacket, Rosenberg, Muir Gray, Hayner, & Richardson, 1996, p. 71). The Canadian crusade steered the adopting disciplines to predicate the term *evidence-based* in describing the shift to evidence-based medicine. However, no record was found identifying the person who coined the term *evidence-based practice*, now the preferred term to describe the new practice paradigm across disciplines.

The U.S. March to the EBP Revolution

The EBP movement in the United States did not gain popular acclaim until the Institute of Medicine (IOM) report "To Err Is Human: Building a Safer Health System" (2000) unmasked the human, social, and economic cost of preventable medical errors. The exposé drew national attention.

In a sequel report, "Crossing the Quality Chasm: A New Health System for the 21st Century" (2001), the IOM made a landmark decision to convene experts from various disciplines to dialogue and configure actionable plans to address the issues of quality care. The report called for the reinvention of healthcare delivery, not only for improvement, but also for innovation. Broad aims and recommendations with simple rules were laid out to serve as catalyst for change: "Rule 5: Evidence-based decision making: Patients should receive care based on the best available scientific knowledge. Care should not vary illogically from clinician to clinician or from place to place" (2001, p. 62); "The unpredictability of behavior in complex adaptive systems can be seen as contributing to huge variation in the delivery of health care" (2001, p. 64); and "effective infrastructure is needed to apply evidence to health care delivery" (2001, p. 145).

The American Nurses Association's watchful vigilance earned the profession recognition as avant-garde in EBP in the United States (U.S.), with its mainstream media publication of "Nursing's Agenda for the Future" (2002). The publication showcased how the association forged ahead to unite U.S. nursing organizations in identifying 10 distinct domains to bring about positive changes for nursing and the healthcare system. Under one domain, delivery systems/nursing models, a strategic objective was to "develop strategic partnerships to advance the use of research findings and EBP to design, implement, and evaluate new integrated practice model" (American Nurses Association, 2002, p. 11). This report has been complemented by a blueprint for action in transforming the nursing profession as a vital force in meeting the future health needs of diverse populations. This blueprint for action is "The Future of Nursing: Leading Change, Advancing Health" (Institute of Medicine [IOM], 2011). The rich corpus of information in the report is a wellspring for continuing dialogue in reframing the role of nurses in a changing and complex healthcare landscape.

Several IOM reports have been published since the chasm was unearthed. In particular, "Health Professions Education: A Bridge to Quality" identified EBP as one of five core competencies of all healthcare professionals (IOM, 2003). The other four competencies include, to provide patient-centered care, work in an interdisciplinary team, apply quality improvement, and utilize informatics. In 2012 the IOM published "Best Care at Lower Cost: The Path to Continuously Learning Health Care in America," further underscoring the complexity of the healthcare system and defining the imperatives required to ensure evidence-based health care (IOM, 2012). The reports served as a catalyst for national institutions and associations to champion the translation of the IOM recommendations into actionable plans relative to EBP.

A stream of policy and program changes relating to EBP was developed in schools of nursing and other venues. In 2001, the University HealthSystem Consortium, in a joint venture with the American Association of Colleges of Nursing, pioneered the development of a standardized national postbaccalaureate nurse residency program for new graduates. Between 2002 and 2003, the University HealthSystem Consortium pilot implemented the standardized curriculum requiring completion of an EBP project in 12 demonstration areas (Goode & Williams, 2004). Over the past 10 years the curriculum has been adopted by members of the consortium across the United States, with feedback that recognized the EBP component as "highly valued by the organizations" (Goode, Lynn, McElroy, Bednash, & Murray, 2013). The American Association of Colleges of Nursing reframed the "Essentials of Baccalaureate Education for Professional Practice" in 2008 and charted Scholarship for EBP as Essential III (American Association of Colleges of Nursing, 2008). The Essentials ushered in the integration of a stand-alone credit course in EBP.

The EBP revolution in the clinical practice setting predated the publication of the IOM's 2000 report. For example, in 1999, a pilot study at the University of Texas Medical Branch at Galveston (UTMB Health), an academic medical center in the southeastern part of the United States, was implemented to evaluate its EBP model, called DCI (Sanares & Heliker, 2002). In fact, the forerunners of other EBP models had been launched in the U.S. nursing landscape as early as 1994. Two examples are Stetler's Model of Research Utilizations and the Iowa Model of Research-Based Practice, both of which were transformed and renamed later as EBP models. By

2000, several EBP models, such as the Advancing Research and Clinical Practice through close Collaboration (ARCC) and the Academic Center for EBP Star model of Knowledge Transformation (ACE Star) were introduced. The purpose of these models was to guide the inquiry and process for implementing EBP (White & Dudley-Brown, 2012).

THE CHALLENGES OF MAINSTREAMING EBP

Nurses' watchful vigilance is constantly challenged to keep current with breakthroughs in biomedical science, new clinical care technologies, and changes in population sociodemographics. The greater challenge is to discern the implications and/or application to nursing practice. Just-in-time access to information is increasingly within reach with quantum leaps in the communication and computer industries.

Knowledge and Skill Gap

Knowledge and skill gaps typically occur at a greater degree among nurses whose basic education did not systematically integrate the principles and application of EBP. As noted earlier, nursing educational programs have begun introducing EBP as a standalone formal credit course in the undergraduate nursing curricula. EBP also became mainstreamed in the graduate levels of nursing education curricula. Although the EBP literature exploded and continuing education opportunities increased exponentially over the past decade, individual and organizational barriers lingered. Lack of time and resources, inadequate knowledge and skills, and technological and financial barriers were identified (Sadeghi-Bazargani, Tabrizi, & Azami-Aghdash, 2014). Organizational factors, such as workload, unsupportive staff and management, lack of authority to change practice, and a workplace culture resistant to change persisted (Williams, Perillo, & Brown, 2015).

Evidence Translation

Evidence translation remains a thorny path. A mere statement that EBP is a key strategic initiative to achieve excellence is not sufficient to create organizational change. True commitment is manifested in the consistent flow and allocation of resources that are interwoven with willingness to disrupt a culture in situ. Rules of engagement need to be transformed into principles of engagement to ensure buoyancy in complex systems. Creativity is warranted in devising new ways to embed EBP in the structure and processes of nursing and health professions. Obviously, new leadership behaviors that combine innovation and EBP competencies are needed to build teams and systems that can disrupt long-held beliefs and practices. Additionally, a new lens is needed to find new methods for outcome measurement in an ecosystem of uncertainty.

The systematic review conducted by Flodgren, Rojas-Reyes, Cole, and Foxcroft (2012) on "Effectiveness of Organizational Infrastructures to Promote Evidence-Based Nursing Practice" indicated that "the problem is not a lack of nursing models . . . but that the studies are at a high risk of bias or have not been designed to generate effectiveness data" (2012, p. 9). A model that not only addresses the process of EBP, but also addresses the EBP literacy of nurses at the bedside and encourages innovative person-centered care EBP, is called for. This model is DCI. The reader is invited to use DCI to determine its effectiveness in setting the stage for building human and organization capacity for EBP and innovation.

DCI: A PLATFORM FOR EBP AND INNOVATION

DCI is an EBP model and a wellspring for idea generation toward practice innovation. DCI guides the nurse's expedition in bringing the best evidence from the realm of probabilities to the realities of practice. The translation of evidence synthesis in the realities of practice sparks possibilities for innovation that transforms what works now to what would work better tomorrow. Along this expedition, DCI provides principles, processes, and pathways for practice inquiry, evidence translation, and idea generation. The uniqueness of the DCI model is the inductive process that was used to engage groups of practicing clinicians to fine-tune the model in a large academic medical center located in the southeastern United States.

The processes and principles of DCI provide the pathways and establish the groundwork for a culture of dialogue to validate, improve, or change practice. According to psychologist and philosopher Donald Polkinghorne, "practices are grounded in understandings people have about the world, and these understandings are, in turn, influenced by the effect of their practices on the world" (2004, p. 5). The precepts of two scholars–consultants in organizational culture and leadership—expand a deeper understanding of Polkinghorne's conception of culture in complex adaptive systems. Bennis (2000) posited that "cultures do not turn sharply with the pages of the calendar; rather, they evolve gradually over time. By becoming aware of what is changing today, we determine what we must improve upon tomorrow" (2000, p. 4). Schein (2010) underscored that "culture is both the *here and now* dynamic phenomenon and coercive background structure that influence us in multiple ways. Culture is constantly re-enacted and created by our interactions with others and shaped by our own behavior" (2010, p. 3). DCI facilitates continuing dialogue among stakeholders about understanding and exploring the reciprocal relationships of practices, culture, and the world.

The DCI model was pilot implemented in 1999 at UTMB Health using participatory action research, which incorporates both quantitative and qualitative approaches that are equally important in understanding the practice of nursing. Participatory action research allowed the extraction of clinicians' perspectives in designing the inquiry approaches, which provided a frame of reference and learning options that resonated with the clinicians. The learning options developed for DCI were designed to be congruent with the process of inquiry being taught. Technology that allowed for interactive and self-paced learning was employed so that each step of the learning experience produced meaningful discovery. Critical theory was applied as the theoretical underpinning, along with the precepts espoused by the following scholars: Lewin (1946), on his work that emphasizes the inclusion of practitioners as local experts on all phases on the inquiry; Habermas (1987), on his work that focuses on critical knowledge based on the principles of collaboration, reflection, and communication; and Freire (1970), on his work that underscores the need for an interactive learner-empowered environment (Sanares & Heliker, 2002).

The DCI implementation system is organized around five cyclical phases (**Figure 9-1**). The first three phases engage nurses in systematic inquiry and evidence

Figure 9-1 The DCI model

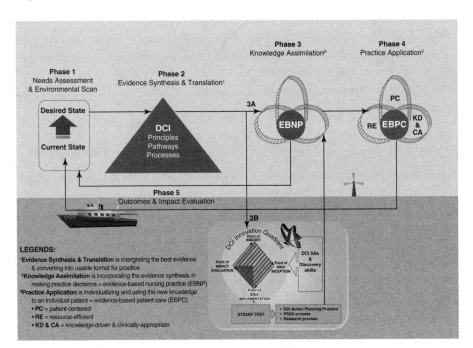

Courtesy of University of Texas Medical Branch at Galveston (UTMB Health)

synthesis, both individually and collectively. The last two phases invite the patients, families, and the other members of the interprofessional team into collaborative conversations about evidence-based patient-centered care and achievement of targeted outcomes. The five phases of DCI operate like a hub with an interconnecting network of inquiries to steer the enculturation of EBP and cultivation of practice innovation.

Phase 1: Needs Assessment and Environmental Scan

Phase 1 is the hub wherein nurses are engaged to reflect upon their level of knowledge, skills, and attitudes in EBP and their proclivity to idea generation. This is complemented by a scan of the organization's capacity to support and encourage knowledge and creative works. The principles of appreciative inquiry, grounded in the seminal works of David Cooperrider as described by Bushe (2012), are melded in the process of contextual scanning to leverage organizational strength and opportunities for change. The positive spin engendered by appreciative inquiry is envisaged to build on facilitative forces instead of overemphasis on barriers and problems. The DCI's foundational theoretical underpinning, critical theory, tempers the undiscerning application of appreciative inquiry principles. The DCI process does not ignore the contextual problems; rather, inquiry is framed around the issue with a focus on the positive outcomes of interest. The marching mantra is: how can we set that stage to bring EBP and innovation to the bedside?

The assessment and scan is completed online and considered individually to guide a personal journey or collectively to map an organizational EBP and innovation expedition. The reflective nature of Phase 1 permits the transportability of the DCI model to other settings. The assessment results are compared with the EBP vision of the stakeholders to move current practice to a desired future.

Phase 2: Learning, Evidence Synthesis, and Systems Development

The results in Phase 1 direct nurses and/or organizations in moving to Phase 2. Phase 2 is the hub for learning the EBP skill set, structuring organizational systems that optimize the application of these competencies, and synthesizing the body of best evidence. The power of Phase 2 is the accessibility of its virtual hub that operates like a marketplace where nurses can purchase goods and products based on their needs and passion (**Figure 9-2**).

Learning EBP Skill Set

The learning process is guided by three principles that emerged from the series of EBP pilot studies conducted at UTMB Health. The first principle focuses on accountability as a prerequisite to achievement. Accountability is defined at the individual nurse level

Figure 9-2 DCI website

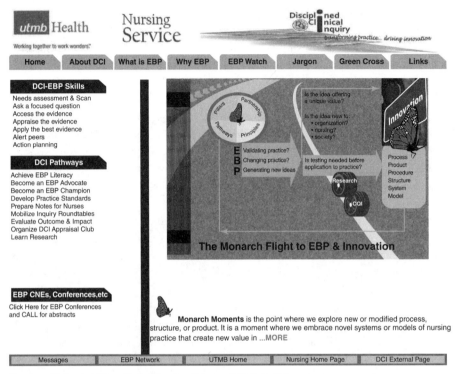

Courtesy of University of Texas Medical Branch at Galveston (UTMB Health)

through performance evaluation tools and clinical advancement criteria that define EBP expectations. At the organizational level, accountability is achieved by structuring evidence-based criteria to assess functions and introduce changes. The second principle specifies that inquiry is an essential dimension of professional nursing practice. This presupposes that nurses are cocreators of practice-based knowledge. To be effective, a nurse must have a sense of inquiry and use evidence in unraveling clinical issues. The third principle portrays EBP as a collaborative endeavor. EBP is shaped by those who create it, use it, and evaluate it. These three principles guided the development, implementation, and evaluation of various self-directed online learning modules and pathways that are accessible in a one-stop dedicated website for EBP (Sanares-Carreon, Waters, & Heliker, 2010).

Systems Development

DCI regards the development of individual nurses' knowledge and skills in parallel with the development of organizational systems that support the application of the learned competency to foster EBP. Five key points guide the success of the process. Each point is highlighted along with the associated leadership behavior it requires. Key point 1 is clear articulation of the value of EBP as reflected in the nursing services' organizational structure, professional practice model, and/or strategic plan (messaging, visioning). Key point 2 is the designation of a dedicated EBP expert or strategist to lead the development, planning, implementation, and evaluation of the EBP program of nursing service (leadership skill matching, diverse team building). Key point 3 is formalization of the accountability structure for EBP that ascribes to a network or matrix-type structure that indicates lines of communication, areas of cooperation, and resource commitment (transparency, information flow, accountability). Key point 4 is recruitment and development of clinicians with varying specialties to form the core EBP team (boundary spanning, relationship building). Key point 5 is authorization of dedicated time, critical resources, and sufficient autonomy for EBP teams to carry out their charges (resource allocation, leveraging opportunity) (Sanares, Waters, & Marshall, 2007). For many organizations these five key points may be new to the system and thus requires leadership that both understands the EBP process and the unique needs and challenges in practice innovation. At UTMB Health, two key systems have been restructured to incorporate the process and principles of DCI: the Clinical Advancement Program (CAP) and the Policy and Practice Standards System. A key feature of the CAP is the designation of EBP as a key domain of nursing practice. To advance to the highest clinician level (expert level), the nurse is expected to demonstrate competency in the five core EBP skill set specified in the DCI model. The other levels in the CAP entail varying degrees of EBP expectations (Sanares et al., 2007).

The Policy and Practice Standards System nested in EBP was instituted in accord with the results of a cross-sectional research study that explored its feasibility at UTMB Health. The EBP expert or strategist served as cochairman of the nursing-wide Evidence-Based Policy and Practice Standards committee to foster the evidence-based system. Nurses saw the value of the investments in learning and knowledge translation, given the clear linkages and applications in the CAP and Evidence-Based Policy and Practice Standards. Consequently, nurses started feeling a sense of ownership on the evolving EBP culture with the visibility of the impact of their contribution and continuing commitment (Sanares et al., 2007).

Evidence Synthesis

Although there is a standardized method for the synthesis of research-based evidence, there is no consensus regarding the method for the integration of the various types of evidence for application at the point of care. DCI offers three sequential steps of mapping, relating, and interpreting as a process for integrating the evidence. Activation of the three-step process is in essence a pretranslation process that bridges Phase 2 and Phase 3 of the DCI cycle.

DCI defines mapping as the process of plotting the evidence in a side-by-side fashion. The goal is quick visual examination of the nature and strength of the relationship of the intervention with the outcomes of interest. The next step is relating the evidence by identifying similarities and differences of the findings and starting to draw inferences or conclusions. The goal is determination of the relative value of the evidence in reference to the nature of the focused question. The third step is interpreting, which involves summarizing and grading the body of best evidence. The goal is to answer the focused question.

Phase 3: Knowledge Assimilation and Practice Innovation

Phase 3 is the hub that transmutes learning in two paths, one is knowledge assimilation and the other is cultivating new insights for practice innovation. Knowledge assimilation is routine application of the EBP skill set as an integral part of nursing practice, thereby referenced as evidence-based nursing practice. Practice innovation, on the one hand, is viewing evidence synthesis generated in Phase 2 with a different lens that sparks or refines creative ideas. The rate and level of knowledge assimilation and practice innovation is not solely a function of an individual nurses' abilities and motivation, but equally a function of the organizational system in which nurses practice.

Knowledge Assimilation: Evidence-Based Nursing Practice

The learning experience in Phase 2 is a catalyst to the emergence of an evidence-based nursing practice culture. This hub engages a community of nurses in reshaping the professional practice of nursing at the bedside. The DCI model acknowledges that evidence-based nursing practice may be demonstrated in varying degrees based on level of clinical practice and education. However, the collective effects of practices that are grounded on EBP behave like a network in creating an evidence-based nursing practice culture.

The true value of knowledge assimilation is its impact on how effectively the users translate this knowledge to person-centered care practices. Of course, it is not reasonable to expect all nurses in every situation to access, critique, and integrate best evidence. As such, instead, DCI offers organized efforts and a medium where sources of best evidence are shared and disseminated. The DCI model offers strategies for transforming new knowledge into an accessible format that nurses can utilize at the point of care as well as pathways that promote knowledge assimilation.

Practice Innovation: Creativity and Generation of Novel Ideas

A new path that is distinct from evidence-based nursing practice emerged in Phase 3. The path is practice innovation. Its emergence grew out of nurses' intense engagement in EBP. The evidence integration in Phase 2 is traditionally used to validate, modify, or change practice. Some nurses were able to view the evidence with a dual lens, an eye that can visualize even the smallest sparks of new possibilities. For example, two nurses in the day surgery units were concerned about nausea and vomiting. Instead of simply improving the status quo, they challenged it. They explored alternative therapies and began to reflect on creative ways of integrating new knowledge gained with innovative methods of preventing nausea and vomiting.

The novelty of new idea occurs at various levels. The idea might already be an innovation elsewhere, but it may be new to the organization. Thus, it can still be valued as an innovation. The goal is implementation, otherwise such ideas will remain untried, as a lost opportunity. Starting small is valued as much as aspiring for a big breakthrough. Even small changes brought about by innovation can have an immeasurable impact in complex interconnected systems.

The DCI model framed the tools for practice innovation by dovetailing the EBP skill set with the discovery skills posited by Dyer, Gregersen, and Christensen (2011). The works of Hill, Brandeau, Truelove, and Lineback (2014) related to setting the stage for innovation were later used as complementary precepts. The section on innovation in this chapter will discuss practice innovation in more details.

Phase 4: Practice Application

Connecting with patients and collaborating with interprofessional teams take place in the hub of Phase 4. With nurses' advancing capacity to bring to the bedside the fusion of new knowledge and innovation, evidence-based patient care becomes the normative culture. Evidence-based patient care is defined in DCI as the optimal interface among patient-centered, resource-efficient, knowledge-driven and clinically appropriate care. Nurses acquired increasing sense of empowerment to collaborate as collegial partners in care with the competency gained in Phase 2 and the evolving evidence-based nursing practice community experienced in Phase 3.

Nursing's Unique Contribution

Evidence-based patient care is a complex process that requires inputs from everyone on board. It is generally hard to pinpoint with precision which contribution made the difference in the care of patients. However, each professional discipline has accountability to specific aspects of care. For example, a patient diagnosed with a metabolic disorder has shown an elevated cholesterol level. The physician will be guided by the results of systematic reviews of randomized control trials (RCTs) in prescribing a medication regimen. The EBP-empowered nurse will reflect on the therapeutic efficacy of the prescribed medication in tandem with the patient's perspectives and circumstances. In essence, the nurse makes a series of decisions based on issues relative to administration and assessment of the patient's actual and potential response to the medication.

The role of patient's family is equally considered, especially on issues of medication adherence and observation of side effects. The complementarity and collaboration of the physician and the nurse in this exemplar exercise or an equivalent word makes evidence-based patient care come alive at the point of service.

Strength of Nursing Contribution

The example illustrates that there is no single system of hierarchy that would be adequate to address all issues in nursing practice, not because there are fewer RCTs available to support the efficacy of nursing interventions, but because patient issues that are sensitive to nursing interventions may not be appropriately addressed using the evidence produced by RCTs alone. The wisdom of one of the global pioneers in EBP clearly describes the practice of nursing:

> *The practice context is complex, people are complex, and clinicians are complex. The best evidence will most probably come in different forms, in different situations, and context ... Knowing how to decipher this complexity... and knowing how to match situation and context with appropriate evidence, will perhaps be the most important requirement of the 21st century practicing nurse. (Estabrooks, 1998, p. 30)*

This perspective reflects that nursing care is not prescriptive, but highly contextual. Nursing practice draws from various sources of knowledge and multiple ways of knowing toward an enlightened understanding of the complexity and the uniqueness of each patient care encounter (Chinn & Kramer, 2011). In recognition of this perspective, DCI offers an evidence wheel wherein the leveling system accounts for the nature of the clinical issue. The evidence wheel is an unfinished prototype that may change subject to advances in emerging sciences, such as pharmacogenomics or proteomics, among many others.

Phase 5: Outcomes and Impact Evaluation

Although named as the last of the five phases of DCI, the hub for measuring outcomes and renewing for best results is not an end point. It occurs at various points and interfaces along the DCI phases. The phases of DCI cascade in a network of hubs that interface in an iterative process. The progressive movement is propelled by built-in evaluation checkpoints that bring the nurse to the hub in Phase 1 if the desired outcomes are not meeting targeted levels.

The iterative evaluation process ascribes to two strategies. The first approach focused on the extent to which DCI has facilitated: competency, acculturation, productivity, and satisfaction. The second approach involves objective assessment of the EBP products developed by individual nurses using an EBP skill set and criterion-based reviews of EBP and innovation projects. The subjective evaluation processes ascribe to empowerment evaluation, adapted from the seminal work of Fetterman, Kaftarian, and Wandersman (1996) which was designed to help people help themselves and improve their programs using a form of self-evaluation and reflection. It has been argued that "to ensure that programs have a lasting effect, they need to be conceptualized, negotiated, run, and evaluated jointly by all stakeholders" (Van Vlaenderen, p. 343). Consistent with these principles, DCI offers self-evaluation tools that build nurses' **capacity** to assume **accountability** for tracking their achievement, recognizing areas for **improvement**, and using **evidence-based strategies**. Empowerment evaluation is utilized alongside other objective measures (Sanares-Carreon et al., 2010). The tools will be discussed in the evaluation section of this chapter.

SURFING THE WAVES OF EBP THROUGH DCI

The DCI model creates footprints for healthcare systems in surfing the waves of EBP. To begin the inquiry process, DCI emphasizes understanding how the dynamics between nurses and the organization set the tone for a personalized and contextualized approach to change (DCI Phase 1). The next footprint is need-based learning and applications in accomplishing the organizational vision. Surfing the waves of EBP at this juncture presents undercurrents and challenges. DCI offers learning packages that prepare nurses and nursing organizations to weather the storms and navigate the surge of barriers both within and beyond the ecosystem (DCI Phase 2). Learning has no meaning unless it is brought to the bedside. DCI offers pathways that tap into the strengths of nurses through self-selection. The DCI footprints are not carved in stone; they are conceived and created as an unfinished prototype to adapt to dynamically changing environments. A new footprint emerges as practice innovation is threaded simultaneously with evidence translation (Phases 3 and 4). No system is perfect. DCI has self-correcting processes that remind nurses that inquiry is a continuous reflective process, much like innovation. At any point along the DCI phases, immediate outcomes are evaluated, and the cycle is repeated (Phase 5).

Regardless of the point at which you or your organization is in the EBP expedition, the footprints of DCI provide tracks and trails toward formation of an EBP community in a changing complex healthcare landscape. The following discussion will share four DCI prime movers that scale up the enculturation of EBP and emergence of innovation. These were uncovered over 15 years of clinical engagement in DCI at the point of service and are presented for your consideration.

Reforming Workforce Development into Self-Renewing Knowledge Force

Two genres of nurses slowly defined the nursing landscape in the past 5 years in reference to EBP competencies. The new cohorts are nurses whose EBP-mindedness has been molded during their academic journey via a formal credit course in EBP. The other cohorts are those who did not have the benefit of a formal academic course in EBP. The DCI process is self-renewing because on one's own accord, a nurse can revisit his or her EBP competency level and self-identify personal areas for improvement. Based on perceived needs, the learning modules can be activated anytime at the nurse's own pace. DCI offers a stepwise method in leading these divergent nursing genres to become one knowledge-force community; these are DCI-EBP Literacy and DCI-5As.

The DCI-EBP Literacy Method

DCI-EBP Literacy fast tracks the acquisition of basic EBP skill set with practical application for bedside clinical decision making. The approach is especially helpful among nurses who did not have an academic course in EBP. The simplification is effected with its focus on filtered or preprocessed evidence. This type of evidence comes in the form of short summaries (e.g., evidence summaries from databases such as DynaMed, ACP Smart Medicine, UpToDate, or Clinical Key-First Consult) that are based on the integration of several research studies that have been preappraised and interpreted by experts in an accessible format for point-of-care application. DCI-EBP Literacy allows nurses to complete a cycle of EBP within a short amount of time because the challenge of sifting through an avalanche of single studies and critiquing each one is eliminated. DCI-EBP Literacy allows nurses to focus more on the value of the outcomes of EBP instead of on the difficulty of learning the process (Sanares-Carreon et al., 2015).

The DCI-5As Method

The complementing method is learning the same five EBP skill set, but with inclusion of unfiltered or unprocessed evidence. The learning modules focus on the five competencies for EBP, called the DCI-5As Method: (1) asking a focused question, (2) accessing the evidence, (3) appraising the evidence, (4) applying the best evidence, and (5) alerting peers of the adaptation of new knowledge. These five competencies are offered in self-directed modules to provide the foundational knowledge necessary for clinicians to develop EBP competencies. The process is both extensive and intensive because it offers interactive exercises that provide opportunities for the immediate application of the concepts and principles. As such, as soon as each discrete module is completed, achievement of the targeted outcome becomes a natural outgrowth. Tools and templates that serve as outlines and guides are made available online for ease of access. Each page on the website provides easy access to a Web master who can answer questions or facilitate a referral to appropriate experts. These learning activities may be completed independently with the option of coaching from an EBP expert (Sanares-Carreon et al., 2010).

Reconfiguring Formal Relationships into Interconnected Networks

Sustainability of EBP at the point of service requires EBP emissaries who are part of the community wherein patient care is provided. The versatility of an informal network structure in tapping expert-level nurses with varied clinical specialties to be unit-based EBP emissaries steered the formation of the EBP network. Three jointly optimizing approaches may be used to form the DCI–EBP network: role models, unit-based champions, and a core network.

Advocates: Role Models

Nurses across nursing services are recruited to participate in several feasibility studies, such as the creation of the evidence-based policy and standard system, development of the DCI-EBP Literacy program, or the pilot of a reformed accountability system for EBP. Although group processes are used in honing the EBP skill sets of program participants, individual assessments can be conducted. Willing and competent participants become members of the network of individuals who role-model, inspire, and peer coach in areas such as the DCI teaching and learning website. Two complementing DCI pathways are available for learning the ropes of becoming an EBP role model or advocate. The take-home message is to consider every EBP project or program as a recruiting venue in spotting a prospective member of the network. Project or program immersion is an excellent setting for building basic competencies.

Champions: Unit-based Coaches and Mentors

The second approach grew out of nurse-initiated personal decisions to advance to an expert-level nurse clinician. This approach is nested in a CAP wherein completion of an EBP product is a requisite for advancement. This provision also applies to all incumbent expert-level nurses to validate their level of practice by conducting an EBP project. The learning process is nurse driven with on-demand coaching and mentoring. Members of the network are expected to serve as EBP mentors at the unit level. The take-home message in this approach is to proactively recognize opinion leaders and those who are pursuing advanced degrees. Invite them to join EBP work teams whose clinical issue matches their area of interest. Engagement in EBP inquiries is a good first step toward becoming unit-based champions.

Core Network: Nursing System-wide EBP Experts

The third approach involves the advanced competency-based education in EBP of a select group of nurse leaders who have advanced degrees. Members of the Core acquire progressive EBP expertise through partnership with EBP scholar/strategist in conducting EBP projects with nursing wide application and implication. The take-home message in this recruitment approach is to identify nurses whose formal position allows for flexibility of time that would allow for on-demand consultation and commissioned EBP works.

Postscript

No two organizations are alike. The academic medical center's (AMC) experiences in the formation of the EBP network is intended to share the strategies for adaptation or to spark new ideas for building a core team of nurses that will help navigate the personalized EBP expedition of organizations moving to an EBP culture. The network, compared to a formalized structure, accords greater opportunity for innovation and flexibility in tapping into the collective intelligence of the nursing organization.

The combined effect of the three approaches populated the UTMB Health EBP network. The role models were nurses who have competency in the simplified version of EBP, called DCI-EBP Literacy. Quite recently, the new genre of nurses who underwent the EBP training during their residency program became de facto role models. These cohorts went beyond DCI-EBP Literacy, but not at the level of a mentor. The AMC looks at this genre as the game changers. Take note that the networks skill set are in EBP. As of this writing, only the members of the Monarch teams (discussed later in this chapter) have been introduced in the DCI approach to innovation.

Synchronizing Segmented Initiatives into Complementing Inquiring Communities

DCI offers several pathways wherein nurses may select one or a combination of options to advance evidence translation. Nurses can choose to become involved by assuming a leadership role or becoming a member of the team. These may seem segmented at first glance, but they can be synchronized toward creating inquiring communities with shared experiences and shared vision. Just as no two nurses are alike, each nursing unit has its own unique culture. The emerging inquiring communities can collectively decide which pathways work well for them considering their own unique memberships. EBP is generally perceived as hard to learn, let alone to sustain, if the medium and strategy employed are out of synchrony with the community's norms. Each community must be empowered to decide and choose approaches that it considers a good fit to optimize acculturation of EBP. The following pathways are web-based with access to on-demand coaching. The tools and processes can be customized in any setting. Consider this a marketplace of ideas wherein you can access and choose based on your passion.

Pathway for Becoming an EBP Champion

There are nurses who are motivated to become EBP champions. These nurses show one or a combination of the following attributes: (1) motivation to become proficient in EBP applications, (2) leadership skills focused on solving problems and improving practice, and (3) teaching and team-building skills. EBP champions play instrumental roles in developing a critical mass of RNs in EBP initiatives. Put simply, they serve as coaches and clinical site resources in EBP. The presence of champions strengthens the EBP infrastructure around critical connections across disciplines. Furthering these inter-professional connections is considered important in the strategic development of evidence-based clinical practice. Champions are expected to help the nursing service reach the tipping point (moment when something unique becomes commonplace) in EBP (Sanares-Carreon et al., 2010).

This pathway requires 40 to 100 engagement hours, depending on the baseline EBP knowledge and skill level of the learner. The engagement period may be conducted in successive days or spread over a period of time, depending on learning style and organizational resources. The benchmark for success is completion of an evidence synthesis with a detailed action plan for evidence translation. This is the pathway for the key members of your EBP network.

Pathway for Developing Evidence-Based Policy and Standards System

There are essential nursing functions whose activities have been traditionally accepted by both clinicians and management as a component of nursing practice. The most notable of these essential functions are the development of practice standards, provision of patient teaching, and quality improvement projects. If the authoritative statements guiding day-to-day nursing practice are not keeping pace with the most current best evidence, potential adverse effects on patient care may arise. Ensuring that nursing practice standards keep pace with the most current best evidence remains an ongoing challenge. The pathway may be completed in 24 to 40 hours, spread over a 1 to 2 month period (Sanares-Carreon et al., 2010).

Adaptation of the Evidence-Based Policy and Standards pathway is woven into the existing organizational structure and process for developing and updating policies and procedures. An algorithm or a flowchart may be used to define the point at which the EBP process is conducted. The predefined outcomes of interest of the policy/standards of care are the focus of the EBP review. The evidence synthesis is consequently integrated in the policy as appropriate with conscientious consideration of the context within which the policy/standards is used. The approach ensures accountability and provides checkpoints for the systematic integration of the EBP principles. Clinical experts at the unit level are the targets for this pathway. The learning pathway can also be used in developing evidence-based order sets, checklists, and other guides for point-of-care service.

Pathway for Organizing an Appraisal Club

The purpose of an appraisal club is to develop and advance nurses' ability to appraise the quality, rigor, and strength of published research studies. A nurse leader facilitates a small group to review and critique a study, and evaluate its implications and application in practice (Sanares-Carreon et al., 2010). If the club sees the potential of an article as a trigger to reexamine current practice, the nurse leading the session is expected to prepare an action plan for the conduct of an EBP review to generate an evidence synthesis. A brief summary using an appraisal club template is prepared and shared to generate community interest on the clinical issue.

This type of session is generally referred to as journal club. In view of the availability of research articles in electronic databases and the increasing number of online publications, the club is renamed more generically as an appraisal club. A variant for the one-article approach is highly advocated. Use at least two articles on the same clinical topic, not only as a reminder that one research article is not sufficient to change or validate practice, but also to provide initial exposure in critically summing up research-based studies. Consider introducing club members to the critique and interpretation of systematic reviews to start immersing them in the process of how research synthesis is systematically conducted.

Pathway for Preparing Notes for Nurses

Notes for Nurses focuses on practices that address the question, why are we doing what we are doing? Nurses engaged in this pathway use the DCI process to systematically summarize the best evidence derived from the integration of research, expert opinion, pathophysiologic rationale, patient perspectives, and other recognized sources of nursing knowledge. The primary purpose of this pathway is to share with peers the most current, valid, and reliable evidence-based knowledge about nursing practices. New knowledge is presented in a concise one-page format that nurse clinicians can quickly peruse in the midst of a high-intensity care environment. The summaries can be published on internal websites or presented in poster format that may be placed on clinical units. EBP projects developed by members of the EBP network can be considered Notes for Nurses. Notes for Nurses is especially important for issues of nursing practice when best evidence is not accessible on vendor-developed evidence summaries (Sanares-Carreon et al., 2010). If you have a nurse residency program, the completed EBP projects that are summarized in poster format can be considered for Notes for Nurses.

Pathway for Mobilizing Clinical Inquiry Roundtables

This pathway allows nurses to reflect on actual care provided for a particular patient. The problems encountered and the successes achieved along the care continuum are identified. Evidence-based data are referenced as nurses engage in the inquiry process, exploring the causes and solutions sensitive to nursing interventions. At the end of the session, nurses are expected to acquire better understanding and practice perspectives. Insights gained in the session lead nurses toward the exploration of opportunities for EBP. The inquiry session serves as a reflective lens using one of three structural formats: (1) patient case presentation, (2) multidisciplinary case review and analysis, and (3) multidisciplinary patient care planning (Sanares-Carreon et al., 2010).

The roundtable approach engages the collective intelligence of nurses in EBP in action. It is ideal that filtered evidence, such as evidence summaries or systematic reviews, be used to answer the clinical inquiry. If not available, at least three recent high-quality research studies are brought to the roundtable in a tabular format that compare and contrast the research design, sample or sampling, significance, and findings. The interactive dialogue will focus on the incorporation of research-based evidence with a particular patient's clinical condition and experience with care. This pathway challenges the experiential knowledge of the roundtable in incorporating the evidence in actual patient care situations.

Postscript

While the learning modules for acquiring the EBP skill set enable you and your organization to start the boarding process on your EBP expedition, the pathways enhance one's capacity to weather the waves and storms for continuing the expedition. Sustaining nurses' engagement is multifactorial. A bundle approach may be needed. This suggests that you may need to choose a string of pathways that meld into the culture to keep nurses interested and energized. You may need to be creative or consider incentive systems. Keep an eye on your target; the processes and strategies can change. You will not know what will work until you take the first step.

Organizing Discrete Resources into a Central Hub for Learning and Communication

Access to resources is vital in setting the stage for an EBP culture. Disparities in access range from frustration in locating available organizational resources to increasing capacity in building new critical EBP components. A central hub for EBP resources is one of the cornerstones of the DCI model. Figure 9-2 shows the portal of the one-stop EBP website. The asynchronous learning modules, self-directed pathways, and one webpage containing all the links for sources of evidence are just a few of the resources to include. This latter feature was instrumental in ensuring access to the central hub directly at the portal of UTMB Health's webpage for use by other disciplines.

Another key feature is a site that inspires and motivates others by featuring and celebrating the accomplishments of individuals who have completed EBP projects. The publication and other medium for sharing new knowledge serve to inform and invite the community to work together. For example, evidence reviews that are published in Notes for Nurses can move forward for translation, research, or fuller dissemination. The shared governance councils are potential venues for collaborative translations of completed evidence syntheses that have nursing-wide application and implications. For example, completed evidence reviews that have rigorous evidence for translation to practice may be presented to the education council for wider dissemination; those that are ripe for translation can be coordinated with the practice council. The research council may be invited to lead the knowledge discovery on evidence that is not strong enough to support a change in practice.

The central hub is operated as a living system. It needs constant updating. A good strategy is to secure an electronic content management system that could create shared ownership on a certain portion of the website, thereby distributing accountability for making updates. Leveraging the advances in computer technology would make the central hub a living and breathing space in setting the stage for an EBP culture wherein innovation emerges and thrives.

FRAMING EBP AS A CATALYST IN SETTING THE STAGE FOR INNOVATION

"Meeting the needs of those cared for by practitioners often requires the invention of new activities as well as creative responses" (Polkinghorne, 2004, p. 3). "It is only through reflection and dialogic interaction with patients that the nurse enhances her/his understanding and becomes aware of new possibilities for care" (Polkinghorne, 2004, p. 151). The process of DCI establishes the groundwork and the background understanding for a culture of care that questions traditional practices that are no longer effective.

Innovation is any idea that is new to an organization and leads to a replacement of an existing process with a new set of activities. The new set of activities may be an administrative, operational, or technical innovation, such as new products, services, or models (Seelos & Mair, 2012). Uncertainties are inherent in innovation. The uncertainties can be technological, market based, regulatory, sociopolitical, acceptance or legitimacy, managerial, timing, and consequence. For example, consequences of innovation cause uncertainty because they cannot be predicted in advance (Jalonen, 2012). Notwithstanding, the call for innovation could have never been more intense than in today's healthcare environment.

There is no simple or single recipe for setting the stage for innovation. The literature, however, is replete with concepts, ideas, and experiments on innovation. The approaches range from examination of the nature of the innovation itself (e.g., Rogers, 2003) to analysis of the behavior or biology of the innovator (e.g., Dyer et al., 2011), or exploration of organizational and environmental factors (e.g., Hill et al., 2014), among many more approaches. The following discussion intends to contribute to the growing perspectives to inspire and keep the dialogue going in nurturing innovation as a way of life in healthcare organizations. The DCI perspectives will cover processes and structures to foster a culture of idea generation and practice innovation that are weaved around the principles of EBP as a catalyst for accelerating innovative behavior.

Weaving the Process for Cultivating Innovation

The DCI model is an innovation in itself. DCI was sparked by a need for practice change, which was refined through insights gained from an integrative review of the literature. The original intent was not to develop a model for EBP, but rather to create a transparent process for nurses in learning and reflecting about EBP. The learning package and other tools and processes were creatively designed and subsequently pilot tested using participatory action research to engage the end users. Staff and management continue to support and invest in DCI for the enculturation of EBP in nursing systems.

Convergence of the EBP–Innovation Interface

DCI offers a paradigm that demonstrates how the footprints of EBP and innovation form a diamond trail. Both EBP and innovation begin with an inquiry and curiosity about something that is causing a clinical dilemma or something that is unknown. From this point, EBP moves forward with an intermediate goal of evidence synthesis, while innovation moves toward creative idea generation. The widest point of the diamond trail is formed when each reaches the intermediate goal. DCI portrays this divergent trail as an opportunity for setting up synergy. As such, DCI builds bridges so evidence synthesis and creative ideas can inform one other. This happens at the cusp between Phase 2 and Phase 3 of the DCI model (Figure 9-1). The symbiosis may spark or refine the creative idea or enrich the evidence synthesis. Irrespective of the results of the interface, both EBP and innovation cascade to the ultimate goal of implementation. This is the other end of the diamond trail wherein EBP and innovation are in unison once again. This diamond trail shows that the true essence of EBP and innovation is implementation. The reconvergence may spark subsequent diamond trails; this is referred to as the DCI diamond principle. Within this dynamic context, DCI becomes an ethic of idea generation in tandem with a willingness to take risks and the capacity for experimentation as essential elements for the emergence of a culture of innovation.

Integration of Innovation in the DCI–EBP Cycle

As a living and breathing EBP model, in 2011 the DCI model incorporated the emergence of practice innovation in Phase 3 on its iterative cycle (Figure 9-1). Along the road to innovation, DCI offers four points, forming an innovation quadrant that highlight the key processes and principles to guide the innovation expedition.

Point of Inquiry

Figure 9-3 shows the location of the cusp of Phase 2 and Phase 3 of the DCI phases, which is labeled Phase 3a. An enlarged diagram of Phase 3a is shown in Figure 9-3, which schematically depicts the key points of the DCI innovation quadrant. Point 1 is the point of inquiry wherein a clinical question is defined, calling for the application of the principles of DCI-EBP Literacy or the DCI-5As Method. After an evidence synthesis is completed, the new knowledge is individualized to patients. In essence, this is the point where the innovative ideas of others are brought to the bedside.

Point of Inception

The point of inception is characterized by the generation of creative ideas that have the potential to benefit the patient and possibly a similar population. The challenge is the capacity to use the principles of looking beyond the obvious and visualize interconnectivity between the new knowledge and the contextual factors in the care environment and beyond its walls. The goal is to unleash creativity and begin to

---

Figure 9-3   DCI innovation quadrant

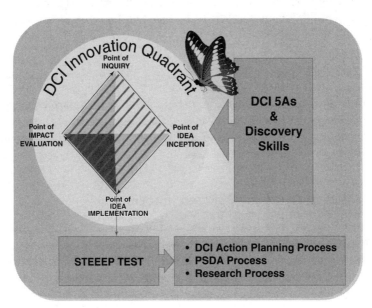

Courtesy of University of Texas Medical Branch at Galveston (UTMB Health)

dream and explore possibilities that would bring better value for patient, nurses, organizations, or the nursing profession. Initiation of dialogue with others is highly encouraged to exchange ideas and conduct an opportunity assessment. It is helpful to communicate with others outside the arena of specialization or discipline. The ideas may come in several forms, such as a new product, a transformed service, a novel learning strategy, a new model, and so forth, that not only improve, but challenge, the status quo.

Point of Implementation

Point of idea implementation is bringing creative ideas to the bedside. A trial run is conducted to observe and understand the factors affecting the viability and feasibility of the creative idea. A rapid analysis and prototyping are advocated with a turnaround time of 4 to 8 weeks. The results of the trial run are used to streamline the implementation of the creative idea in the practice setting. Take note of the arrow pointing to the activation of the STEEEP test, based on the six key dimensions of care delivery that are advocated in the IOM's "Crossing the Quality Chasm" report (2001): safe (avoids injury), timely (can be implemented without harmful delays), effective (with clear parameters about who would best benefit), equitable (does not vary in quality when applied in different groups), efficient (avoids waste), and patient centered (can be individualized based on needs and values). If the STEEEP test is not satisfied or if there is a problem making the evaluation, three forms of inquiry are recommended: DCI action planning, further research, or a quality improvement approach. The trial run requires investments in time and other resources. The need to engage unit leadership to bring the idea to the bedside is key.

Point of Evaluation

The point of impact evaluation is the point of assessing beyond the immediate results to identify long-term effects and any unintended effect of the innovation. This is the point of measuring observable results instead of counting activities. The measures are focused on assessing if the innovation works and works well, and gauges the tangible benefits in the real world of practice.

Carving the Structure for EBP and Innovation

Comparatively, it may appear that the introduction of new processes for EBP and innovation sails smoother than reconfiguration of structural arrangements. Both are equally challenging because process and structure are weaved together to achieve results. As mentioned earlier, EBP ascribes to a network structure that operates as a web of experts, champions, and advocates who carry the torch for EBP with continuing support from institutional leadership.

Devolution of Accountability to Operational Level

The need to locate accountability for EBP where it is received by patients is a novel frontier in achieving true enculturation. The interweaving of EBP and innovation as reflected by the DCI diamond principle calls for an accountability structure that mirrors both. Building self-managing teams, leveraging the power of connectivity in harnessing bedside talents, and incentivizing EBP work and creative ideas, are the powerhouse for the devolution of the accountability for EBP and innovation. The cornerstone of the conjoined EBP–innovation accountability structure leverages the shared commitment among strategic and operational leaders in concert with a critical mass of RNs with strong foundational knowledge, skills, and willingness to engage in EBP and innovation. Within this emerging culture, both staff and management make an investment.

As mentioned, a network structure for EBP is advocated. A viable structure for innovation is undergoing a trial run in the AMC. With a convergence of EBP and innovation, as reflected in the operationalization of the DCI diamond principle, it is prudent to hypothesize that some members of the EBP network may become innovation trailblazers. A more detailed discussion is provided in the section on the Monarch project later in this chapter.

Incorporation of EBP and Innovation in Nursing Professional Practice Model

The nursing professional practice model is the structure that schematically defines what nurses believed about nursing practice. The professional practice model incorporates the care delivery system which provides the structure on how care is provided across the continuum. When EBP and innovation are explicitly identified as one of the core elements or values of the professional practice model, nurses will tend to reflect and inquire about everyday practice from a perspective of EBP and practice innovation. This mindset will eventually become hardwired, and the desired practice ethic emerges.

Keeping an eye on the professional practice model will cascade to keeping an eye on a target linked to achieving everyday excellence. While the focused question in EBP is precisely defined, creative ideas may be free-floating and are encouraged to build-up without the restraint of boundaries. Setting targets that align with the vision and strategic plans of the organization is advocated. The targets are focused on those that have the potential to benefit patients, nursing, and the organization. For example, targets for patient-focused innovation are issues on decreasing risks and/or complications, enhancing patient experience, or increasing adherence to treatment plans. Nurse-focused innovation, on the one hand, may cover targets on advancing competency, raising satisfaction levels, or improving compliance and adherence. The targets for organization-focused innovation consider issues about decreasing cost, increasing marketplace visibility, or gaining competitive edge. The details are left for the would-be innovator to figure through freedom of creative expression.

Institution of Incentives and Rewards

In complex interconnected systems, small pockets of change matter in making a difference. Big or small, creative ideas have to be encouraged to reach the innovation stage. For example, to best understand that EBP emerges from translation of evidence synthesis and not from the critique of one journal article, the DCI proponent used the hand as a metaphor to visually show the sources of evidence. The little finger was used to represent local knowledge, such as policies and other organizational data. The ring finger, customarily the choice for a wedding or engagement ring, represented the relationship with the patient, acknowledging their values and perspectives. The middle finger, generally the tallest, represented expert opinion, reminding nurses that this is only one of the many sources of evidence. The forefinger represented research-based evidence because it points with a relative degree of precision to what works, but this is only one of the sources of evidence. Lastly, with the thumb pointing toward the self when held up in a handshake position, it is assigned as the nurse's experiential knowledge and serves as the integrator of all four major sources of evidence. This is taught with a caveat that before nurses touch a patient, they have to look at their hands and ask, in reflection, if the nursing action is grounded on integration of best evidence.

The example is a very small idea but, as a learning tool it has demonstrated great impact, giving inspiration about how small ideas can make a difference. As nurses find enthuse in the treasure hunt for evidence to validate and/or change customary practices, they are inspired to be proud of any creative ideas. UTMB Health introduced a chief nursing officer (CNO) ADMIRE award in 2012. ADMIRE is an acronym for advancing, developing and modeling innovation, research and EBP. The CNO ADMIRE award is the reward system component of the Nursing Services' Monarch Moments Initiative to promote a culture of innovation. It is a celebration of nurses' contributions to the science of nursing practice toward the achievement of enhanced patient care quality, advanced nursing practice, and strong marketplace presence.

Dovetailing DCI–EBP with the Skills of Disruptive Innovators

Figure 9-4 illustrates how DCI dovetails the five EBP skills with the five skills of the disruptive innovators posited by Dyer and colleagues (2011). Consistent with the paradigm wherein EBP was grounded, the EBP skills are demonstrated following a systematic process. On the other hand, the skills of the disruptive innovators (discovery skills) may not necessarily follow an ordered pattern congruent with the creative component of innovation. The following discussion will bring to the healthcare setting the five discovery skills of Dyer and colleagues (2011) as each one is dovetailed with the DCI-5As. The synergy of the DCI–EBP and discovery skills was used in the implementation of the UTMB Health Monarch Moments Initiative with permission from the lead author.

**Figure 9-4   Dovetailing the DCI–EBP skills and disruptive innovators'
discovery skills**

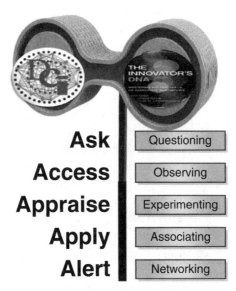

Courtesy of University of Texas Medical Branch at Galveston (UTMB Health)

Ask a Focused Question: Questioning

DCI-Ask is inquiring about a clinical issue by identifying the patient, intervention, comparator intervention, and the outcomes of interest using a Patient-Intervention-Comparator-Outcome (PICO) format. DCI advocates to build on Ask and follow it with provocative Questioning, which was described by Dyer and colleagues (2011) as a strategy to question the unquestionable and to question what if to impose or eliminate constraints or challenge common wisdom. Questioning is the gateway to the generation of creative ideas.

Access the Evidence: Observing

DCI-Access involves a comprehensive search of all the sources of evidence to find the answer to the focused question. Mastery of this skill sharpens the nurse's ability to be thorough and pay attention to all the relevant evidence. The immersion in DCI-Access is an excellent breeding ground for developing observation skills. Dyer and colleagues (2011) explained Observing as watching (not just visually) intensely, carefully, intentionally, and consistently to look for surprises, anomalies, or the unexpected. Disruptive innovators look for cues, pay attention, or take notes about everyday experiences with the goal of finding new ideas.

Appraise the Evidence: Experimenting

DCI-Appraise is the critical appraisal of the evidence to weed out the faulty evidence and identify the level of evidence of those that were found good. Engagement in Appraise exposes nurses to the actual conduct of research by other scholars. The exposure is especially impactful if the research design is evaluative. Constant engagement in Appraise builds nurses' sense of how intuitive hunches are tested. This vicarious experience can serve as a starting or leaping point for developing Experimenting behavior. Dyer and colleagues (2011) argued that while scientists work in the laboratory or under some controlled condition, the world is the laboratory of the innovator. The behaviors of experimenters include unceasing exploration of the world, both intellectually and experientially, forming h*ypotheses along the way. While* Observers *are intense watchers,* Experimenters are intellectual explorers in piloting new ideas or products. (Dyer, et al, 2011). DCI advocates that nurses who have generated evidence synthesis as a product of Appraise are now situated to use the new knowledge in Questioning, Observing, *and* Experimenting.

Apply the Body of Evidence: Associating

DCI-Apply refers to using the evidence synthesis in answering the focused question and translating the new knowledge in practice. While Appraising is considered most challenging by nurses, Apply is actually more challenging because one must connect the value of the new knowledge to an individual patient situation. True mastery of Apply requires a blend of experiential, intellectual, and behavioral skills. This is one reason why evidence translation has been a bottleneck for EBP—finding the right blend is no simple endeavor. Even a beginning skill in Apply is a good starting point in developing the Associating discovery skills. Associating is pattern recognition across seemingly unrelated questions, concepts, or ideas. This is the only cognitive skill in the Dyer and colleagues (2011) typology. The more diverse the prior knowledge, the more connections can be made. This calls for mixing and matching quite different concepts and the zooming in and zooming out of different ideas (Dyer et al., 2011). DCI advocates that teams are used in the discussion of application and translation of new knowledge and encourage the group in Associating with unrelated or unlikely application or translation to generate creative ideas.

Alert Peers: Networking

DCI-Alert is sharing and spreading new knowledge to peers, other disciplines, patients, and their families. Regular demonstration of Alert actually builds a network. The discovery skill Networking is finding and testing ideas with a network of people with diverse backgrounds and perspectives to elicit varied responses. In essence, Networking leverages on the creative ideas of the crowd. Networkers, according to Dyer and colleagues (2011) are actively searching for new ideas by seeking people with the propensity to offer a radically different perspective.

THE MONARCH MOMENTS INITIATIVE: THE COURAGE TO BLAZE NEW TRAILS

Complexity thinking considers metaphors as a medium that communicates the message of dynamism and practice transformation (Doll & Trueit, 2010). The UTMB Health Monarch Moments Initiative ascribes to a metaphor wherein catching caterpillars enables nurses to identify practices that are crawling and slow to achieve desired outcomes but can be transformed into monarch butterflies by leveraging on EBP skill sets as take-off point for engagement in idea generation. The metaphor inspires inquiry toward creating multiple interpretations and engaging collectively to blaze new trails in challenging current practice. The structure agenda is to devolve the accountability for EBP and innovation to the place it is expected to occur; while the process agenda is to engage the collective intelligence of nurses in conducting evidence synthesis as a catalyst for idea generation. The challenge is transforming the creative idea into actionable plan and the courage to move forward for a rapid analysis and/or prototyping with commitment and passion to meet predetermined targets amidst complexity and uncertainty in the local environment.

Testing and "Thinking Different"

"The best creative thinking happens at the frontlines" (Martin, 2011, p. 82). The healthcare environment is ripe with issues and situations that present problems, questions, or difficulties in the course of providing nursing care. These are fertile breeding grounds for creative EBP moments; a moment of finding answers, seeking verifications, or gaining new knowledge. These moments present opportunities that lead beyond standard application of evidence toward creative ideas.

Monarch's twin goal is to cultivate innovation mindedness that builds readiness to provide patient care in a dynamically changing ecosystem. The complexity viewpoint is embedded in the change strategies as nurses engage in continuing dialogue to recognize uncertainties and uncover approaches of handling everyday challenges. As *EBP mindedness* becomes the normative culture, *Monarch moments* begin to emerge. A *Monarch moment* happens when the new knowledge gained from an EBP query and/or EBP review sparks new insights about new possibilities over and beyond what the current evidence describes. It is a moment that stirs the challenging of the status quo with provocative questions. The concern is not only about improving existing processes to make it a little better. Instead, the mindset is rewired to think in terms of possibilities that create new values to enhance the patient experience, clinical outcomes, or organizational capacity. These are *Monarch moments* because they are transformational experiences, similar to how a caterpillar prepares itself (comparable to learning the EBP skill set) to evolve into a butterfly. From crawling like a caterpillar to its metamorphosis into a butterfly with newly developed wings (e.g., acquired knowledge and EBP skills), the monarch is now capable of navigating new horizons and plot a course to the future at a far more accelerated rate than that of the crawling caterpillar.

Leveraging the Synergy of the Monarch Quad

Monarch capitalizes on the results of evidence synthesis to spark or refine creative ideas. This is achieved by installing four interfacing prime movers to maneuver the flight of the Monarchs in the academic medical center. Collectively called the Monarch quad, the prime movers are pillars, partnerships, principles, and pathways. In Figure 9-3, the schematic diagram of the flight of the monarch to innovation, depicts the collective power of the Monarch quad to direct its flight toward innovation. The pillars include the DCI model and professional practice model that are already in place in nursing service. Flanking these models are two new structures: the accountability platform and the CNO ADMIRE awards, both of which were described earlier. The second prime mover is partnerships between the operational managers and bedside clinicians. The partnership is expected to be the precursor of engagement leadership style expected to drive formation of a network of Monarchs in a weblike structure. A principle-based approach that is nonprescriptive provides the flexibility in interpretation and application in the context in which these will be used. The principles directly address how engagement in EBP and innovation is going to occur in terms of the engagement of operational managers, planned dedicated time, team formation across the network, and lifelong learning. The pathways are the prime movers toward achieving the desired outcomes and monitoring the return on investment (Sanares-Carreon, in press).

Connecting and Building Self-Managing Teams

Monarch was designed to explore the process and structure for devolving the accountability for EBP and idea generation such that care is provided and received by patients. The vision is to evolve Monarch teams in forming weblike interconnections with other teams in the system. The expedition intends to uncover the operational managers' openness to account engagement in EBP, and practice innovation as integral part of nursing workflow. The following are milestones of the flight of one Monarch team as an example. The Monarchs are nurses from various units of a clinical cluster under the umbrella administration of a nursing director. The team was initially led by an operational nurse manager who fostered partnerships among the members but was later substituted by an assistant nurse manager in view of workload issues. The EBP program manager coached the Monarch nurse leader who was directly engaging the team. The approach was used to slowly form a self-managing team at the operational level. The blended learning approach during the Monarch onboarding session was complemented by self-directed learning modules in EBP and innovation from the DCI website to further advance individual skills. The partnerships among the Monarchs generated creative ideas, which were targeted to enhance the patients' experience across their area of practice. The collective intelligence of the Monarchs was tapped to complete the evidence synthesis. The synergy of the newly acquired DCI–EBP skills and the discovery skills of disruptive innovators posited by Dyer and colleagues (2011) accelerated the Monarch's quest for unexplored possibilities in the AMC. The original clinical issue was focused on uncovering creative educational strategies to foster breastfeeding. The change in leadership led to a shift in interest to rapid analysis of strategies that may decrease anxiety levels of postpartum mothers who are unable to physically be with their infants. Integration of evidence suggested the potential of virtual presence through mobile communication technology.

The viability and strength of the team lies on their collective spirit to use the skills and insights they gained in their Monarch expedition to become the building blocks toward a culture that values EBP and innovation. The Monarchs are role models who share their new knowledge and experience with their respective units. The Monarch team is envisioned to continue to regroup and evolve as the core to take accountability for setting the stage for EBP and innovations as the normative culture of the clinical cluster. The Monarch teams from various clinical clusters are envisioned to connect like a network to share successes and challenges.

Postscript

Monarch is the first DCI project that did not use the research method to pilot test the viability of a new initiative. It used the DCI action planning approach that provided the teams with flexibility to self-navigate their respective EBP–innovation expedition. Accountability for the achievement of patient-centric outcomes is within the purview of the Monarch leader; the goal of the EBP program manager or expert is observing, and influencing to ensure that the Monarch thrives in a dynamically changing ecosystem. Tracking the collective ability of the team in completing the evidence synthesis and the translation plan was challlenging. A simplified, yet less directed, monitoring mechanism is being introduced (Sanares-Carreon, in press).

CRUISING THE METRICS OF EVALUATING FOR VALUE

There is an avalanche of data about the past and the present, but none about the future. Scholars in both research and practice arenas have designed and used methods of extrapolating past trends to predict the future. The approaches served well under stable conditions. The complexity and uncertainties of the current healthcare landscape markedly limits the precision of the current tools. The rules of engagement become restrictive. A resurgence of the principles-based approach is gaining ground.

The 21st century is an era of accountability. In the arena of EBP, there is limited guidance related to assessing the effectiveness of its implementation. The current measures are focused on specific clinical outcomes in terms of what is achieved and not achieved. Issues of sustainability and behavior change had not been considered (Bick & Graham, 2010). While a certain level of precision is warranted to ascertain the true value of the results, in most instances the practice is studying the observable and easily measurable, or those factors that can be counted (Porter-O'Grady & Malloch, 2010). The bigger challenge, however, involves outcomes emerging in complex systems that are often nonlinear and unpredictable, requiring new tools for tracking results in real time (Davidson, Ray, & Turkel, 2011), otherwise the information is rendered antiquated. The web of relationships that nurses build within and across the care continuum to provide the desired level of care in concert with the holistic nature of nursing, further complicates the evaluation process. The following concepts and approaches are presented to serve as discussion points for continuing the conversations on evaluating the value of EBP and innovation in healthcare organizations.

Knowing the Key Areas to Measure

The first area of reflection is, what are we measuring? The immediate outcomes may include awareness of the current and potential EBP abilities of stakeholders. As level of awareness increases, readiness to learn new knowledge and skills are important triggers for launching a training program for EBP and innovation to targeted individuals who will bring about the greatest return on investment. At this juncture, the key areas of evaluation are levels of abilities and competencies. Attitudes are important aspects that beg attention. Phase 2 of the DCI cycle (Figure 9-1) is the point where learning outcomes are measured. Learning has marginal value until the new knowledge is applied in the real world of practice. The evaluation may focus on the point of view of the care provider, the recipient of care, or the organization relative to the outcome and impact of knowledge translation. Phase 3 of the DCI cycle points to the evaluation of the assimilation of evidence-based nursing practice and innovation as a routine part of everyday practice. The primal goal is evidence-based patient care. Phase 4 points to evaluation of patient-centric outcomes. These evaluations are carried out by asking when, how, and whose perspectives. The DCI model may therefore be used as a frame of reference for identifying the various points of conducting evaluation.

Choosing Analytic Models for Evaluation

The goal of evaluation is appraisal of the value of an intervention or program in supporting or advancing the organizational mission and vision. In its most generic terms, the results are used as information in making decisions for resource allocation. This is one reason why most analytic models for evaluations are called decision-making models. Alemi and Gustafson (2007) provide a discussion of several decision analysis models that may be considered in health care. Some examples are rapid analysis, decision trees, cost-effectiveness clinics, modeling and measuring uncertainty, modeling preferences, program evaluation, and benchmarking clinicians, to name a few (Alemi & Gustafson, 2007). Another perspective is looking at evaluations to assess the degree to which predetermined targets are met and using this information to make informed decisions about the next step. In this instance, the objective is to improve a process or product to achieve the outcome. Either way, the choice of the analytic model is crucial.

An analytic model worth exploring is the EBP decision-making process. In asking the question, the aim of the evaluation explicitly identifies the expected effect of the variables (interventions) to the outcome of interest on a defined population. To find the answer to the evaluation question, data that are collected mirror the accessing the evidence phase of the EBP process. The data are methodically analyzed just as evidence is systematically appraised. When appraisal is completed, the data are synthesized and the findings are presented to the decision makers in a decision analysis format for appropriate action. The actionable plan is developed and implemented as in applying the body best evidence. Stakeholders are alerted about the actionable plan for optimum uptake.

Defining the Timing and Data for Evaluation

The value of the evaluation method is a function of its appropriateness as a tool for measuring the outcomes of interest and the validity of the results it generates. In essence, evaluation of EBP and innovation ascribe to the principles of appraising the evidence. Traditionally, evaluation can be formative, midstream, and summative. One area of inquiry is determination of data or program maturation so the evaluation is conducted not too early or too late to generate optimum data for analysis.

The other related issue is the meaningfulness of the results for decision makers relative to resource allocation. Current tools range from rigorous statistical results from research to run charts from quality improvement reports. Vendor-prepared benchmark data are also available upon subscription, as well as reports from regulatory bodies such as The Joint Commission. Tapping into these reports provide rich sources of data for evaluation. The promise of translating real-time data such as those related to the aggregation of clinical data from electronic medical records into clinical intelligence (healthcare counterpart of business intelligence) that make sense to clinicians would lead to making point-of-service patient care decisions.

Balancing Quantitative and Qualitative Measures

The debate over the argument that numbers speak louder than words faded when the patient experience started becoming a metric of care. A purist and highly polarized approach on either side of the debate is not tenable. The goal is striking a balance where value holds the fulcrum. The DCI tools are summarized in the following discussion as take-off points for the exploration of equivalent objective tools for evaluation.

Evaluating the Culture

The evolution–revolution of an EBP–innovation culture is evaluated based on nurses' perception about the factors that facilitate or hamper the desired practice ethic using a five-point Likert-type scale. Objectively, the evolving culture is considered to be actualized when nurses routinely embed the principles and processes of systematic inquiry to identify problems, create solutions, and strategically initiate evidence-based action plans and/or test creative ideas that were sparked or refined by evidence synthesis. One major limitation of the self-report approach to evaluation is an embedded bias on account of the nature of personal experiences and beliefs about a perceived threat and the consequence of a disrupted status quo.

Evaluating Competency and Productivity

The expected competencies correspond to a defined skill set and their consequent application during the EBP–innovation expedition. A Likert-type scale that ranges from awareness, beginning skills, independence, and mentorship is used to self-assess competency level. Productivity, on the other hand, is self-assessment that is based on both the amount and depth of the contribution or participation. The role of the leader and the member is appraised in parallel streams. This means that one has to make an evaluation based on the role that one assumed during the engagement.

Evaluating Satisfaction

This evaluation is intimately tied up with the evaluation of culture in view of personal impact of the DCI–innovation expedition. The evaluation is highly dependent on the degree to which present personal goals are met and the perception about implications to one's future plans. This area of evaluation may be likened to an assessment of patients' satisfaction and experiences with care, wherein the most recent experiences have the potential to cloud the true level of satisfaction. Nurses are therefore cued to engage in deep reflection about the overall experience, with the goal of communicating the areas that require improvement for a smooth sailing expedition.

REFLECTIONS

This chapter describes an approach for setting the stage for an EBP–innovation expedition. As EBP becomes the normative culture, the emergence of innovative behavior was observed in a number of nurses in the EBP community. DCI capitalized on the observed phenomenon and began setting the stage for activating EBP as a catalyst for accelerating innovative behavior. Along the expedition, the true enculturation of EBP and innovation in the nursing system and work flow continues to be challenged by various barriers.

A collective mindset that looks beyond barriers and sees through windows of opportunities to challenge the status quo is empowering for setting the stage for EBP and innovation. This creates a culture of openness and a community commitment to work together. In this community bedside nurses are tapping into the knowledge of genres of new graduates with academic preparation in EBP. Clinical experts are forging partnerships with DNP and PhD-prepared nurses. Operational nurse leaders are taking accountability in engaging clinical nurses in EBP. Executive nursing leaders are prioritizing resource allocation for EBP and innovation initiatives.

In a capsule, EBP is evidence synthesis plus implementation, whereas innovation is the generation of creative ideas plus implementation. The current focus of discourse and analysis has not always succeeded in implementation. The issues affecting evidence synthesis and generation of creative ideas begs equal attention. One of the biggest innovation challenges that remain, therefore, is creating a process to exploit the collective intelligence and creativity of not only the nursing community, but also the entire healthcare and broader community to identify possibilities and reveal openness for untried solutions. We need to set the sail and navigate a course on a fast track of an EBP–innovation revolution—from the crawl of the caterpillar to the flight a monarch butterfly.

REFERENCES

Alemi, F., & Gustafson, D. H. (2007). Introduction to decision analysis. In F. Alemi & D. H. Gustafson (Eds.), *Decision analysis for health care managers* (pp. 91–116). Chicago, IL: Health Administration Press.

American Association of Colleges of Nursing. (2008). Essentials of baccalaureate education for professional practice. Washington, DC: Author. Retrieved from http://www.aacn.nche.edu/education-resources/BaccEssentials08.pdf

American Nurses Association. (2002). Nursing's agenda for the future. Retrieved from http://infoassist.panpha.org/docushare/dsweb/Get/Document-1884/PP-2002-APR-Nsgagenda.pdf

Bennis, W. (2000). *Managing the dream: Reflections on leadership and change.* Cambridge, MA: Perseus.

Bick, D, & Graham, I. D, (2010). The importance of addressing outcomes of EBP. In D. Bick & I.D. Graham (Eds.). Evaluating the Impact of Implementing EBP. (pp. 1-14). Oxford, UK: Wiley-Blackwell

Bushe, G. (2012). Foundations of appreciative inquiry: History, criticism and potential. *AI Practitioner,* 8(14), 8–20. Retrieved from http://www.gervasebushe.ca/Foundations_AI.pdf

Chinn, P' L., & Kramer, M. K. (2011). Integrated theory and knowledge Development in nursing (8th ed.). St. Louis, MO: Elsevier.

Claridge, J. A., & Fabian, T. C. (2005). History and development of evidence-based medicine. *World Journal of Surgery, 29*(5), 547–553.

Davidson, A. W., Ray, M. A., & Turkel, M. C. (2011). *Nursing, caring, and complexity science: For human-environmental well-being.* New York, NY: Springer.

Doll, W.E. & Trueit, D. (2010). Complexity and the health care professions. *Journal of Evaluation in Clinical Practice, 16,* 841-848.

Dyer, J., Gregersen, H., & Christensen, C. M. (2011). *The innovators DNA: Mastering the five skills of disruptive innovators.* Boston, MA: Harvard Business Review Press.

Estabrooks, C. A. (1998). Will evidence-based practice make practice perfect? *Canadian Journal of Nursing, 30,* 15–36.

Fetterman, D. M., Kaftarian, S. J., & Wandersman, A. (1996). *Empowerment evaluation: Knowledge and tools for self-assessment and accountability.* London, UK: Sage.

Flodgren, G., Rojas-Reyes, M. X., Cole, N., & Foxcroft, D. R. (2012). Effectiveness of organizational infrastructures to promote evidence-based nursing practice. *Cochrane Database of Systematic Reviews, 2012*(2), 1–46. doi:10.1002/14651858.CD002212.pub2

Freire, P. (1970). *Pedagogy of the oppressed.* New York, NY: Seabury.

Goode, C. J., Lynn, M. L., McElroy, D., Bednash, G. D., & Murray, B. (2013). Lessons learned from 10 years of research post-baccalaureate nurse residency program. *Journal of Nursing Administration, 43*(2), 73–79.

Goode, C. J., & Williams, C. A. (2004). Post-baccalaureate nurse residency program. *Journal of Nursing Administration, 34*(2), 71–77.

Goodman, K. W. (2002). Foundations and history of evidence-based practice. In K. W. Goodman (Ed.), *Ethics and evidence-based medicine: Fallibility and responsibility in clinical science* (pp. 1–10). Cambridge, UK: Cambridge University Press. Retrieved from http://assets.cambridge.org/97805218/19336/excerpt/9780521819336_excerpt.pdf

Habermas, J. (1987). *The theory of communicative action* (Vol. 1). Boston, MA: Beacon.

Hill, L. A., Brandeau, G., Truelove, E., & Lineback, K. (2014). Collective genius. *Harvard Business Review, 6,* 94–102.

Institute of Medicine. (2000). *To err is human: Building a safer health system.* Washington, DC: National Academies Press.

Institute of Medicine. (2001). *Crossing the quality chasm: A new health system for the 21st century.* Washington, DC: National Academies Press.

Institute of Medicine. (2003). *Health professions education: A bridge to quality.* Washington, DC: National Academies Press.

Institute of Medicine. (2011). *The future of nursing: Leading change, advancing health.* Washington, DC: National Academies Press

Institute of Medicine. (2012). *Best care at lower cost: The path to continuously learning health care in America.* Washington, DC: National Academies Press.

Jalonen, H. (2012). The uncertainty of innovation: A systematic review of the literature. *Journal of Management Research, 4*(1), 1–47. Retrieved from http://www.macrothink.org/journal/index.php/jmr/article/view/1039/958

Lewin, K. (1946). Action research and minority problems. *Journal of Social Issues, 2,* 34–46.

Martin, R. L. (2011). The innovation catalyst. *Harvard Business Review, 89*(6), 82–87.

Polkinghorne, D. (2004). *Practice and the human sciences: The case for a judgment-based practice of care.* Albany: State University of New York Press.

Porter-O'Grady, T., & Malloch, K. (2010). *Innovation leadership: Creating the landscape of health care.* Sudbury, MA: Jones & Bartlett Learning.

Rogers, E. M. (2003). *Diffusion of innovations* (5th ed.). New York, NY: Free Press.

Sacket, D. L., Rosenberg, W. M. C., Muir Gray, J. M., Hayner, R. B., & Richardson, W. S. (1996). Evidence based medicine: What it is and what it isn't. *British Medical Journal, 312* (13), 71–72 .

Sadeghi-Bazargani, H., Tabrizi, J. S., & Azami-Aghdash, S. (2014). Barriers to evidence-based medicine: A systematic review. *Journal of Evaluation in Clinical Practice, 20,* 793–802. Retrieved from http://www.ncbi.nlm.nih.gov/pmc/articles/PMC2349778/pdf/bmj00524-0009.pdf

Sanares, D., & Heliker, D. (2002). Implementation of an evidence-based nursing practice model: Disciplined clinical inquiry. *Journal for Nurses in Staff Development, 18*(5), 233–240.

Sanares, D., Waters, P., & Marshall, D. (2007). Mainstreaming evidence-based practice. *Nurse Leader, 5*(3), 44–49.

Sanares-Carreon, D. (in press). From caterpillars to butterflies: Engaging nurse leaders in EBP reform. *Nursing Administration Quarterly.*

Sanares-Carreon, D., Waters, P., & Heliker, D. (2010). A framework for nursing clinical inquiry: Pathway toward evidence-based practice. In K. Malloch & T. Porter-O'Grady (Eds.), *Introduction to evidence-based practice in nursing and heath care* (2nd ed., pp. 31–56). Sudbury, MA: Jones & Bartlett

Sanares-Carreon D., Comeau O., Heliker D., et al. (2015). An educational pathway to fast track evidence-based practice at the bedside. *Journal for Nurses in Staff Development, 31*(1): E1-E6.

Schein, E. H. (2010). *Organizational culture and leadership* (4th ed.). San Francisco, CA: Jossey-Bass.

Seelos, C, & Mair, J. (2012). *What determines the capacity for continuous innovation in social sector organizations* (Rockefeller Foundation Report: Stanford PACS Center of Philanthropy and Civil Society). Retrieved from http://www.christianseelos.com/capacity-for-continuous-innovation_PACS_31Jan2012_Final.pdf

Smith, R., & Rennie, D. (2014). Evidence-based medicine: An oral history. *JAMA, 311*(4), 365–367. doi:10.1001/jama.2013.286182

Van Vlaenderen, H. (2001). Evaluating development programs: Building joint activity. *Evaluation and Program Planning, 24,* 343–352.

White, K. M., & Dudley-Brown, S. (2012). *Translation of evidence into nursing and health care practice.* New York, NY: Springer.

Williams, B., Perillo, S., & Brown, T. (2015). What are the factors of organizational culture in health care settings that act as barriers to the implementation of evidence-based practice? A scoping review. *Nurse Education Today, 35*(2), e34–e41.

Recognizing Pattern Changes as Evidence for Innovation Work

Sandra Davidson

CHAPTER OBJECTIVES

Upon completion of this chapter, the reader will be able to:

1. Compare and contrast the mechanistic and conversational perspectives of organizational structure.
2. Understand the philosophical basis for taking a complex relational view of health-care organizations.
3. Identify individual, team, and organizational patterns that can be useful evidence to inform innovation work.
4. Describe key relational strategies and activities that can enhance organizational conversations.

INTRODUCTION

Bernard Baruch once said, "if all you have is a hammer, everything looks like a nail." In large part, the industrial revolution, modernism, and scientific management (Taylor, 1911) shaped the structure of our organizations for most of the 20th century. Organizations were built and managed like machines. This mechanistic thinking permeated every aspect of organizational life, right down to the kinds of conversations held: we talk about pulling the lever, moving the needle, scaling down, and re-engineering (Booth, Zwar & Harris, 2013; Laloux, 2014). Indeed, to rephrase Baruch, if all we have is a machine, everything looks like it can, and should, be automated. However well-intentioned this efficiency-driven view may be, we know that organizations are made up of people, not cogs. In health care, we can go even further to say that our organizations are made up of people whose work it is to help and heal other people. Many of us have experienced firsthand the perils and pitfalls of working within mechanistic systems inherited and perpetuated by the status quo of the 20th century. Is it any wonder that such workplaces can feel cold, impersonal, and isolating? Or that our patients can feel that they are treated more like a number (or a diagnosis) than a person?

Thanks to paradigmatic plurality and the postmodern movement (there is more than one right worldview; there are multiple truths) we now have a wide range of organizational metaphors, theories, and models that may be more useful and helpful for leaders in health care. I might also add that there is a growing evidence base that can inform our application of organizational and leadership theory into practice. This chapter will focus on describing and exploring healthcare organizations from the relational and complexity informed perspective that we will call the organization as conversation (Booth et al., 2013; Gergen, 2015; Suchman, 2011). This emerging perspective is rooted in social construction theory, complex responsive processes, and pragmatism. From this perspective, paying attention to dialogic patterns that are formed within the organization can be useful evidence to both inform and evaluate innovation work. Strategies and behaviors, that leaders at every level of the organization can use to support innovation from a complex relational stance, will also be shared.

WORLDVIEWS: IF WE BELIEVE IT, WE SEE IT

Our perspectives and beliefs about organizational life are predicated on our overall worldview. A worldview is a connected set of beliefs and assumptions about the form and function of the world coupled with beliefs about how best to investigate it (Kuhn, 2007). The predominant paradigm and habits of thought about organizations are still largely rooted in the mechanistic, empirical, and rational ways of being. As such, objectivity and linearity also form the ways we conduct research as we seek to understand the world around us. This has implications for what we believe counts as useful or strong evidence. One of the clearest examples of this is the well-known levels of evidence pyramid (**Figure 10-1**).

Now, I must be clear here. I am not taking an antiempirical stance in this chapter. Far from it. There are many clinical and research questions that are best answered by the use of rigorous quantitative and empirical methods. And indeed, the levels of evidence pyramid does provide a useful framework for clinicians to use in appraising and making evidence-informed decisions about patient care. We will further explore the concepts of evidence and evidence-based practice (EBP) later in the chapter. For now, let us acknowledge that EBP is always enacted within an organizational context (primary care office, hospital system, public health district). Often, in such complex organizational settings, initiatives fail and preferred outcomes are not achieved, even when the evidence initiatives were based on suggestions

Figure 10-1   Pyramid of evidence

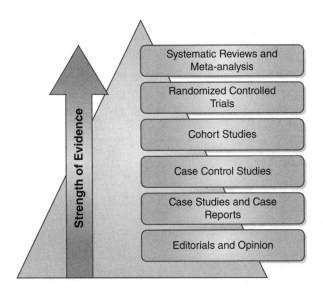

that improvement should occur. From a complex relational perspective, there is much more to EBP than simply following the steps outlined in the latest clinical practice guideline. However, given our proclivity for viewing the world as linear, rational, and mechanistic, we seek to control and minimize the extraneous factors that constantly confound our plans. We often do not pay attention to the ever-present relational dynamics that seem to defy our best planning. Hassan (2014) used an excellent analogy for why empirical, rational, and predictive methods often do not work in complex adaptive contexts. "Imagine the difference between throwing a rock and throwing a live bird" (2014, p 19). To take this a step further to the complex relational view, imagine releasing a flock of doves from a box, like at an outdoor wedding (**Figure 10-2**).

Each dove is an individual, but it also relates to all the other doves. They must negotiate and coordinate their movements and actions as they take to the sky. There is no predetermined, predictable path that every dove follows. Granted, they may all share the goal of returning safely to their roost, but each dove takes its own path. There are the doves that are first out of the box and lead the way home, and others that might need encouragement to take flight and leave the box. So too are our organizations made up of individuals that are in relation to each other. We must negotiate and coordinate our actions to reach our common goals. Personality, free will, and choice are ever present as we go about our day-to-day work together.

Figure 10-2 Relational complexity takes flight

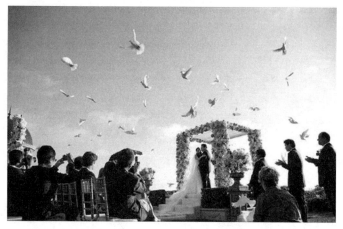

Courtesy of Pamla Wright

The Value of Seeing Differently

For every complex problem, there is an answer that is clear, simple, and wrong.

—H. L. MENCKEN

Widening our perspectives to consider more than just the dominant worldview presents different ways of thinking about human experience, and this often counters many of our taken-for-granted habits of thought. Because of this, it can be met with skepticism and scrutiny in both practice and research communities. However, it is precisely this novelty that makes complexity informed and relational perspectives useful frameworks for innovation in health care. As Kuhn suggests, "That complexity counters many commonplace assumptions means that there can be a re-noticing of ourselves and our world: a re-thinking and questioning of taken for granted, no longer tested assumptions" (2007, p. 160).

Many analogies have been used to describe and explain what happens in organizations. As we mentioned previously, the predominant view of the 20th century was organization as machine. **Table 10-1** presents an overview of three different organizational perspectives. Organization as organism is a popular perspective that has been applied and developed in the latter part the 20th century and early 21st century. I have included it here as a midpoint perspective between the machine and conversational perspectives because it illustrates the incremental shifts toward embracing organizational complexity rather than controlling or ignoring it. However, this perspective still retains many of the linear and rational characteristics of the machine model. The third view is organization as conversation. The remainder of this chapter will focus on this perspective.

Table 10-1   Comparison of Organizational Perspectives

	Organization as Machine	Organization as Organism	Organization as Conversation
Theoretical perspectives	Newtonian physics, industrialization and scientific management	Complex adaptive systems, biological sciences, behaviorism	Social construction theory, complex responsive processes, pragmatism
Structural characteristics	Linear, hierarchical, closed system	Boundaried, organized functionally, aim is homeostasis, open system	Cocreated, pattern making, socially constructed and shared
Change is . . .	Controllable, introduced to a system from outside (cause and effect)	Evolutionary, adaptive, observable, and measurable	Local, emergent, participatory, and pragmatic (getting things done together)
System is . . .	Simple	Complex	Complex and relational
Leadership is . . .	Top-down, positional, exerted from outside the system, strategy and plan driven	Decentralized, formal and informal, enacted from various positions but still considered outside the system, outcome driven	Reflexive, enacted in participation with others in day-to-day interactions, relationship driven

ORGANIZATION AS CONVERSATION

In this section we will set the stage for thinking about and working within organizations using a complex relational perspective. The foundations of this perspective are found in complexity science (specifically complex responsive processes). The complexity principles of emergence and self-organization are the basis of understanding organizations as formed by patterns of meaning and patterns of relating (Stacey, 2012; Suchman, 2011).

Patterns of meaning are specific themes that exist in an organization. For example, an organization's mission and vision serve as a pattern of meaning that informs the collective organizational identity. A mission driven by fiscal responsibility and profitability would influence the priorities and actions of every individual within the organization in a way that would be very different than an organization with a mission focused on patient safety.

Patterns of relating, or how people interact with each other, form an organization's culture (Suchman, 2011). There may be habits of relating, such as a preference for e-mail communication, that result in specific patterns of relating that are different from that of an organization with a preference for face-to-face conversations. Maybe there are rituals around meetings (the unit manager always sits at the head of the table, or it is taboo to be late for a team meeting). These examples of patterns of relating illustrate culturally embedded understandings about power dynamics that are ever present in organizations (Davidson, 2015).

Emergence is an important aspect for leaders to understand. The patterns just described are emergent and evanescent. That is, they are enacted in the moment-to-moment interactions among people as they go about their work. As such, patterns must be perpetually re-created in each interaction or they cease to be. The flipside of this is that with every interaction or conversation, there is an opportunity for a new pattern to emerge. The living present is filled with potential—to re-create and perpetuate existing patterns or to bring into existence new ones.

To summarize, an organization can be understood as a temporary stabilization of themes and habits that serve to organize the experience of being together that takes place locally and in the living present (Fonseca, 2002). Organizations are paradoxical places where ideology and values-based human relating can manifest both stability and the potential for transformation (Booth et al., 2013). Making sense of what happens within organizations from a conversational stance necessitates a very different view of leadership. If leadership does not reside in the realm of planning, command and control, or otherwise exerting power to effect change in the system, what is the role of leaders?

Relational Leading

Just as the mainstream mechanistic, linear, and rational ways of being have shaped our organizations, so have they shaped our concept of leadership. A leader is traditionally thought of as an individual who is separate and stands isolated from others. From this perspective, a leader is an individual who possesses internal knowledge about how to be a leader or the personal ability to apply leadership skills to a given situation. Much of the discourse and literature on leadership is based on this perspective. Of course, there is the long-standing premise that leaders are made, not born, and its corollary, some people just have "it" and are born leaders. Both of these arguments are based on rationalist or bounded assumptions that "leadership potential resides within the individual person" (Gergen, 2009, p. 331). As I asserted in previous sections, if we choose to look at our world from the lens of relational complexity, we find different answers. Exploring the concept of leadership is no different.

Gergen observed, "None of the qualities attributed to good leaders stands alone. Alone, one cannot be inspiring, visionary, humble or flexible. These qualities are achievements of a co-active process in which others' affirmation is essential" (2009, p. 331). Fonseca (2002) suggested that an organization is a temporary stabilization of themes or habits that serve to organize our experience of being together. In essence, an organization creates the context in which the relational process of leadership happens. From the complex relational stance, leadership patterns emerge in the relational process that occurs among people in the living present, where the potential for novelty and change always exists (Walker, 2006).

If leadership is a relational or conversational process that emerges in the living present, then the essential role of the leader is to be present and participatory from moment to moment in his or her interactions with others. Leadership becomes improvisational in nature, rather than adhered to learned tactics or skills. Walker (2006) suggested that it may be more appropriate to speak of leadership potential rather than skill; potential carries with it a sense of movement, whereas skill seems to be a static construct.

New language is a powerful tool for creating the potential for novelty and change. If we want to transform leadership into something beyond our mainstream, mechanistic, and boundaried understanding, a change of language may be useful in generating new ways of leading. Gergen suggested that we consider replacing leadership with relational leading:

Abandoned are the endless and often contradictory lists of what it takes to be a good leader. In their place we find increasing emphasis on collaboration, empowerment, dialogue, horizontal decision making, sharing, distribution, networking, continuous learning and connectivity . . . While leadership denotes the characteristics of an individual, relational leading refers to the ability of persons in relationship to move with engagement and efficacy into the future . . . To be sure, individuals may be designated as leaders, but the process of leading is ultimately relational. (Gergen, 2009, p. 333)[1]

---

[1] By permission of Oxford University Press, USA. www.oup.com

If we start with this perspective of relational leading, what are the patterns of meaning and patterns of relating that generate the conditions for relational leadership? How do we individually and collectively engage relationally in ways that move us toward the preferred future of health care?

COMPLEX RELATIONAL BEING

This section will present an overview of the philosophical roots and key concepts that support the complex relational way of understanding organizations. These iconoclastic ideas provoke us to reconsider and reimagine our organizations and the ways in which we contribute (or not) to the themes and habits that constitute them. Taking a relational perspective of healthcare organizations is a bit like putting on X-ray goggles. We may be looking at the same people, environment, and challenges, but suddenly we see new focal features and aspects that were previously obscured from our sight. The beneath-the-surface view opens new possibilities and the potential for transformation.

Ways of Being Together and Making Meaning

The complex relational viewpoint builds on the theoretical foundations set forth by American sociologist and pragmatist George Herbert Mead (1863–1931). Mead's concepts of gesture and response are important in understanding the process of meaning making within organizations. Meaning is born out of the experience of conversation that occurs in the living present. The abstractness of human interaction can be more fully understood if we choose to view human interaction as the unit of analysis rather than viewing the system or its agents as the unit of analysis, as is the case in systems thinking. Meaning arises in the living present, as do choice and intention (Stacey, Griffin, & Shaw, 2000). Our choices and intentions in the present moment are shaped by our past experiences.

Meaning, then, is a social construction. According to Mead (1934), meaning arises in the gesture–response interactions among people that occur in a medium of symbols. A gesture is a kind of symbol (an emotion, personal reflection, or explanation, for example). Mead understood the word *symbol* to be derived from the Greek words *symbolon* (a mark or token) and *sym-ballein* (thrown together). A gesture made by one person that is responded to by another is a symbol (Mead, 1934; Stacey, 2001). Meaning is created in the *response* to the gesture. This triadic relationship of gesture–response–meaning arises out of the social act of communicating (**Figure 10-3**). As such, any collaborative human interaction is made possible through the use of symbols. Together, the gesture and response symbolize or constitute a meaning.

Figure 10-3   Gesture, meaning, response triad

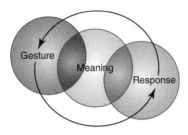

In this way of conceptualizing meaning making, knowledge is not something that resides in the minds of individuals; it is created through the social act of relating. As such, knowledge is perpetually created by people interacting with each other in the living present. From a complex relational perspective, knowledge is simply the thematic patterns that emerge to organize the experience of the ongoing process of relating (Stacey, 2001). Mead purported that the self and society are always co-occurring. If this is so, it becomes pointless to ask whether organizations learn or people learn because the process is the same (Stacey, 2001). Human interaction or the process of responsive relating is simply people weaving together their actions to accomplish joint endeavors successfully (Stacey, 2001).

Power Dynamics: Complex and Relational

All human interactions and processes of relating include elements of power. Drawing on the work of Elias (1998), Stacey (2006) viewed power not as something possessed by any one person, but as a feature of all human relating: "In order to form, and stay in, a relationship with someone else one cannot do whatever one wants. As soon as we enter into relationships, therefore, we constrain and are constrained by others . . . we also enable and are enabled by others" (2006, p. 134).

Power is this enabling and constraining way of relating. The balance of power is often tilted in favor of one person based on the need the two individuals may have for one another, and this may shift over time or vary by context (Stacey, 2006). If we frame power relations in terms of Mead's idea that the individual and social are at once forming and formed by each other, there is no distinction between I and we identities (individual and social). Power relationships form groupings or patterns in which some are included and others are excluded. These patterns evoke a powerful feeling of belonging in which an individual identifies and resonates with the we of the group (Elias, 1998). Again, if the I and we are inseparable, then the larger patterns of inclusion and exclusion reflect the complex, conflictual, and cooperative patterns of power relating (Stacey, 2006). Understanding power relating within an organization as the patterns of inclusion and exclusion that create and sustain relationships is key.

If organizations are temporary stabilizations of a set of themes and habits (Fonseca, 2002), then the patterns of power are always present within organizations. Elias (1998) suggested that power figurations are sustained by ideologies, which in turn are sustained by gossip and processes of shame. Furthermore, power relationships and an organization's dominant patterns are made to feel natural and are stabilized by the unconscious and underlying ideology (Stacey, 2006). Ideology is a patterning process in which themes of inclusion and exclusion are perpetually reproduced. It follows, then, that "ideology exists only in the speaking and acting of it" (Stacey, 2001, p. 153). Often, the speaking of ideology takes the form of gossip in day-to-day interactions, as described by Stacey:

> *The gossip builds layer upon layer of value-laden binary pairs such as clean-dirty, good-bad, honest-dishonest, energetic-lazy and so on. In less obvious form, the same point applies to the "in-out" dynamic created by particular ways of talking, for example, talking in terms of complexity, in terms of psychoanalysis, in terms of management control, and so on. Such gossip and other ways of talking attribute "charisma" to the powerful and "stigma" to the weak, so reinforcing power differences. (2001, p. 153)*

Within organizations, the enabling and constraining forces that people use often take the form of emotions. Shame, jealousy, empathy, and compassion are all interwoven into the complex pattern of themes that make up organizations. Cooperation, conflict, politics, and negotiation are all elements of ordinary everyday communication that are lived out moment to moment (Stacey, 2006). Paying attention to the ordinary watercooler conversations and sidebar comments at staff meetings provides a way to understand the patterns of power and ideology within organizations.

Case Example: Paging Dr. Frick

Organizations are defined by the stories that are told. Stories are expressions of our shared culture that can either stabilize (perpetuate) or potentially transform an organization. I see this clearly represented and supported by the organization as conversation perspective. Humans are, by nature, social beings, and storytelling is a powerful means to communicate, share, and perpetuate the values and norms (ideology) of any given culture. I first remember experiencing the power of stories to shape culture when I was a new nurse.

As many beginning nurses do, I worked on a casual basis on several different units within the same hospital. One weekend I picked up a Friday evening shift on a medical unit and then a Saturday evening shift on the adjacent surgical unit. Back in the early 1990s, overhead paging was still one of the most effective ways to contact physicians and surgeons who were on rounds throughout the hospital. In this particular hospital, nurses and other staff members who needed to reach a physician would call down to the switchboard, and the operator (who had a lovely English accent, by the way) would then page the physicians overhead along with the extension numbers that they were to call.

On Friday evening, two physicians, Dr. Frick and Dr. Hebert, were needed by staff of the same unit. The operator announced, "Dr. Frick and Hebert please call 4295." Of course, to the casual listener it sounded like she was paging Dr. Frick'in Hebert! I happened to be at the nursing station on the medical unit writing in a patient chart at the time. Several of my nurse colleagues and the unit clerk were also there. After hearing the page, we all looked at each other and laughed. One of the nurses said, as she continued smiling, "I know Dr. Hebert seems serious, but he has a great sense of humor—I bet he's getting a good laugh out of that!" Several others at the desk nodded in agreement, smiling, and then we went about our work.

The next evening, I was waiting for report to start on the surgical unit. One of the nurses burst into the room and said, "Did you hear that overhead page last evening?" She went on to say, "I heard that Dr. Hebert was so mad that he went down to the switchboard and told that poor operator off!" She continued by saying, "He's still on call this evening, so we'd better be careful not to tick him off!" I was stuck by the two very different interpretations of this event. On the medical unit, it was a story of an honest mistake, which anyone with a sense of humor could easily laugh off. On the surgical unit, the story was of retaliation, belittlement, and fear of being the next person to incur the wrath.

As I continued to work on both units over the next 6 months, I came to realize that the interpretations of this event were emblematic of the overall culture of each unit. On the surgical unit, everyone always felt on edge, and there was an intense fear of making mistakes. When a mistake inevitably happened, it meant that humiliation and shame followed for the unfortunate perpetrator. In contrast, the medical unit was a place of teamwork, camaraderie, and learning. If a mistake happened, the entire team supported the people involved, and it was an opportunity to improve our communication and processes. Eventually, I was offered a regular position on both units. I bet you can guess which one I chose.

Questions

1. Do you have an example organizational story that you have experienced? What is it?
2. Think about the last time you were in the cafeteria or lunch room with colleagues. What were the themes of the conversations? What might this tell you about the culture?
3. How might you change the story within your work unit, organization, or group? Think about how you could purposefully use patterns of relating, patterns of meaning, and new language to introduce ways of being (for the better!).

Living Present: Here and Now

From a complex relational perspective, the future is unknowable and therefore unpredictable (**Figure 10-4**). This means that many of our traditional ways of planning and communicating within organizations (such as long-range planning; setting carefully projected targets; and executing detailed implementation guides) are not particularly useful or relevant from a complexity view. Rather, the point of impact and influence that we have in organizations occurs in the living present (here and now). The living present provides a starting point for conceptualizing causality differently. Rather than thinking of causality as we ordinarily do, in a linear way (such as an organization moving toward a mature state or realizing a prechosen goal), from a complex relational aspect the future is under perpetual construction rather than predetermined. This means that human interaction that takes place in the living present perpetually modifies and shapes the future based on the more-or-less immediate past. The past, present, and future are all mutually enacted in the living present. Although the future may be unpredictable and unknowable as our day-to-day conversations move us into the future, it becomes somehow more recognizable (Stacey et al., 2000).

Strategic Plan or Conversation Guide?

As discussed previously, our individual choices in everyday dialogue that build upon organizational patterns of meaning and relating are the crux of organizational change and potential. Taking up this premise (that relationships and coaction that take place in the living present are the inflection point for organizational change) means that we must reexamine the utility and value of long-range and strategic planning.

Almost every organization is engaged in some type of long-range or cyclical strategic planning process (e.g., 5-year plan). This practice is deeply rooted in our linear and mechanistic view of organizations. Of course, from an organization as machine stance, it is reasonable to have a group of managers, operators, and leaders set targets and, with some degree of certainty, be able to predict outcomes. Imagine that a line manager in a factory wants to produce a million widgets in the next 3 years. Based

Figure 10-4   The future emerges as we move toward it

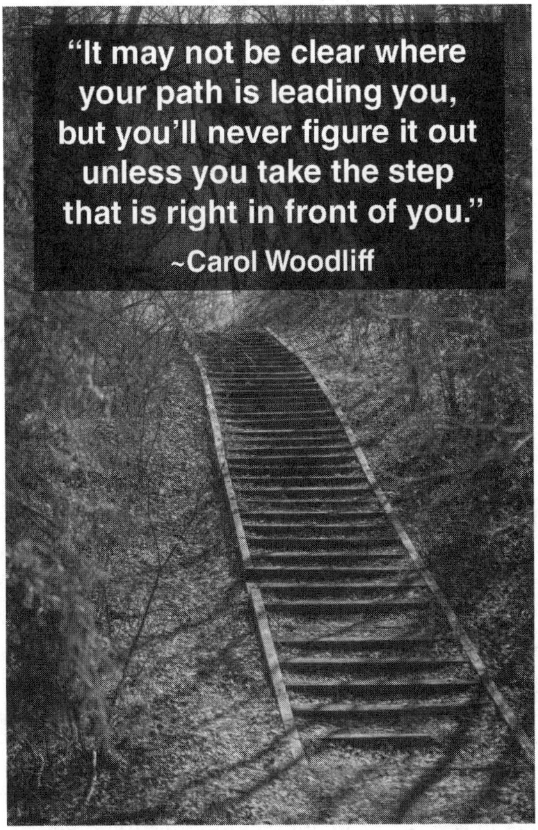

"It may not be clear where your path is leading you, but you'll never figure it out unless you take the step that is right in front of you."
~Carol Woodliff

Used with permission. Photo credit: James Davidson

on the number of widget machines available and the speed (rate of production) and availability of raw materials, she determines that each machine will need to run for at least 12 hours per day with a production rate of 10 widgets per hour to meet this long-range target. The application of this type of mechanistic planning to human organizations is the legacy we retain from Taylor's *Scientific Management* (1911). Complex human organizations are not predictable, nor are they linear, yet we still feel compelled to create 5- and even 10-year strategic plans born of a management theory that is more than 100 years old.

Stacey (2006) proposed that from a complex relational stance, strategic plans are grand organizational fantasies that function primarily as social defenses against the anxiety of not knowing and not being in control. Managing our collective human anxieties and fears about the unknown and the uncontrollable provides a very plausible rationale for why strategic planning has endured. From the organization as conversation stance, at best, strategic plans can function as an organizational conversation guide. That is, the goals, strategies, benchmarks, and projections of the organization that are detailed in such a plan may be taken up by local teams and form the basis for dialogue about how the local team will contribute to and act in ways to move the organization closer to the future aspirations. At worst, strategic plans can blind individuals and teams to the possibility of more generative and improvisational behaviors that might emerge. Recall that design and planning at an organization-wide scale (generalizations) can only ever be enacted in local, specific, and particular contexts (Stacey, 2006).

Grand organizational plans often come in conflict with local emergent themes, expectations, and intentions, and thus strategic planning, when taken too seriously or enacted militantly, can hamper team functioning. The conflict that can arise between the strategic plan (what we are supposed to do over the next 5 years) and the on-the-ground realities (what is really happening here and now) must then be negotiated by the team, and this can mean precious time and energy are wasted on figuring out what to do when things do not go according to plan. The question that begs is how do we organize and coordinate our work if not through planning? Stacey suggested that grandiose planning does not mean abandoning purposeful actions and movement toward organizational improvement. "It simply means taking a humbler stance and working realistically in our own local interactions to improve what we can" (2012, p. 127).

Our ways of talking together can enliven and engage us or control and alienate us. Becoming more aware of our organizational habits, patterns, and norms enables us to purposefully choose the ways in which we talk, listen, and attend to each other. The next section will introduce ideas that can help us focus on local interactions in the living present.

The only thing we know about the future is that it will be different. Trying to predict the future is like trying to drive down a country road at night with no lights while looking out the back window. The best way to predict the future is to create it.

—PETER DRUCKER

WORKING LIVE: IMPROVISATION

Our ability to pay attention to our experiences with others in the living present becomes a critical skill in organizational life from a complex relational stance. The capacity to dwell in the present moment and to respond in emergent ways to what is taking form is something we can all develop. To many of us, this way of being is commonly understood as the ability to improvise. In organizational contexts, improvisation is perhaps less theatrical in nature than the metaphor of jazz musicians or an improv comedy performance. Rather, it is more the distinction between the raw and honest quality of witnessing a live (real-time) interview and watching a prerecorded and skillfully edited interview (Shaw, 2006). The latter has a hollow and rehearsed quality to it that is less authentic.

In any organization, there are well-used and routinized scripts (patterns of meaning and relating) that organize and stabilize our day-to-day ways of being together. This might take the form of a standardized clinical pathway, for example. In some instances, we may not want novel patterns to be created. In health care there will always be situations where precision, replicability, and a high degree of reliability are warranted and valuable (Suchman, 2011). One example is the surgical sign-in, time-out, sign-out checklist (World Health Organization, 2008). Such standardized scripts are imperative for patient safety. However, we must also realize that each time a script is enacted, there are subtle differences because of the unique emergent and contextual conditions. This means that team members are paying attention to the present moment and adapting and modifying their interactions in a way that is appropriate to the unique current situation. This is different than the dogmatic (unthinking) adherence to a protocol that becomes robotic and acontextual.

Imagine that a surgical team is in the midst of the presurgical time out, and they are introducing themselves (and their roles) to Mr. Johnson (the patient). The nurse begins to pick up on nonverbal cues from Mr. Johnson (he looks confused and does not seem to understand what they are saying). The nurse then realizes that Mr. Johnson has already removed his hearing aids and cannot hear the team members. The nurse adapts to this context by handing Mr. Johnson his hearing aids so he can put them in for a moment to ensure that he hears and understands what is being said to him. This is different than a surgical team that is simply going through the motions and introducing themselves to the patient, per the checklist, and failing to pick up on Mr. Johnson's cues that he does not understand what they are saying.

Discussion

Improvisation is very commonly linked with creative and artistic endeavors, such as jazz music and improvisational theater. How might you learn from and adopt best practices and strategies from these genres and use them in your own conversations and relationships?

Reflect on the concepts that have been discussed in this chapter, such as the following:

- Organization as conversation
- Working live (present moment)
- Innovation
- Relational leading

(*continued*)

What opportunities do you see in your own practice for integrating these concepts and practices? What challenges might you face in adopting such practices? What are some ways you might mitigate these challenges?

Paying attention to and discerning the most appropriate patterns (stabilizing or emergent) for any given situation is a form of improvisation. It simply means that we need to tap into the present moment (the gestures being made) and respond in a way that creates resonant meaning for those involved. This is the essence of working live; there is no rote or automatic default setting or response. Instead, is it about actively sensing the future as it emerges in the present moment. Sometimes that calls for perpetuation of existing patterns in our meaning making; other times we are called to break a pattern and open up the possibility for new ways of being. Our capacity for this type of improvisation is enhanced as we seek to develop and use practical judgment (Stacey, 2012). Practical judgment is made possible by reflexivity.

The goal of reflexivity is to be able access and use knowledge and situational awareness in real time to respond to the emerging present moment. Over time, and with practice, our ability to be in the moment and respond improvisationally within it (reflexivity) becomes familiar to us, and we begin to build practical judgment.

This is similar to what has been described as *habitus* in healthcare settings—the situated use of tacit knowledge within an emergent and complex clinical situation (Benner, Sutphen, Leonard & Day, 2010; Bourdieu, 1990). Likewise, Benner, Hooper-Kyriakidis, and Stannard (1999) described the concepts of thinking in action and reasoning in transition as essential components in the development of clinical expertise. Thinking in action is the pattern of thought in action that is directly tied to responding to the demands of a changing situation and noticing the nuances of the interaction in the present moment (Benner et al., 1999). This is again similar to the ideas of working live and developing practical judgment that are being presented here, although we are extending and connecting these ideas beyond clinical experiences to a wider organizational and leadership context.

The work of relational leaders is to use practical judgment and to be able to distinguish among situations where stability and reliability need to be assured and other situations that call for novelty and creative emergence, then to be able to act accordingly.

Otto Scharmer's *Theory U* (2007) is an excellent resource for anyone seeking additional description and guidance about how to do and be in complex relational organizations. **Table 10-2** summarizes Scharmer's five movements that in essence move us through the U. An additional column highlights some of the concepts and relational competencies from this chapter that resonate with each of Scharmer's movements.

In the previous discussion we have talked about improvisation within complex relational organizations. In essence, working live is a particular way of being and relating in our day-to-day interactions that opens up the potential for meaning to emerge from the

Table 10-2   Scharmer's Five Movements

Theory U Movements	Descriptions (Scharmer, 2007)	Complex Relational Competencies and Activities
Coinitiating	Listen to what life calls you to do, connect with people and contexts related to that call. Convene constellations of core people then coinspire common intention.	• Mindfulness and reflection • Relational leading • Creating new local patterns of relating • Enacting generative ways of talking and making meaning
Cosensing	Teams take deep-dive learning journeys that bring them to places of greatest potential. Observe and listen with an open heart, mind, and will.	• Relational leading • Dwelling in the living present • Cocreating new local patterns of meaning • Reflexivity, practical judgment
Copresencing	Dwell in a place of individual and collective stillness. Open up to creativity and presence, and link to the future that wants to emerge.	• Relational leading • Dwelling in the living present • Mindfulness • Improvisation and reflexivity
Cocreating	Build landing strips for the future by prototyping living microcosms to explore the future by doing.	• Creating and experimenting with novel patterns of meaning and relating locally • Innovation through emergence and improvisation
Coevolving	Codevelop a larger innovation ecosystem that connects people and actions beyond boundaries. Seeing and acting from the whole.	• Relational leading • Moving local innovation to the wider organization • Stabilizing new themes and patterns of meaning and relating (become the organizational ways of being)

living present. In the sections that follow, we will delve deeper into two aspects of relational being that influence how patterns of relating emerge: ways of talking and ways of listening.

Ways of Talking

As we have previously discussed, our ways of speaking in organizations are patterns that can reinforce and stabilize culture. Social norms and values are taken up and become the ideology of the larger social group. However, humans possess the wondrous capacity for free will and choice. This means that each conversation presents an opportunity for reinforcing existing group values and norms, or for novelty and change.

Over time, the choices we make in daily conversations result in a pattern of speech or habitual ways of talking.

How aware are we, from moment to moment, of how we are speaking? It is easy in the busyness of our work to fall into familiar and comfortable language and to then perpetuate and reify patterns we may not consciously intend (or want). By contrast, by being aware of our words and choosing language intentionally, we can purposefully perpetuate themes and ideology that are resonant and useful to us; or we can take up new language and new ways of speaking with others that are more authentic and meaningful. Language serves to form, and can transform, meaning. Emergent new meaning can transform our ways of being.

From a traditional mechanistic view of organizations, language is used in particular ways. Skilled leaders have always used language to persuade, motivate, and even control. The art of rhetoric has been employed in a vast array of contexts, from political campaigns to marketing a new breakfast cereal to large-scale social change initiatives. Even the daughter of friends skillfully used rhetoric to sway her parents in her quest to acquire a family dog.

"Rhetoric may be understood as the techniques of prose composition or speech which enable one to influence the judgment or feelings of others. It is the art of using language effectively" (Stacey, 2012, p. 119). So, then, what does rhetoric look like when we view the organization as conversation? Here are some rhetorical devices for consideration (**Table 10-3**).

Table 10-3   Rhetorical Devices in Organizations

Rhetorical Device	Traditional Hierarchical	Complex Relational
Influence the path of a conversation	Let's stay on target here	What might that look like?
Destabilize	There is no appetite for this	Does this process add value?
Construct urgency	There is a short turnaround	The faster we share this with other teams, the sooner all patients will benefit
Metaphor	Organization as machine	Organization as conversation
Irony	Doing more with less	Focusing on what works, helps us find energy to fix what is wrong
Influence beliefs about what is true or real	Evidence shows	This worked for us

Modified from Stacey, R. (2012). *Tools and techniques of leadership and management: meeting the challenge of complexity.* New York: Routledge.

These examples serve as a starting point to assist us in being more aware of the language we choose and how we use rhetoric in our organizations. If we take up the complex relational view of organizations, the power to transform our workplace comes from the quality of relationships that we engage in. We are at once formed by and forming the future as we talk about it together.

Ways of Listening

Communication is a collaborative process. It is enabled by both gestures (speaking and nonverbal cues, such as facial expressions and hand movements) and responses to those gestures. Taken together, gestures and responses create a kind of collective understanding, or shared meaning. Listening, attending to the conversation, and generally paying attention is, of course, an important aspect of this collaborative communicative process. Recall the earlier discussion of meaning that emerges out of the communicative process of gesture and response. To offer our response, we must be attuned to the gestures that another person (or group of people) is making. Gestures include nonverbal cues and verbal communication. Sometimes it as crucial for us to listen between the words as it is to listen to the words themselves to fully apprehend the meaning that is being put forth.

Just as we can choose the way in which we talk and make use of language, we can also purposefully choose how we listen and attend in conversations. We all know how it feels when we have another person's full attention and to have them listen to us intently and without distraction. We also know what it is like to be in conversation with someone who is preoccupied and only half listening to what we might be saying. The quality of these interactions is distinctly different. As such, the possibility of what might emerge from them is also divergent.

Table 10-4 illustrates a variety of ways of listening that can dramatically change the way in which meaning emerges in interactions. Of course, certain ways of listening may be more appropriate in some situations than others. We can work to develop practical judgment around our ways of listening by purposefully choosing to attend to conversations with a particular quality.

Mindfulness

Much of this chapter has discussed and stressed the importance of developing the capacity of dwelling in the living present. I am sure many readers have already been thinking about mindfulness because this is indeed a practice that focuses on being present moment to moment.

Mindfulness is described as the energy of being aware and awake in the present moment. To be mindful is to be present and at one with those around you and with

Table 10-4 Ways of Listening

Ways of Listening	Characteristics/Quality	Example
I already know that	Downloading. We listen to reconfirm habitual beliefs, judgments, and values. We deny or discount what does not fit with what we already know.	The evening news program reports that more stringent gun laws reduce violent crimes.
Wow, look at that!	Object-focused listening. Paying attention to facts and novel data that disconfirms current ways or thinking/doing. Empirical and cognitive in nature (objective).	A clinical expert is talking about the results of a new study that suggests a new treatment is beneficial.
I know how you feel	Empathic listening. Real dialogue; we are less aware of our own agenda and are focused more on connecting with the other person.	A patient is sharing his or her difficult but hopeful story of recovery from a life-threatening illness.
I cannot describe it, but I feel I am part of something larger	Emergent listening. Generative and focused on the emerging edge of the present moment. Listening from a state of flow or grace. Authentic, coming into being.	In a team meeting, you and your colleagues are in the zone and on your way to developing a shared vision for a patient-centered culture.

Modified from Scharmer, C. O. (2007). *Theory U: Leading from the future as it emerges.* Cambridge, MA: Society for Organizational Learning.

what you are doing (Plum Village, 2015). Developing one's mindfulness practice is an excellent opportunity to cultivate the ability to participate and contribute to the organization as conversation, not to mention that the significant physical and emotional benefits of mindfulness practice have been well researched and documented (Brown & Ryan, 2003; Grossman, Niemann, Schmidt & Walach, 2004).

Learning Activity: Exploring Meaning and Cocreation

1. Take a few minutes for each person in the group to individually read William Stafford's poem "A Ritual to Read to Each Other."
2. Reflect on the poem and try to relate it to the main concepts in this chapter, such as the following:
   - Organization as conversation
   - Patterns of relating

- Patterns of meaning
- Ways of talking, listening, and being
- Innovation
- Other concepts and ideas that emerge for you

3. If you wish, make a few notes about your reflections (there is no right or wrong here; focus on the personal meaning you make from the poem).

4. Have a volunteer from the group read the poem aloud as everyone else listens.

5. Take another moment for self-reflection. Did hearing the poem read aloud by another person change the way you experienced the words and meaning? If so, how? If you were the reader of the poem, what was your experience of reading the poem out loud to others?

6. Now invite group members to share in a discussion about the experience. Here are some questions that might guide the sharing:
   - What concepts from the chapter did individuals find reflected in the poem?
   - What past experiences, emotions, images, or questions surfaced in the reading of the poem?
   - Was it difficult to fully listen or attend to the person who was reading the poem aloud? Why or why not?
   - What is our experience (right now) of talking about this activity? What meaning are we making? How are we talking together? Are themes and patterns emerging?
   - Has the individual meaning we found in the poem shifted as a result of the group dialogue? How? Why?

"A Ritual to Read to Each Other"

If you don't know the kind of person I am
and I don't know the kind of person you are
a pattern that others made may prevail in the world
and following the wrong god home we may miss our star.

For there is many a small betrayal in the mind,
a shrug that lets the fragile sequence break
sending with shouts the horrible errors of childhood
storming out to play through the broken dyke.

And as elephants parade holding each elephant's tail,
but if one wanders the circus won't find the park,
I call it cruel and maybe the root of all cruelty
to know what occurs but not recognize the fact.

And so I appeal to a voice, to something shadowy,
a remote important region in all who talk:
though we could fool each other, we should consider—
lest the parade of our mutual life get lost in the dark.

For it is important that awake people be awake,
or a breaking line may discourage them back to sleep;
the signals we give—yes or no, or maybe—
should be clear: the darkness around us is deep

Source: William Stafford, "A Ritual to Read to Each Other" from Ask Me: 100 Essential Poems. Copyright © 1960, 2014 by William Stafford and the Estate of William Stafford. Reprinted with the permission of The Permissions Company, Inc. on behalf of Graywolf Press, Minneapolis, Minnesota, www.graywolfpress.org.

In this section we have explored the improvisational nature of working from a perspective of organization as conversation. To be present in the moment and to purposefully choose how we speak, listen, and generally show up in conversations are competencies that we can all work to cultivate. Earlier in the chapter we discussed the overall implications of what it means to take up a complex relational view in our day-to-day work, such as how this view leads us to think differently about leadership and planning. Now we will turn our attention to specific topics of EBP and innovation. Building on the ideas presented earlier in this chapter and our growing understanding of what it means to take up the complex relational perspective, let's explore further.

COMPLEX RELATIONAL HEALTH CARE: BEYOND INSTRUMENTALITY AND EITHER/OR THINKING

One of the critiques of the EBP movement is that it leads to cookbook medicine or overly prescriptive guidelines that do not leave room for consideration of context, patient preference, and other local conditions (Romana, 2006). Yet many of us who work in the area of complexity and innovation are often asked to provide tools or recipes to assist leaders and practitioners to make changes in their organizations (Patton, 2011; Stacey, 2012). The pull of our habitual mechanistic and empirical ways of talking and acting is strong. Indeed, part of the conundrum is language based (Gergen, 2009). What commonly understood language do we have that allows us to communicate to others that we are seeking guidance about how to do things differently? We ask for tools, guides, manuals, or instruments. The organization as conversation perspective can create an opportunity to introduce new ways of talking together and to create a new vernacular that move beyond tools to something else that resembles relational processes or ways of being, for example. What would it look like to be an evidence-based healthcare team? How can a complex relational lens assist us in this process?

Evidence and EBP

Clinical decisions should be informed by evidence, but it is the role and responsibility of the clinician to critically appraise and then apply that evidence in a manner that is contextually appropriate.

The application of evidence within a specific context brings us back to an earlier point about practical judgment. Recall that in practical judgment, two aspects are brought to bear. First, our past accumulation of knowledge (including research-based evidence), experience, and praxis provide us with an array of possible actions. Second, the unique contextual tapestry of the present moment must be sensed and discerned. Practical judgment happens at that point of convergence between the past and the emerging future in the living present. This way of understanding contextual appropriateness is intensely particularized (local). Before we move on to discuss how EBP happens in teams and organizations, let us take a step back to consider what counts as evidence?

What Counts as Evidence?

Kuhn (2007) reminds us that our predominant worldview is constituted of a connected set of beliefs and assumptions about the form and function of the world coupled with beliefs about how best to investigate it. As previously discussed, our Western habits of thought are still largely rooted in the mechanistic, positivistic, and rational ways of being. As such, objectivity and linearity also form the ways we conduct research as we seek to understand the world around us. This has implications for what we believe counts as useful or strong evidence.

We largely believe that measuring things (such as blood cells, antigens, outcomes, effects) means quantifying them. We seek to isolate, control, and randomize in an effort to ensure validity and rigor. In other words, the predominant discourse about evidence and what is good or bad, weak or strong, is based in rationalism, positivism, and linear thinking. This either/or way of thinking coupled with a strong affinity for valuing positivistic inquiry as strong, sets us up for a false dilemma between quantitative and qualitative inquiry. The false dilemma becomes this: if quantitative evidence is strong or good, then qualitative evidence must be weak or bad.

A more balanced view of these two types of inquiry is that they both have merit and value, and depending on the question or phenomena we seek to investigate, one may be more appropriate than another. Again, we arrive back at the issue of contextual appropriateness. Just as it would be considered inappropriate to design a phenomenological study to discern the efficacy of a new proton-pump inhibitor in an adult population, it is likewise as ludicrous to use a randomized control trial to determine the usefulness of an innovative care delivery model implemented in a multihospital care system. What might be more beneficial in addressing our complex, multifaceted, and often chaotic healthcare system is a healthy dose of both, and thinking.

This means that we are open to the idea that there may be more than one right way—multiple right answers. It provides a basis for synergy among ways of thinking. **Table 10-5** presents an array of research methods that align with two of the perspectives we have discussed in this chapter (organization as machine and organization as conversation). The table is meant to illustrate the value of both and thinking when it comes to evidence. Rather than falling prey to the false dilemma and feeling pressed to choose one or the other, imagine the possibility of holding both perspectives as different but useful and valuable.

To use a comfortable (albeit mechanistic) analogy, imagine that you are using a computer program, and one window provides you with a spreadsheet view of data with raw numbers and averages. Another window presents this same data organized by theme and category. Both views use the same data but portray it in very different (and useful) ways. The most complete understanding of the data or phenomena comes from being able to toggle between the two screens.

Let us return for a moment to the issue of language and specifically how it relates to evidence. Any one of us who has read research articles can attest that quantitative and qualitative researchers use different language. Many of us are fluent in one language, and some of us may even be bilingual. For discussion purposes, let us suppose that quantitative is the predominant language spoken in health care. How much more varied, challenging, interesting, and inclusive would our conversations be if we challenged ourselves to learn a new language? Granted, we may not become fluent, but seeking to understand, or at the very least appreciate, a different way of speaking can be very enriching.

EBP

A publication is a complex abstraction of the actual activities that were undertaken to address a research or clinical question. Based on the aims and focus of the journal, the

Table 10-5 Worldviews and Research Methods

Worldview	Resonant Research Methods
Modernism, rational, positivistic, empirical EBP Organization as machine	Rational scientific inquiry, such as experimental and quasi-experimental studies, randomized control trials, meta-analysis, case controlled studies
Complex relational Practice-based evidence Organization as conversation	Qualitative inquiry, such as grounded theory, action research, metasynthesis, phenomenology, narrative inquiry, organizational ethnography, authoethnography

value judgments made by the authors about what data and results are most important or salient, and the assessment of the peer reviewers and editors about the overall quality and merit of the study, the reader finally receives a 15–20 page glimpse into the complex undertaking of the original study.

After a study, systematic review, or meta-analysis is completed, published, and finds its way into the hands of practitioners, it enters a complex milieu of health care. There is a wide array of unpredictable and highly relational dynamics that influence the dissemination, implementation, and local value judgments about the usefulness and value of the evidence.

From a complex relational perspective, EBP is a specific theme that serves to help us organize our work together in health care. Specific patterns of relating and patterns of meaning emerge as the generalized theme of EBP is taken up. Here are some examples:

- Patterns of relating in EBP:
  - Journal clubs
  - Clinical practice guideline implementation committee
  - Latest clinical practice guidelines are embedded in electronic medical records
  - Dedicated computer on each unit for database searching (CINAHL, MEDLINE, and other EBP-related resources, such as clinical practice guidelines)
  - Shared governance monthly meeting agenda has a standing item for EBP updates
- Patterns of meaning in EBP:
  - Organizational vision is adapted to include a statement about high quality, evidence-informed care
  - Award is developed to recognize teams that exemplify or demonstrate excellent patient outcomes based on the use of EBP
  - Clinical staff who have completed an intensive 2-day training session about EBP are given unique lapel pins that identify them as EBP champions
  - EBP expert is invited to be keynote speaker at organization-wide clinical care conference

The specific patterns of meaning and relating are taken up (or not) in local clinical settings. Recall that the organizing theme and patterns are enacted or perpetuated only in the speaking and doing of them. What conversations happen at the local level that might stabilize the theme of EBP? Perhaps a well-respected nurse practitioner enthusiastically shares a new meta-analysis that supports the use of cognitive behavioral therapy as an effective secondary prevention strategy for patients with coronary heart disease. The team may then decide to explore cognitive behavioral therapy programs they could use in a pilot project.

All of the constituent aspects of complex responsive processes come into play in the complex, conflictual, relational activities of day-to-day organizational life. Consider the potential influence of the following aspects of complex responsive processes in relation to EBP:

- Ideology (organizational values and norms)
- Power dynamics (in group versus out group dynamics; processes of shame)
- Dance between stability and transformation of patterns and themes

Figure 10-5 illustrates evidence generation and the flow of evidence into a healthcare practice that eventually may be taken up and form EBP. The bottom half of the diamond represents the pyramid of evidence that we generally use to appraise, and make sense of condition-specific evidence. After this accumulated high-quality evidence reaches practice environments, it becomes the basis for practice (the floor of evidence).

Figure 10-5   EBP diamond

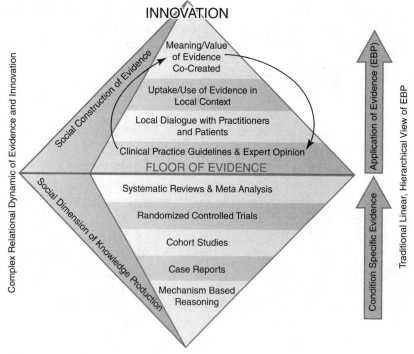

Data from Lefkowitz, W., & Jefferson, T. C. (2014). Medicine at the limits of evidence: The fundamental limitation of the randomized clinical trial and the end of equipoise. *Journal of Perinatology*, *34*(4), 249–251. doi:10.1038/jp.2013.172

What occurs, then, is the complex relational process that I have called the social construction of evidence. In other words, this is the process of making sense of evidence in local interactions, which is iterative and ongoing. Sometimes the sense-making process results in the introduction of novelty (local tweaking of evidence to better meet the needs of patients and providers) or stability (the adoption of EBP that the team experiences as valuable and useful).

In some instances, the process of meaning making may result in the identification of a gap in the evidence or a misalignment of the evidence to the practice setting. This may result in the introduction of novel conversations, themes, and patterns that can lead to transformation and innovation. Innovation, then, can represent practice-based evidence (Gergen, 2015). The creation of new knowledge and practices emerge as novel patterns and serve to organize our way of working together differently.

INNOVATION AS TRANSFORMATIONAL CONVERSATION

Earlier in this chapter we discussed both/and thinking as an alternative to the either/or false dilemma. Both and thinking can also enable innovation. The both of the statement recognizes the need and value of holding multiple perspective as useful and viable. The and is innovation. And represents the yet-to-be-formed idea, process, or product that may emerge from ongoing conversations and the introduction of sufficient novelty.

Fonseca (2002) suggested that innovation is the emergence of dissipative structures of meaning and that a certain level of misunderstanding (redundant diversity of meaning) is required for innovation to occur. Different ways of talking or new patterns of relating can lead to misunderstanding. In the ensuing conversations, people probe and question each other to attempt to stabilize meaning and understanding. In this process, new (shared, coconstructed) meaning may emerge that becomes a new pattern. This is the complex relational process of innovation.

Of course, there are a myriad of organizational dynamics that can either coalesce to enhance the potential for innovation or dynamics that conspire to minimize the potential for novelty and change. **Figure 10-6** illustrates the hurly-burly blend of relational dynamics from which innovation may emerge.

If I were to ask you to name someone you know who is innovative, you would probably quickly come up with a name. It might be someone from popular culture, like Steve Jobs or Mark Zuckerberg, or a historical figure such as Thomas Edison or Leonardo da Vinci. It might just as easily be Dr. Jones who works in the office two doors down from you. Whoever it is that came to mind, we could agree that innovators have a capacity or habitual ways of being that emancipate innovation. From a complex relational perspective, people who are skilled in innovation have habituated ways of talking

Figure 10-6   The mess of healthcare innovation

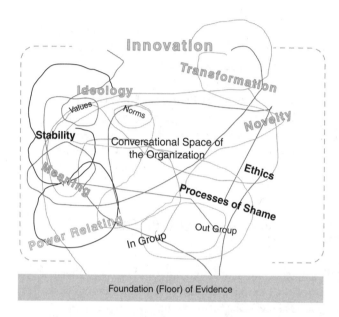

and attending in conversations. Further, they may leverage or create novel patterns of relating that bring together a constellation of coconspirators in a way that introduces sufficient novelty, misunderstanding, and diversity to produce innovation. Each one of us can build our capacity for innovation, for leadership, for improvisation. Many ideas for this have already been highlighted in this chapter (such as ways of listening and talking, and dwelling in the present moment). In the final section, we will discuss several ideas that relate specifically to our capacity for innovation.

SAY YES TO THE MESS

Frank Barrett wrote a wonderful book, *Yes to the Mess: Surprising Leadership Lessons from Jazz* (2012), that brings together his experience in organizational behavior and development and as a jazz pianist. In the book, he provides helpful perspectives and insights that leverage the capacity for improvisation in the service of relational leadership and innovation. Many of the principles in Barrett's book resonate with what we have discussed in this chapter.

Figure 10-6 illustrates the messiness of healthcare organizations as conversations. Looking at the figure may induce anxiety, uneasiness, and even panic in some readers. Often our initial reaction (based of our habitual mechanistic and linear ways of thinking) is to simplify, control, and organize. Stacey (2012) suggested that this craving for order and planning are a very human reaction to the anxiety evoked by not having control. Innovators, however, have developed a capacity to say yes to the mess and to dwell in the disorder and see the potential that emerges.

I am reminded of a technique that is used in improvisational theater. When a fellow actor leads with a line that you have no idea how to respond to initially, actors use the rhetorical device "yes, and . . .". This values and honors the creation from the other actor and allows an addition to the scenario without derailing, controlling, or closing off the potential for what might emerge from the collaboration. Yes, and . . . can be a useful way of talking together that invites emergence and allows us to build on the ideas of others.

Another attribute of skilled innovators is their ability to build and maintain trusting relationships. For people to be okay dwelling in the messy present moment, not knowing and even misunderstanding, there must be a sense of trust (Fonseca, 2002). Trust is the relational antidote to our anxiety of not knowing. Creating a sense of relational safety and trust allows people to stay engaged in the evolving conversation, and the ebb and flow of misunderstanding and new meaning.

Curiosity is also a potent tonic for innovation. In my experience, taking up an attitude of curiosity has allowed me to move beyond downloading and object-focused listening in challenging conversations. Rather than dismissing what someone is saying or looking for only the facts, curiosity keeps us engaged and we are able to attend to the conversation at a higher level. The next time you are in a conversation and you feel anxiety mounting, or if you find you are switching into download mode, try moving beyond the emotion of anxiety by asking yourself a curious question: why would someone think that way or do what they did? Pursue the answers with a curious attitude.

Brené Brown is a shame and vulnerability researcher. One of her most recent publications is *Daring Greatly* (2012). In it, she explores shame and vulnerability within organizational contexts. In her book she recounts a conversation with a silicon valley CEO, in which she asked him what he believed the greatest barrier to innovation was. He replied, "I don't know if it has a name, but honestly, it's the fear of introducing an idea and being ridiculed, laughed at, and belittled" (2012, p. 186). What this gentleman is describing is shame. In our earlier conversations of complex relational organizations, we have identified that processes of shame are a powerful social sanction enacted to maintain stability and the dominant organizational ideology. He goes on to say that "the problem is that innovative ideas often sound crazy and failure and learning are part of revolution" (2012, p. 186). Brown identified that for innovation and creativity to flourish and create positive change, there is a need to rehumanize our workplaces—to invite and welcome vulnerability as an essential element of innovation.

The concept of rehumanization brings us full circle to the two metaphors of organizational life that we began this chapter with: moving away from the organization as machine and toward a vision of organization as conversation (what is more human than talking together about our day-to-day work?). This means having the courage to have honest conversations about shame and daring to shine a light into dark corners that we would rather leave unexplored or ignored. Brown (2012) calls these kinds of conversations disruptive engagement. What wonderful new language for creating patterns of meaning that move the conversation forward.

REFERENCES

Barrett, F. J. (2012). *Yes to the mess: Surprising leadership lessons from jazz.* Boston, MA: Harvard Business School Publishing.

Benner, P., Hooper-Kyriakidis, P., & Stannard, D. (1999). *Clinical wisdom and interventions in critical care: A thinking-in-action approach.* Philadelphia, PA: Saunders.

Benner, P., Sutphen, M., Leonard, V., & Day, L. (2010). *Educating nurses: A call for radical transformation.* Stanford, CA: Jossey-Bass.

Booth, B. J., Zwar, N., & Harris, M. F. (2013). Healthcare improvement as planned system change or complex responsive processes? A longitudinal case study of general practice. *BMC Family Practice, 14*(51), 1–12.

Bourdieu, P. (1990). *The logic of practice* (R. Nice, Trans.). Palo Alto, CA: Stanford Press.

Brown, B. (2012). *Daring greatly.* New York, NY: Avery.

Brown, K. W., & Ryan, R. M. (2003). The benefits of being present: Mindfulness and its role in psychological well-being. *Journal of Personality and Social Psychology, 84*(4), 822–848.

Davidson, S. J. (2015)). Shifting the balance: relationship as power in organizational life. *Nursing Forum, 50*(4), 258-264.doi:10.1111/nuf.12115

Elias, N. (1998). *On civilization, power, and knowledge.* Chicago, IL: University of Chicago Press.

Fonseca, J. (2002). *Complexity and innovation in organizations.* London, UK: Routledge.

Gergen, K. J. (2009). *Relational being: Beyond self and community.* New York, NY: Oxford Press.

Gergen, K. J. (2015). *An invitation to social construction* (3rd ed.). Thousand Oaks, CA: Sage.

Grossman, P., Niemann, L., Schmidt, S., & Walach, H. (2004). Mindfulness based stress reduction and health benefits: A meta-analysis. *Journal of Psychosomatic Research, 51*(1), 35–43. doi:http://dx.doi.org/10.1016/S0022-3999(03)00573-7

Hassan, Z. (2014). *The social labs revolution: A new approach to solving our most complex challenges.* San Francisco, CA: Berrett-Koehler.

Kuhn, L. (2007). Why utilize complexity principles in social inquiry? *World Futures, 63*(3–4), 156–175.

Laloux, F. (2014). *Reinventing organization: A guide to creating organizations inspired by the next stage of human consciousness.* Brussels, Belgium: Nelson Parker.

Lefkowitz, W., & Jefferson, T. C. (2014). Medicine at the limits of evidence: The fundamental limitation of the randomized clinical trial and the end of equipoise. *Journal of Perinatology, 2014*(34), 249–251. doi:10.1038/jp.2013.172

Mead, G. H. (1934). *Mind, self and society.* Chicago, IL: Chicago University Press.

Patton, M. Q. (2011). *Developmental evaluation: Applying complexity concepts to enhance innovation and use.* New York, NY: Guilford Press.

Plum Village. (2015). The mindfulness bell. Retrieved from http://plumvillage.org/the-mindfulness-bell/

Romana, H. W. (2006). Is evidence-based medicine patient-centered and is patient-centered care evidence-based? *Health Services Research, 41*(1), 1–8. doi:10.1111/j.1475-6773.2006.00504.x

Scharmer, C. O. (2007). *Theory U: Leading from the future as it emerges.* Cambridge, MA: Society for Organizational Learning.

Shaw, P. (2006). Introduction: Working live. In P. Shaw & R. Stacey (Eds.), *Experiencing risk, spontaneity and improvisation in organizational change: Working live* (pp. 1–18). New York, NY: Routledge.

Stacey, R. D. (2001). *Complex responsive processes in organizations: Learning and knowledge creation.* London, UK: Routledge.

Stacey, R. D. (2006). Complex responsive processes as a theory of organizational improvisation. In P. Shaw & R. Stacey (Eds.), *Experiencing risk, spontaneity, and improvisation in organizational change: Working live* (pp. 124–138). New York, NY: Routledge.

Stacey, R. (2012). *Tools and techniques of leadership and management: Meeting the challenge of complexity.* New York, NY: Routledge.

Stacey, R. D., Griffin, D., Shaw, P. (2000). *Complexity and management: Fad or radical challenge to systems thinking?* New York, NY: Routledge.

Suchman, T. (2011). How we think about organizations: A complexity perspective. In A. L. Suchman, D. J. Sluyter & P. R. Williamson (Eds.), *Leading change in healthcare: Transforming organizations using complexity, positive psychology and relationship-centered care.* London, UK: Radcliffe.

Taylor, F. (1911). *Scientific management.* New York, NY: Harper.

Walker, D. (2006). Leading in the moment: Taking risks and living with anxiety. In P. Shaw & R. Stacey (Eds.), *Experiencing risk, spontaneity and improvisation in organizational change: Working live* (pp. 97–123). New York, NY: Routledge.

World Health Organization. (2008). *Implementation manual: Surgical safety checklist.* Retrieved from http://www.who.int/patientsafety/safesurgery/ss_checklist/en/

CHAPTER 11

Failure and Resilience: The Lifeblood of Innovation

Tim Porter-O'Grady and Kathy Malloch

Genius is 1% inspiration and 99% perspiration.

—THOMAS EDISON

CHAPTER OBJECTIVES

Upon completion of this chapter, the reader will be able to:

1. Examine the elements and characteristics of failure in the innovation process, and appreciate its contribution to sustainable success.
2. Identify the recovery strategies related to managing failure on the trajectory toward successful innovation and its implementation.
3. Use particular strategies and processes directed to managing the landscape of failure and utilizing failure as an incremental measure for success.

UNDERSTANDING FAILURE

During the space shuttle program, in what was later called the Challenger incident, a rocket carrying astronauts into space blew up in midair. The Rogers Commission report explored the decision-making processes leading up to the accident and concluded that there was a serious flaw in the process that led to the disastrous launch of the shuttle on January 28, 1986. The report found that management practices were at odds with many of the system needs, and failure to communicate with all parts of the system led to a breakdown in understanding and communication, both of which were identified as major contributors to the cause of the accident (U.S. Congress, Senate Committee on Commerce, Science, and Transportation, Subcommittee on Science, Technology, and Space, 1986).

The report of the Nuclear Regulatory Commission's assessment of the Three Mile Island disaster also found a failure in communication and misunderstanding with regard to processes and procedures and the level of mutual understanding among leaders and the system related to those processes, policies, and procedures (Sills, Wolf, & Shelanski, 1982).

Both of these disasters reflected common, ordinary failures in operating processes that can be replicated in many organizations and systems around the world. Failures such as these occur daily in organizations in every place on the globe in ways that reflect errors arising out of routine activities.

Enormous numbers of activities are undertaken in routine and ritualistic ways every single day in every workplace in the world. These ritualistic and repetitive activities are often quickly noted, briefly addressed, then placed in the historical dustbins of the organization, long forgotten while anticipating and addressing the next opportunity with its associated error. Failure, however, is central to the human experience. Failure is a requisite on the journey through life, learning, and adaptation. Indeed, without failure there is simply no measure for success (Bennis, Sample, & Asghar, 2015). Success then can be said to be the appropriate aggregation of sufficient error. Failure can serve as both a stimulus and a deficit, depending on how it is approached and perceived. Regardless of perception, the action of error is a productive and important part of all or any of the elements of innovation. In fact, innovation depends on failure and error as a way of both discerning and delineating where one is in the innovation process and what works and what does not work (**Figure 11-1**). Without this demarcation,

Figure 11-1 Understanding failure

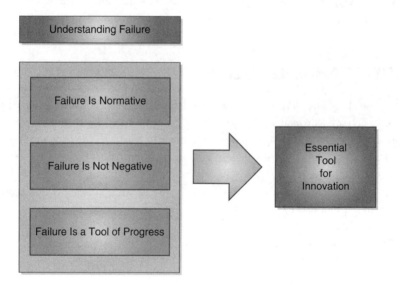

there is no way to ascertain progress, or lack of it, toward the creation of the new, the different, and the previously unconceived (Akintoye, Goulding, & Zawdie, 2012). As James Joyce suggested, "Mistakes are the portals of discovery" (Cleary, 2014). Innovators stimulate reflection and recalibration, suggesting new tweaks or approaches or ways of undertaking an issue or finding a solution to a problem. The millions of silly and even monumental errors that one will confront on the journey to innovation serve as the highway to the seminal or significant failures that provide the demarcation between the major movements or processes, or lack of it, on the journey to producing an innovative outcome.

Most of the time errors and failures are essential constituents of the journey of innovation. Indeed, the landscape and processes associated with successful innovation requires embracing error and failure and incorporating them into the operational mechanics and processes associated with successful innovation dynamics. Good leadership of innovation counts on the utility of failure and uses it as a part of the measurement mechanism essential to determine the viability and validity of decisions, choices, and processes associated with the positive movement toward successful innovation.

THE TRUTH ABOUT FAILURE

Innovation research consistently shows that most systems, organizations, and innovation processes are not terribly comfortable with accepting and valuing failure (Anderson & Costa, 2010). Indeed, most leaders are uncomfortable with failure because it is often seen as a reflection of one's competence, capacity, success, or lack of it. Historically, failure was used as a template to assess whether companies or individuals were successful in their undertakings and efforts. Failure, of course, was deemed unacceptable. This attitude created a perception about failure that alienated it as a legitimate part of organizational dynamics and clearly enumerated it as a deficit when assessing leadership behavior. In short, organizations and their leaders abhor failure. The emotional response and reaction to the presence of failure is so palpable in leaders that any mention of failure as a value generates a sense of incongruence, contradiction, and disbelief. In the history of leadership, there is only horror and negative reactions to the remotest suggestion that error and failure have value.

At a personal level, the deep pain associated with the negative notion of failure leaves a lasting imprint on both mind and experience. Because the negative impulses create much more reactive pain and depth of feeling than do pleasure and success, failure is deeply remembered and recalled with only the darkest of images. The intensity of these memories creates a painful psychodynamic relationship to the concept of failure and error that any belief that it could be used as a positive force and an essential measure of success simply strains individual credulity. Therefore, from every place in the organization, from personal to collective experience, the notion of error and failure as a positive dynamic creates such cognitive dissonance that it is virtually impossible to overcome and creates an organizational psychology that makes embracing failure inconceivable and unlikely. Simply, learning to love failure violates every part of our organizational and professional understanding.

The conceptual and actual vision of failure is as a bitter pill that, at best, is taken as bad-tasting medicine and, at worst, considered a terminal event. Therefore, organizationally and personally, failure is to be avoided at all costs, whether in our thoughts or in our deeds. Any notion of incorporating it into our legitimate operating processes or using it as a measure of progress goes way beyond the realm of possibility and creates a cognitive and organizational noise that makes it impossible to explore error and failure with any level of objectivity or intentional examination in a way that can make it useful and viable as a learning tool.

There are five basic scenarios or circumstances within which organizations and leaders approach the notion of failure that are negative and nonproductive but are common and consistent with contemporary management practices:

1. The organization completely rejects mistakes as legitimate. In this case, the organization finds mistakes completely unacceptable, rejects them, and does everything possible to eliminate them, hide them, ignore them, sweep them under the rug, or simply let them fall into oblivion. The organization has no mechanism for engaging or addressing error or failure, and undermines its capacity to create the milieu that provides the opposite: a perception of success, good choices, and positive attribution for all its processes and accomplishments. The failure-evading organization creates a leadership climate that is only superficially positive and reacts strongly to failure in any of its forms.

2. The organization can acknowledge error and failure, but works diligently to hide and cover it. In this scenario, leadership in the organization recognizes that error and failure do occur but consider them, at their foundation, exceptions, unusual circumstances, and unacceptable. Because they do occur, it is important in these systems to identify error, not to give it value but to find where the blame needs to be placed to isolate it, eliminate it, or punish it so it will not raise its ugly head again. In these organizations and management cultures, error and failure are to be feared, and those who are associated with it are to be hated and/or punished in a way that leaves a message to the organization and its people that error occurs, but it is unacceptable, and failure is not a strategy that leads to rewards or positive relationships in the organization.

3. The organization recognizes that error occurs, and that it occurs regularly, and it can be generated at any time and any place in the organization. Still, in this organization, error and failure remain unacceptable—an anomaly to which leaders

must object. If the error is found, it is to be analyzed and studied deeply to find out its characteristics and genesis, why it arose, what it means, what went wrong, and how to eliminate it from the processes and functions of the organization so it will not have an opportunity to arise again. In this case, error is seen as a necessary but present deficit that, if studied carefully and deeply, can be managed and eliminated from processes in a way that minimizes it and hopefully, over time, diminishes or eliminates it. Here again, error and failure are seen as deficits, but if studied appropriately, they can be acknowledged as part of identifying the root cause in an effort to diminish or eliminate it and replace it with positive and successful processes that reduce the chance of error or failure arising again.

4. Error and failure is recognized as a part of any process of implementation and is present in unrecognized forms in every design and project. Here again, error and failure is seen as a deficit, an uncontrolled outlier or variance that invariably rises to the surface because of the imperfection of planning, strategizing, or acting on an initiative or undertaking. Error or failure in this case will always arise and must be accommodated and expected as one of the normal vagaries of any human undertaking. Still, the accommodation of an error is not the engagement of it. In this scenario, failure is still visualized as an arc of unaccepted variants that must be accommodated because it invariably appears not because it is a tool of measure that may indicate specific viable and valuable data regarding process and decision making. Here again, the accommodation of the organization leads to an effort to reduce the impact of error and failure and to manage it in a way that reduces its risk and negative influence. If not for the error or failure, the situation is seen as an otherwise positive and successful process.

5. A standard of behavior in many organizations is the consideration that there are some people in the organization that are either personally committed to the failure of a project or do not actively embrace it, ultimately leading to its failure. Here again, failure and error are seen as deficits, in this case, personal and intentional ones, where stakeholders do not invest or commit to the strategy or undertaking of the organization in a sufficiently robust way to assure that an innovation or initiative will be successful and sustainable. This lack of engagement and embracing the strategic imperative or design trajectory of the organization causes or creates error and failure, thus affecting the organization's viability and measures of success. In this case, it is believed that if the leaders in the organization can obtain sufficient engagement and embracing of a project or initiative by all the impacted stakeholders, they can diminish the potential for failure and accelerate the potential for success. Here the notion of error and failure is invested in the insight regarding whether individual commitments or participation operates at a sufficient level of intensity to minimize the chance for failure and maximize the opportunity for success. The belief of leadership in this

scenario is that engagement and embracing the initiative or activity is positive. The risks of error and failure are minimized because of the offsetting energy of the collective commitment, ownership, and engagement of stakeholders in the work of the initiative or innovation. In this perception, it is believed that this full sense of engagement and empowerment creates a critical mass that itself inherently diminishes or eliminates the potential for error and failure in the organization (von Held, 2012). And, of course, it does not.

> **Discussion**
>
> How has your organization historically approached the issue of failure? How is it affected your own attitude toward failure as a member of that organization?

These five examples demonstrate how fear of error or failure becomes entrenched and embedded in the culture of the organization. This occurs in a way that facilitates and expands individual fear, uncertainty, and downright opposition to the presence of error and failure in the dynamic processes of the organization. These sentiments create an operating milieu where the role of failure is significantly diminished. In truth, the chances of accelerating the potential for failure are enhanced simply because the organization itself fails to recognize failure as an elemental and positive force on the trajectory of good design, implementation, and outcome.

PREDICTION AND FAILURE

It appears that the survival rates of natural organisms and companies are about the same. This complexity phenomenon was studied by Paul Ormerod, who found that the trajectory of the extinction rate of species over time matches the extinction rate of companies when measured over the same period of time. No matter the intensity of the effort, most companies tend to fail over the long term (Ormerod, 2010). As pointed out in Tim Harford's best-selling book *Adapt* (2012), the long-term success of companies and their ability to survive extinction had nothing to do with their degree of success in strategic planning. Although some companies, like Shell and General Electric, survived over the decades, the vast majority of companies did not. Therefore, we should be suspicious of any predictions of long-term success for companies, ventures, or initiatives in our current age.

This same data, with regard to the predictability of the survival of companies, applies to almost every other prediction one can make. The predictions of so-called experts appear to produce no more accurate certainty than the prediction of the life trajectory of a company. In fact, one cannot safely predict whether anything will succeed or fail. This understanding drives the notion that failure is deeply embedded in all dynamics and endeavors at every level of nature and human enterprise. Our efforts cannot protect us from the vagaries of failure and uncertainty, nor are we able to predict and anticipate sufficiently to be able to prevent or control failure. The real issue is to demonstrate resilience in the face of inevitable and inherent failure, and to successfully manage the realistic eventuality of failures in the course of our experiential journey.

STRUCTURAL FAILURE: AN IMPEDIMENT TO INNOVATION

Among others, there are two deterministic characteristics that have a direct impact on failure management. They are structural failure and intentional (design) failure (Kale, 2015). Of the two, structural failure is the most dangerous because it impedes the mechanics of innovation and operates in opposition to the activities necessary to stimulate innovation. Structural failure is deeply embedded in the traditional hierarchical design of most organizations and companies, and it operates in a way that opposes the dynamics essential to facilitate and stimulate the innovation process (Davila & Epstein, 2014).

Structural innovation is a metaphor for organizational hierarchy. The more rigid the organizational hierarchy, the less likely it can make room for innovation. Hierarchy acts against innovation insofar as it is structured to support strategic, operational, and functional alignment within the narrow parameters of planning and acting. These structural impediments facilitate failure before any definitive action can be taken leading to any measurable level of innovation. Structural impediments embedded in the hierarchy create such a narrow locus of control and such rigid process protocols that the potential for innovation, with all the vagaries necessary to support it, makes it impossible for innovation to succeed. The notion that the entire organization is driven structurally solely through its strategic trajectory and its associated processes strangles any potential for innovation before it even arises.

The creativity, discourse, openness, and collateral character of the innovative environment simply has no room to thrive in a rigid hierarchy, and therefore all the elements that would contribute to the potential for innovation are skewed or missing. Almost all healthcare organizations are designed in a way that provides a structural impediment to the potential for innovation. The only work-around is the construction of some unique forum, compartment, department, or institute that demonstrates a vehicle to get around the existing rigid parameters in a way that supports the innovation dynamic. In other words, when rigid structures and processes define the organization, innovation is either compartmentalized into a specific team, or innovation exists in the shadows, waiting to be found and stopped.

As a result, there is precious little evidence in these organizations of the action of innovation. Their structural framework does much to contribute to the long-term sensitivity of the organization to the negative vagaries of change to which organizational leadership has precious few resources to respond. The convergence of these negative forces works in concert to contribute to the decline or demise of a system (**Figure 11-2**).

Structural failure provides no infrastructure that allows for the possibility of trial and error and the quirks associated with the multidirectional and multilevel processes inherent in the innovation dynamic. Without a direct relationship to the strategic imperatives and permission from the structured management leadership or the functional mechanisms that support the operation of the bureaucracy, innovation simply has no place to grow. The constraints and rigidities of a clearly defined hierarchical infrastructure represent the supposition that failure and errors are simply unacceptable. This strong insulation from the risks and possibilities of experimentation and failure insulate leaders from the potential that is entangled in accommodating failure and instead offers the stability and organizational rigidity that often cloister its leaders from change and keep the organization from anticipating, predicting, and creating its own future.

Sustainable innovation is never driven from the top of an organization and is therefore anathema to a hierarchical decision-making framework because innovation is stimulated and sustained the closer it generates and operates to the point of service or productivity that energizes and sustains it. The more involvement and interaction for stakeholders and the looser the rigidities of control and organizational permission giving, the more likely an environment for thriving innovation can be created. Structural rigidities are the enemy of innovation and create both an attitude and a disposition toward the essential elements of innovation, including failure, that create a context that makes it impossible for innovation to operate.

Figure 11-2 Structural failure

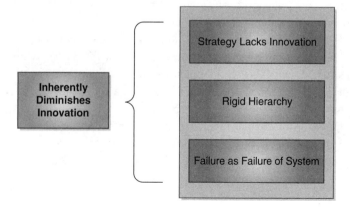

Case Example: Failure

The Blue Ridge National Health System has a long and storied history of success as a major health provider for a multistate region. It has been well noted for its high-quality, excellent physicians, wonderful nursing care, and its clinical model that has been identified as one of the best in the nation. This health system has always been identified as a unique provider, constantly out front in all measures of care and quality. In the past, its clinical model has been touted as one of the best in the country and has been broadly covered by every television network in America.

Rebecca Brown, RN, DNP, has recently been appointed as the new chief executive officer of this very successful health system. She was hired because of her major success in another health system across the country and had been identified as a strong up-and-coming, young administrator capable of providing strong and innovative leadership. When Becky arrived, she found an organization that was traditional, conservative, proud of its accomplishments, and firmly standing on its laurels. She also found many structures and systems that were highly entrenched, many medical and departmental silos, highly compartmentalized patient care services, high cost per unit of service, and leaders with a history and experience of protecting their turf from threat or encroachment.

In addition, the medical system is beginning to experience challenges from competitors who are slowly chipping away at their clinical model and patient population, and are busy innovating new kinds of care delivery systems driven by the demands of the Patient Protection and Affordable Care Act. Many of their competitors are decentralizing health care, emphasizing ambulatory care, and growing community-based services. On the other hand, the Blue Ridge National Health System is highly institutional, with many buildings on a fixed site, a number of related clinics, and very little dispersed community presence. Becky also noticed that there is not much community outreach, representation, or involvement in the strategic or tactical decisions of the organization. Furthermore, much of the decisions are controlled by a handful of powerful physicians with little engagement of other disciplines and the staff at the point of service. Becky identified that what she is confronting is a structural failure in the health system, and she saw that she had much work ahead of her to create a culture of innovation and engagement, which is essential to the health system's future success.

Discussion

We clearly see here an organization with a long history of success. The organization has embraced its success as its permanent identity in a way that ultimately insulates it from the realities and vagaries of a new, different, challenging, transforming, and relevant system prepared to create its future organization. Many of the structures in place are clearly unsustainable, requiring that leadership undertake a full 180-degree shift in strategy, culture, design, behavior, and impact.

Questions

In a team of four to seven members, discuss Becky's role and emerging priorities that will help the system confront its structural impediments (failure) to innovation.

1. What makes this health system structurally unable to engage in impending and necessary innovation?
2. How does an organization's history act to position it to fail in responding to overwhelming indicators of the need for change and innovation?
3. What specific challenges must Becky confront as she assesses the organization's capacity to change its structures to support innovation at the strategic (governance), operational (senior leadership), functional (departmental and unit), and individual (professionals and employees) levels of the organization?
4. As you consider Becky's role, what would be the initial steps or activities you would suggest she take to begin the process of removing the structural impediments to innovation in the health system?
5. How will the organization need to be different, and what will be the new leadership roles that will exemplify the organization's capacity to embrace innovation and engage the staff in transforming the health system?

It is important to note that hierarchical structures are currently threatened by the emergence of complexity science in organizational contexts and the implications of network realities. The leadership of predominantly relational systems and the intersections that describe how these networks operate has served to change the very dynamics of leadership and the organization of work. In health care, the emergence of value-grounded processes and the move from volume-based models to value algorithms has served to shake the organizational landscape, flatten hierarchies, and empower decisions and actions operating at the point of service. This move to more point-of-service configurations and the requirement for decisions and actions generating from these places has rewritten the script for health services, and driven systems to confront their vertically controlled organizational designs. In the face of the need for entrepreneurial, evidence-grounded, and just-in-time decision and action models, leaders now have no choice but to test and experiment with new models of organizing work and structuring for innovation. The demands of collective wisdom and team-based action in the exercise of integrated clinical activity across the continuum require more local leadership, planning, and decision making to assure clinical relevance and efficacy. All these emerging circumstances serve to create the conditions where it is less of an option to maintain rigid hierarchies in the face of growing demand for nimble, mobile, just-in-time clinical decisions and actions, all within a digital infrastructure. The hierarchy in a well matrixed and networked organization does not seek to maintain its formal control of the work, but rather the hierarchy provides guiderails, energy channels, and catalysts for innovation. The structure in innovative organization helps innovation thrive. The structure challenges innovation at the edge of chaos, helping to maintain information feedback loops associated with success and failure, ensuring that the organization can evolve and thrive

INTENTIONAL FAILURE: ESSENTIAL FACILITATOR OF INNOVATION

Intentional failure is simply a metaphor for a context or environment that is, by design, supportive of the dynamics and processes associated with sustainable creativity leading to useful innovation (Bolman & Deal, 2013). Intent implies a level of understanding regarding the structural facilitators and requisites necessary to advance the elements and products of innovation. Innovation demands a high degree of interaction, relationship, communication, experimentation, and trial and error. An environment that facilitates all the characteristics and processes supporting these dynamics is the essential underpinning leaders provide to support sustainable innovation. Intentional failure implies that the organizational constructs have been carefully thought out and the relationship between sufficient organizational structure and the work of innovation has been just as carefully constructed and operationalized in a way that assures the presence of the structural underpinnings supportive of innovation (Hoque & Baer, 2014).

Intentional failure suggests a level of understanding of the role failure plays in innovation. In this understanding of failure, leaders recognize the central and essential value of the role it plays in the innovation trajectory and in the assessment of progress and the determination of success. The recognition is that through experimentation, trial and error, and the incorporation of the risks associated with failure, the innovator and innovative system can actually innovate (Talukder, 2014). Within the paradigm of intentional failure, leaders can construct and use the tools of assessment and progress evaluation to better determine what is and what is not working. Clear to the leaders in intentional failure is the recognition that the delineation of both progress and failure serve an equal role in explaining and measuring the elements of progress in determining what is and what is not working. In this case, innovation leadership embraces failure in equal measure to other indicators of progress recognizing that all of them are important determinants of points of reference on the innovation trajectory. Furthermore, the judgment of failure is no different from the judgment of progress. Each serves as an objective measure of movement and provides a specific demarcation of the development and progress of any innovation. With dispassionate approaches and objective yet definitive tools, innovation leadership can harness the measures of failure as an evaluation of progress and, from it, strengthen choices, change them, and/or adjust the trajectory in any way that can facilitate the potential for positive outcome or impact (**Figure 11-3**).

Figure 11-3 Intentional failure

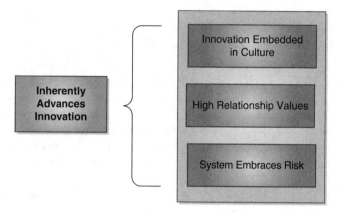

HARNESSING FAILURE AS A STRATEGY OF SUCCESS

Understanding the role of failures in innovation is to understand the dynamics of innovation. Failure through the lens of innovation is an operational element, as much a part of the processes of innovation as any other element. The purpose and work of failure is directed to the following:

- Failure is a tool and component of trial and error in which measurement of progress is essential. Error (thus, failure) is a metric that serves to identify where one is in the process of design or implementation. Failure tells the innovator where he or she is in the process and where the trajectory leads or does not lead. Knowing where not to go or what not to do in the innovation dynamic is equally important to knowing what is affirmed or validated in the innovation trajectory.

- Failures serves as a data point, a source of information, a point of reference that helps the innovator know where he or she is in relationship to other activities associated with the innovation process. Success in innovation can be said to be the sufficient aggregation of appropriate error. This acknowledges that the role of aggregated failure is helping to ascertain the demarcations of progress and the sum of the activities necessary to determine success.

- Failure serves to help identify the critical points of change in trajectory or direction. A failure becomes seminal when it indicates the need for a major reconceptualization or reconfiguration of the innovation process. While innovation is a process, it is not a straight line. Points of failure lead to moments or revolution that may require new thinking or processing and thus completely revamp the dynamics in a way that leads to new thinking or a new direction.

- Failure serves as a vehicle for disruption in a way that may actually cause a stop in a process or create conditions that may completely alter the path of an innovation. The disruption is usually significant enough to invalidate the current trajectory or work, and is a cause for shift or change so significant, that it can be said that it is essentially not the same process. In these cases, the products of innovation may become different and the disruption may be so complete that the product of innovation may be entirely different from that originally conceived.
- Finally, failure may act to invalidate the value and the process of a particular innovation effort. The significance of the failure may be such that the innovation itself is invalidated, making further progress on it purposeless. In this case, failure serves to inform the innovator of the complete nonviability of the innovation or demonstrate that conditions have eclipsed the value or relevance of the innovation in a way that ultimately stops it in its tracks. The positive take on this traumatic realization is that further expenditure of time, energy, and resources are halted, and those efforts can be transferred to other initiatives or innovations.

In each of these cases, failure is a positive tool for the innovation leader (**Figure 11-4**). It serves as a strong metric at every point in the innovation process that relays important data regarding progress and the movement toward success. Free of negative emotion and stigma, it serves as simply another tool, a metric for determining progress, priority, or change.

Figure 11-4   Failure as a positive tool for innovation success

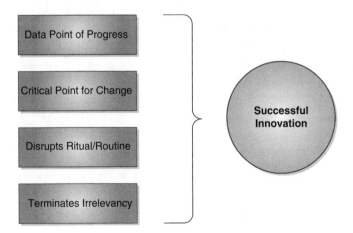

TRIAL AND ERROR: PARTNERING FAILURE AND INNOVATION

All innovation uses mechanisms of trial and error. Different from an improvement that advances something that already exists, innovation is primarily the creation of something that does not exist. Innovation mostly begins with an idea. However, an idea is not an innovation. An innovation is always the product of the work of translating an idea into action or a product. Keeping in mind that in any health system or organization, an innovation must ultimately add value in a way that affects care, service, outcome, or price, the innovation is itself the product.

Because design is the discipline or the work of innovation and is essentially a process of creation, the ultimate product of innovation is usually not fully known. The innovation process is filled with the elements of discernment, discourse, and discovery. Through the collective wisdom and processes of the stakeholders of the innovation, it slowly unfolds and takes shape. That shape forms as a result of small tests, experimentation, and trails along its trajectory. Deeply embedded in this process are all the indicators of progress and failure, each doing its part in validating and moving the innovation process along. Tests of utility lead to further refinement or enhancements or abandonment—shifts or changes in the innovation course. Accomplishment and success validate process, failure stimulates redesign or change. Trial and error contains equal measures of both. The veteran innovator knows that there will be a good measure of both success and failure, and each will do its part to inform the process of innovation and help make the necessary responses to keep the innovation process on track.

Failure also serves to mature the innovator and deepen his or her discernment and reflective process. Many an innovator has suggested that the most important and definitive moments in the innovation process were driven out of a spectacular failure that was so precise and devastating that it caused a dramatic demand for reflection and rethinking. In the time following a failure, new synapses, connections, and ideas are often generated in a way that serves as a tipping point such that the whole innovation hinged on the work done after failure. Indeed, for many an innovator, failure was the catalyst that served as the generator that ultimately redefined the innovation and served to spark a new genesis along its trajectory toward realization and success.

Discussion

How safe is it in your organization to experiment, test, and explore new approaches or different methods of solving a problem, influencing patient care, or advancing the patient experience? What are the boundaries or barriers to keep you from using trial and error as a tool for innovating practice?

Failure acts as a discipline in the dynamic of innovation. Failure is often the sobering point in the process that salts the excitement of ideation and creativity with the reality and sobriety of truth or reality, countering the realm of fantasy that fuels the dreams and hopes that stoke the energy and spirit of the innovation process. Creativity takes the innovator to the heights of possibility, failure provides the sobering foundation that supplies the stark truth about progress and the substance of the innovation in a way that helps inform the reality of the journey. In short, failure is a vital tool in assessing progress and informing the innovator about the realities and potentials of the innovation process itself.

FAILURE AS A TOOL SET FOR EFFECTIVE CHANGE

When failure is recognized in its role as a part of all of the elements and processes of the innovation dynamic, the leader's attention shifts from failure as error to failure as a tool for advancing the innovation process. The degree of utility and vitality brought to the use of failure in the dynamic of innovation determines the veracity and the effectiveness of adaptation, adjustment, or a radical change in course. The use of the tool of failure calls the leader to understand the mechanisms associated with it and to bring intentionality to the use of failure as a normative management strategy. Some of the issues related to the utility of failure are as follows:

- Identify the potential for failure early: If failure is to prove useful, the leader must first have dealt with personal attitudes and dispositions toward the notion of failure. Structuring failure as a normative component of the innovation process seems inherently counterintuitive. Each individual's developmental history informs the attitude toward failure by virtue of how failure was both perceived and handled in the individual's own life journey. Most of us have seen failure either as a challenge, at the minimum, or a devastating occurrence, at the maximum. On either end of a continuum, failure is identified as personal, having both an intimate and a relational impact.

  These personal notions related to perceptions of failure inform the mental model the innovator and the innovation leader bring to their roles. The positive and contributing characteristics of failure operate successfully only after having recognized that the occurrence of failure is a normative circumstance deeply embedded inside the innovation journey. It is important to surrender attachment to the past notions and sentiments regarding failure and equally important to recognize it more objectively as a positive tool set that helps assess points of reference, positive metrics, and potential decisions affecting the innovation process.

As the leader moves more confidently into an objective assessment mental model with regard to the innovation process and embedded error, the utility and value of failure become increasingly obvious. In this more objective framework, the only values that count in managing failure are early identification and early engagement. Much like conflict, the ability to respond positively to the failure in process, approach, strategy, or effort depends on the earliest possible identification and engagement. The sooner an emergent failure is recognized by the innovation leader and the earlier this leader predicts both the content and impact of the failure of effort, focus, strategy, or process, the easier adjustment and recalibration there is in addressing its implications. The more positive the notion and attitude toward the dynamic associated with failure in the innovation process, the more alert the leader is for the potential contribution and value emergent failure provides in informing and managing the innovation process.

- Failure is an indicator of the veracity of the idea: Many ideas generate excitement and enthusiasm in people who generate them and those who are affiliated with them. Often, this excitement and enthusiasm helps inform the conceptual frame of reference with regard to the value and potential of the idea going forward. While this enthusiasm is essential to generate the energy necessary to stay the course in the innovation process, it is also a trap. This conceptual trap serves to create the conditions where the energy itself is the driver leading to sidelining some of the basic tenets of logic, rationality, measurement, value, and sustainability.

Besides its association with creativity, openness, and free association, innovation is also a discipline. It has stages with definitive activity identified with them and specific measures and mechanisms that test the innovation potential and viability (LaRusso, Spurrier, & Farrugia, 2015). Good innovation leaders recognize that if the products of innovation are to be achieved, faithfulness to this process will be critical to success. While the enthusiasm associated with the generation of ideas and the subsequent innovation process is important in keeping it going, the more rational and dispassionate phases of the innovation dynamic provide the more rigid and systematic template and tools essential to move it to successful completion. Failure of an element, component, stage, phase, or notion associated with the innovation serves as a point of measurement where the innovation leader can undertake some objective assessment of the meaning and value of any particular failure and its impact on subsequent decisions and actions related to the innovation. In this case, failure sometimes reflects the lack of veracity or relevance of the innovative idea itself and causes the leadership and innovation team to reflect and to discern the appropriateness of the originating idea and the substance of innovation going forward, should that be a rational decision.

Equally as possible is the determination that the innovation idea is not viable, relevant, or doable. Knowing when to stop an innovation or the innovation process to reevaluate the value equation, is a key leadership behavior that is equally as important as fostering the innovation itself. Whether it is or is not viable should be the product of these more rational processes that subject the innovation in the moment of failure to a more rigorous, rational, and focused assessment using objective metrics that inform and effectively advise correct decision making related to the innovation.

- Value failure for its role in destructive creativity: The leader's assessment of potential or impending failure does not necessarily need to lead to the consideration of the innovation as a terminal event. Failure serves a range of purposes. While one of them is certainly an indicator of the viability of the innovation, there are other factors associated with a particular failure that do the opposite. Sometimes failure is simply delivering the message regarding either choices made or the trajectory of the innovation. Examination of the failure can lead the innovation leader to reflection regarding strategies or processes chosen and their effectiveness in leading to the intended innovation or outcome.

  Sometimes the failure merely calls attention to errors in strategy, process, trajectory, or individual actions. In this case, a reexamination of any or all of these factors and their impact on the lack of positive progress can call the leader to reconfiguration or recalibration of decision, effort, trajectory, or priorities. Having made the necessary course correction, the innovation leader may thereafter create conditions where better convergence around successful innovation processes emerge and, for the next stage or phase, the more successful progress can be noted. Here, failure serves simply as a demarcation for measurement, a moment of reflection, and an opportunity for the innovation team to reconfigure its efforts in a way that better addresses issues leading to the moment of failure and helps the team push past that moment with renewed insight, tools, and tactics that better align with the innovation's trajectory.

- Failure is a tool for redefining the innovation itself: When an innovation process or the trajectory of innovation is clearly not working and the options for success following the planned trajectory are limited or nonexistent, this failure, again, may not necessarily lead to a termination of an innovation. In complex adaptive processes, often what might appear as a terminal event may actually be the ground floor of a more emergent circumstance leading to an innovation or change not previously conceived or visualized in the originating innovation process.

  Often, out of the ashes of a clearly failed innovation process are born the seeds of a new innovation. This new innovation is often better, more viable, and potentially more significant than the failed innovation out of whose ashes it emerged. Indeed, in the innovation dynamic, the death of an innovation may cause the innovators to turn a corner, look sideways, dig deeper, and clear the conceptual decks in a way that makes space for a different conception and a much more viable trajectory leading to something not previously conceived, but now demonstrates a value for which there was simply no vision while pursuing the previous innovation process that unwittingly led to its conception and generation. Here again, the circumstance is a reminder to the innovation leader that in the innovation dynamic, closing the door to a failed effort does not end the work of innovation; often it simply changes its course. Faithfulness to the discipline of innovation helps create the conditions where destruction, deconstruction, and termination can actually serve as a rich medium out of which new and more viable innovation emerges.

- Failure acts as the catalyst for evaluation of the effectiveness of the innovation process: Failure in the pursuit of a particular innovation may actually have nothing to do the innovation itself. Often the failure in the innovation is a symptom rather than effect. Such a failure calls the innovation leader to review the dynamics and processes associated with the discipline of innovation. Through review of the stages and phases of the innovation process and the resources and mechanisms supporting it, the innovation leader often finds points of challenge that lead to an understanding of brokenness and failure in the process itself.

Because innovation is both a dynamic and a process, the failure to achieve the desired outcome may have more to do with inadequacy in the process than in the potential veracity and value of the innovation. Here again, when failure is recognized as normative and serves as an objective tool of assessment or evaluation, information of significance regarding the dynamic is obtained. This information can then yield more effective or aligned elements or processes supporting the innovation trajectory. Indeed, a regular and focused examination of the characteristics and elements of the innovation process and its appropriate support structures helps innovation leaders to further refine the process in ways that makes it more predictable, dependable, and trustworthy. Although each innovation has its own developmental characteristics, all innovation has a common frame of reference within which the foundational set of processes and parameters routinely operate to support and facilitate the innovation dynamic.

Flaws in the process, missing elements, irregular flow, and limits on effective evaluation all converge to create conditions that negatively affect the discipline and processes of innovation. For the innovation leader, the best predictor of flaws in the innovation process are the degrees of repetition in the occurrence of patterns of failure over time. Failing to address these or lack of awareness of their operation can often cause the leader to focus on the innovation rather than on the mechanisms that advance it. More often than not, the failure lies in the mechanics of innovation, not the idea driving it.

Objectively managed, failure is clearly a viable and useful tool in refining and advancing any innovation toward success. However, it takes a manager or leader with

Figure 11-5   Failure as value versus failure as deficit

Failure as Value	Failure as Deficit
• Objective	• Subjective
• Assessment	• Unsafe
• Measurement	• Terminal
• Influence Direction	• Negative
• Set Trajectory	• Destructive

an adjusted attitude and insight toward failure to use these objective tools to success-fully traverse the landscape of innovation. Careful and serious use of the tools of the discipline of innovation help facilitate and enhance the dynamic of innovation. This more balanced and realistic insight about the processes of innovation and its effective-ness grounds the leadership of innovation and increases the likelihood of its successful movement through all stages of development (**Figure 11-5**).

MINIMIZING THE POTENTIAL FOR UNNECESSARY FAILURE

Although it is clear in this chapter that we have emphasized the fact that failure is a fundamental, indeed a necessary, element of the innovation process, it is important to suggest that not all failure is necessary. Sometimes failure occurs because of inap-propriate decision making, inadequate processes, or poorly constructed innovation support structures. Each of these failures is conditional, meaning it can be addressed and managed, and when it is fixed is no longer acts as an impediment affecting the innovation process. Keep in mind, however, that correcting structural flaws in the innovation process does not necessarily diminish the potential emergence of other errors and failures inside the innovation dynamic. Operational flaws are separate cir-cumstances and create different conditions. Structural errors embedded in the process can always have a strongly negative impact on the innovation process and therefore on the innovation itself. Errors of this type operate in a different way from operational error and failure that more simply reflect problems with the processes of innovation.

Innovative organizations are just as intensely human as any other organizations. Essentially, this means that the potential for mistakes, misjudgments, poor planning, bad choices, and uninformed decisions and actions can be just as apparent in the in-novative organization as they are in the other system. With an awareness of this reality, the leader recognizes that he or she is constantly assessing the environment for their presence and evaluating, learning, adjusting, and correcting systems to keep them on course and to support effective innovation processes.

Leaders of innovation can exhibit several behaviors to help minimize unnecessary failure:

- Be bold: Voicing concerns about the alignment, trajectory, and evolution of the innovation is part of the process. Laissez-faire leadership in innovation can lead to value-negative outcomes. The inaction of team members in the innovation dialogue about value, process, and alignment can lead the innovation to lose adaptability and stagnate or cause the innovation to spin into more chaos. Leaders of innovation must both speak up and facilitate speaking up.
- Bridge structural errors: As discussed, many organizations have structural and cultural foundations that can minimize or inhibit innovation. Leaders of innovation can work to bridge these structural gaps through building strong networks of conspirators, external contacts, and linkages to fellow innovators. The network of agents will always be stronger than any hierarchal force. Building a network of innovation is key to minimizing unnecessary error caused by rigid structures and culture.
- Focus on the outcome: Although it is easy to become fixated on the process of innovation (brainstorming, ideation, prototyping, etc.), leaders of innovation must equally focus on the outcomes the innovation will achieve. Many times the innovation morphs and shifts through the process, and teams can lose sight of what they are trying to accomplish. Keeping the vision of the outcome visible to the team will help maintain alignment of the process and minimize errors associated with wasted time, unnecessary iterations, and lack of focus.

INNOVATION FOR VALUE

Perhaps one of the most significant shifts in recent history in health care is the current move from a volume-driven system to one based on value. Currently, the most significant contextual failure that innovation leaders will need to contend with is that related to the move from volume to value. Almost any innovation that emerges today needs to represent the emergence of value-based realities driving much of the strategic work of organizations. No innovation will have any sustainable meaning or even succeed over the long term in its implementation from idea to product if it does not in some way anticipate, facilitate, or advance the engagement of value. The entire arena of health services must now reflect value drivers in a way that now fulfills the obligations of the Tripe Aim.

As mentioned previously, innovation should relate to organizational purpose and strategic imperative. Although there is a challenge in the contest between the unique characteristics of an innovation and the opportunity it provides to undertake something that is new and/or different, the innovation still needs to reflect the major purposes of the organization. In health care, regardless of the changes that are occurring, any innovation that seeks to thrive in the healthcare environment in some way or another needs to advance the service, quality, or price interests of the healthcare organization. A sound element of the discipline of innovation is the assurance that innovation undertakings, regardless of their creativity, somehow directly relate to advancing the healthcare enterprise. In this case, it is the role of the innovation structure to provide that framework, the discipline, if you will, that keeps the generation of resources supporting any innovation undertaken within the framework of the value of the organization. Failing to do so robs the organization of its resources and its capacity to exercise good judgment and action in a way that advance its purposes and value. The following are some critical factors influencing the success of innovation:

- Innovation and strategic relevance: There are all kinds of innovations that are important, meaningful, valuable, creative, and relevant. To the innovation leader, none of them matters if all these elements do not in some way lead to advancing the interests, viability, and sustainability of the organization within the context of its purpose and the service it provides. In health care, supporting innovation activities need to demonstrate how they uniquely contribute to advancing the interests of the organization and provide a foundation for the quid pro quo essential to advancing a thriving health service environment. The significant failure to do so relates specifically to the nonalignment of the innovation efforts with the purposes and roles of the health institution and the efforts necessary to advance the health of those it serves.

  The failure to align strategy and innovation at the systems level creates a critical condition for the organization with its larger environment. Health systems are directed within the contemporary value equation to advance the health of the communities within which they live and operate. Essential to this exercise is the appropriate and careful use of organizational, financial, and human capital in ways that serve that essential purpose (Owens & Fernandez, 2014). In the value equation, evidence of having done so is delineated by the organization's capacity and success in advancing metrics that demonstrate a high level of user satisfaction, strong performance on quality metrics, and competitive pricing of the services and products of the health system. The innovation priorities of the organization that advances performance in these arenas of value measures, and indicates strong alignment among the priorities and activities of the organization and its strategic positioning for success.

● Failure and inadequate resourcing for value: Perhaps the most significant anticipated and predicted failure in the innovation process is the lack of organizational and financial support for innovation activities. Often what occurs in organizations regarding innovation is the provision of a great deal of verbal and personal support with no structural and financial infrastructure to sustain it. For many leaders, innovation is the generation of ideas and thus never lifts off toward a structure for change. As a result, organizations are inundated with ideas related to technological, process, and product innovation with precious little progress toward producing something that matters or makes a difference for the health system.

Innovation projects or processes that are inadequately funded generally die on the vine. These innovations have no way to develop or thrive simply because the most obvious indicator of support—financial resources—is either inadequate or missing. Making appropriate resources available for innovation is the most visual witness of the organizational support for that innovation. Leaders indicate significant value for any undertaking through the medium of the number of dollars devoted to move the innovation toward product or impact. Lacking that, no amount of verbal and personal support for the work of innovation will ever move the innovation anywhere near the fulfillment of its potential.

● Failure of an adequate infrastructure to support the discipline or process of innovation: As clearly identified throughout this text, innovation is specifically defined as an enumerated process with identifiable elements, stages, and metrics that elucidate its properties. In the popular press and in the imaginations of some leaders, innovation is often seen as a series of loosely defined, highly variable, often unstructured dynamics and processes that relate more to idea management than to any definitive and disciplined process that could ultimately produce a product or create an impact on the life of the organization. However, more often than not, nothing could be further from the truth.

Innovation, like any process of production, has elements and stages through which it grows that are necessary for its implementation. Ultimately, an innovation must produce something: either a change or a product. None of this can occur without the capacity to do what is necessary to produce something. Structures related to idea management, knowledge generation, product refinement and development, experimentation and small tests of change, integration of effort, resource management, intellectual property and legal issues, production, evaluation, marketing, and so forth are embedded within the processes and functions essential to the long-term viability and ultimate success of the proposed innovation.

With all of these components and stages essential to the success of an innovation, it comes as no surprise that few innovations make it anywhere near completion. If organizations are to be successful in managing their innovation processes, the essential tools, infrastructure, metrics, resources, and processes must be carefully constructed and aligned to assure all appropriate and necessary efforts converge to positively facilitate the innovation toward successful completion. This essential infrastructure provides both the frame and the glue that enables innovators and associates on the positive trajectory to accessible supports necessary to accelerate the opportunity to succeed. Failure to build this essential infrastructure is failure to equip both the innovator and the innovative process with virtually everything they will need to thrive within the process and to move positively and successfully toward fulfilling the potential of the innovation. It is important to remember that even with the right set of factors energizing the innovation, failure still may occur. For example, even the most successful venture capital firms have about a 10% success rate in funding innovative startups.

- Failure of relevance: Leaders have an obligation to the organizations they lead to make sure that the activities and priorities of the organization best represent three critical elements: (1) the driving characteristics and demands of the larger environment within which the organization lives and operates; (2) the trajectory of the organization is traveling in a way that best demonstrates its response to the environmental and contextual demands within which it lives; and (3) the appropriate decisions and actions that represent the best response to the demands of the environment and the requisites of the trajectory.

Any organization that seeks to thrive must attend to its capacity to be relevant. Relevance represents the characteristics and activities of individuals, groups, or organizations in a way that best exemplifies the broader social, political, technological, and economic forces converging to influence their capacity to thrive. Leaders must demonstrate the essential skills that help them forget inevitable and emerging shifts in reality brought by each of these forces and the impact of those shifts on the decisions and actions of the organization in a way that is timely and appropriate. This predictive and adaptive capacity is a fundamental skill set of leadership within the context of innovation; it is no longer optional if the changes in an organization will represent a goodness of fit between the larger demand for change and growth and the organization's capacity to meet that demand, translate it, and give it form and substance (**Figure 11-6**).

Figure 11-6 Two major leadership capacities

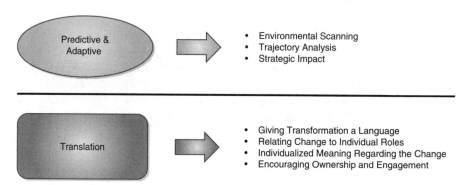

THE CAPACITY TO BE RELEVANT

As the digital environment expands its influence on human and organizational life, the response to it creates a new level of leadership demand, especially with regard to innovation. Because of the breadth of big data and the increasing speed and utility of the information infrastructure, just-in-time responses to the demand for change are now the normative pattern of organizational and team behavior. Unlike traditional changes impacting health service in clinical practice, where changes in policy, procedure, and practices could transition over weeks and months, evidence-based practices now operate within an immediacy where data aggregation, evaluation, and information now impact practice instantaneously, with the expectation that change in practice will occur as soon as we know what that change should be. This milieu creates a new understanding of relevance. The capacity to be relevant depends exclusively on the organization and the individual's ability to predict, adapt, and change. Failure to do so now constrains the organization's opportunity to thrive in a sustainable way and its members' ability to adapt their work to meet the accelerating demands of excellence and the accelerating levels of competitive performance spiraling upward and continually challenging all to improve performance.

A FAILURE OF LEADERSHIP

Fundamental to all delineations and management of failure is the role of the leader. At the end of the day, in all human dynamic organizations, the role of the leader has the greatest significance in impacting the culture, characteristics, work, and outcomes of the organization (Erickson, 2013). Leadership failure usually encompasses areas of awareness, insight, competence, process, and execution. Each of these arenas demonstrate the critical viability of the substance of leadership and challenges leaders to be continuously aware of their capacity to lead in complex dynamic human systems, perhaps most intensively evidenced in the healthcare arena (Porter-O'Grady & Malloch, 2016).

Discussion

Have you ever personally experienced what you considered a failure of leadership? What were the circumstances that led you to that conclusion? What do you feel was missing in the leader's role? How would have you addressed the particular issue differently with what you have gained from reading this text?

With regard to innovation, there are several areas where leadership capacity can affect the successful process and trajectory of innovation work. Like every other area of organizational undertaking, leadership of innovation is as critical as is the innovator's own efforts at producing an innovation. Leaders are predominantly responsible for creating a context that facilitates the creativity and work effort leading to successful innovation. Without this context and structural and relational encouragement, the innovation process can often starve. Strong innovation leaders are advised to be aware of the critical indicators of the failure of leadership. Although they are many and varied, there are a few significant arenas of leadership that have the broadest impact on either facilitating or constraining effective innovation in an organization:

- Failure to predict: As previously outlined, the ability of the leader to demonstrate predictive and adaptive capacity is critical to the success of an innovative organization. Organizations live within a broader context. This context exemplifies a constant vortex and continual shifting and change in ways that represent the constant, undifferentiated, chaotic convergence of the larger sociopolitical, technological, and economic forces affecting every human system.

  Leaders, recognizing this constant and complex pattern of shift and change, continuously read the environment, looking deeply at the contextual issues influencing the organization in the broader setting with a lens directed to determining meaning and impact on the organizational system. These leaders devote particular and specific energies to this predictive activity as a way of translating environmental concerns and influences with a language that translates them into content that has meaning and value for health leadership and organizational members. This is especially true within the frame of innovation. Because innovation represents a relevant response to contemporary and future demand for enhancement, advancement, and transformation of process and product, it requires that there be a goodness of fit among the changing characteristics of the environment and its impact on the culture and life of the organization, and the organization's innovative response to those demands.

In this framework, leaders validate their capacity to manage the vagaries of shift and transformation through the mechanism of good translation. This is demonstrated by their own capacity to be available to the changes generated from the environment, to recognize their meaning and impact on the organization and its people, and to respond specifically and particularly in a way that operates in the best interest of the organization and its ability to thrive. This predictive capacity of the leader is central to assuring the organization's viability and continuous response to environmental and contextual shifts and as a way of assuring that the organization remains relevant, engaged, and busy constructing the positive creation of a preferred future.

- Failure of effective communication: Most people who work in organizations are busy fulfilling the activities to which they are assigned. What encompasses their attention, for the most part, is the work that they do, the people that they serve, and the impact their specific energies and activities effect. Generally, most of the work they do encompasses their full attention and occupies all of their energies in a way that reflects a focus on the present, current working capacity and the functional activities that complete the obligations of the day. Because work is so demanding in real time for most workers in organizations, their ability to be aware of the future, critical shifts in the environment, the emergence of the new and different, and the changing environmental and social circumstances affecting their long-term work is severely limited.

Recognizing this reality, leaders are constantly aware of the need to translate to the organization and its people the conditions and circumstances generating from the larger context or environment that will impact their role. To do this, the leader assures that there is an effective and continuous mechanism for communicating the environmental and contextual demands for currency, change, adaptation, and refinement of contemporary practices into new frames and models that best address the emerging issues moving the organization into its future. These mechanisms of communication are defined and structured in a way that make it easy and accessible for organizational members to access what they need to know, be able to incorporate that information into their practices, and collectively challenge contemporary work functions with emerging realities in ways that encourage them to engage and embrace these potentials for change as a fundamental part of their work.

The system of communication facilitated by the leadership includes opportunities for organizational members to participate in environmental scanning, translation, and application of those dynamics. This means workers have an impact on the work world and affect their own efforts and that of their teams in the exercise of the work of the organization. An effective communication system in a responsive organization is exemplified by broad-based participation, ownership, and engagement by all stakeholders who play a role in translating and adapting environmental demands for change into effective work processes and products in the organization.

Leaders create the communication network and pathways within which this information and organizational response processes can be channeled in a way that demonstrates an effective impact on the organization. This effort continues to make innovation viable and sustainable over the long term. Indeed, organizations that have sustained over generations have done so through the mechanisms of engagement and ownership at every level, using open communication models and mechanisms for assuring that meaningful and important decisions and actions and deliberations about potential innovations have both a voice and a place where ideas are acted upon. Here is where the innovator's voice can be legitimately heard and responded to with appropriate supports throughout the organization. Good communication pathways around the innovative process also help facilitate and support the various structural mechanics in the organization.

Sound communication gives form to the innovation, disciplines the process, and assures that both the mechanics and means that advance the innovation are in place and positioned to accelerate the opportunity for the innovation to thrive. Demonstrated here is the capacity of the organization to continually enable innovation confirmed by its open and interactive communication infrastructure in a way that encourages, supports, and advances the innovation through its various phases and stages to completion and impact.

- Failure to engage risk: So much in health care depends on the capacity of its leaders to manage risk. Historically, emphasis on danger and threats to the safety of patient care have resulted in organizations that are in many ways fundamentally risk averse. This constant focus on assuring that patients remain safe and that harm is avoided and prevented at all costs creates a mental model in an organizational milieu that sees risk as a threat and endangerment to the viability of patient care and the stability of the healthcare organization. While it is important for patients to remain safe and for the work environment that generates the highest-level potential for patient safety, that environment of patient safety should not be confused with the capacity of the organization to engage essential and necessary risk as it addresses constructing of its future.

Risk cannot be eliminated. While risk can be effectively managed, in the course of human events there is always a measure of risk and the potential for that risk to influence decisions, actions, and impacts (Shaw, 2014). Good leaders recognize the value of risk. Embedded deep inside of risk is the potential for improvement, enhancement, and creativity. Indeed, the future of the organization depends on its ability to engage risk, manage it well, and use its dynamics as a generator for creativity and innovation in a way that enhances the organization's opportunity to thrive. For the organization's capacity to succeed over the long term, its members' ability to identify, manage, and utilize risk in decision making, planning, and executing innovation processes is critical (Sundheim, 2013). The leader provides mechanisms and methods for the safe engagement of risk at every level of the organization, with an emphasis that 90% of the engagement of risk needs to occur at the point of service where most of the opportunity for creative insight and innovation occurs.

Good leaders use risk management tools, such as scenario planning, as a way of helping to create a safe environment for exploring, experimenting, and challenging the potential deeply embedded in risk in ways that can be translated to the benefit of the organization. Through the use of case and scenario activities at every level of the organization and in ways that reflect the obligation of strategic, operational, tactical, and functional roles in the organization, patient care is ultimately positively impacted throughout the organization.

Leaders make sure that through scenario or case-based work, external drivers and influences are clearly outlined and articulated, financial and economic indicators and implications are thoroughly vetted, the veracity and strength of a strategy and/or tactic is tested in safe conditions, new possibilities are considered, and process mechanisms can be generated and safely tested to determine their viability and efficacy. The leader providing this kind of a platform in the innovative process assures that innovation is incorporated as a regular expectation of the work of everyone in the organization and is structured in the organization in a way that assures its utility and viability as a fundamental and functioning part of the work of the organization.

● Failure to admit failure: As this chapter clearly attempts to emphasize, failure is a normative, functioning part of the role of leadership in assessing the viability and effectiveness of the innovation process inside the system. Failure is not a deficit for either the organization or the individual if managed properly and with careful leadership wisdom.

Failure serves as a metric, helping leadership know precisely where they are on a specific trajectory related to any innovation. Incremental failure lets the individual and innovation team know about the veracity and appropriateness of any particular element in the innovation dynamic. Failure helps leaders understand, through the use of specific enumerated evaluation elements, where the innovation is currently and its potential along with the choices and actions that can facilitate that potential. Failure also helps leaders identify what does not work, what is no longer appropriate, when a change in course needs to occur, or when a process or project has reached a terminal point in its current trajectory. All of these are objectives and viable tools that suggest to the leader subsequent choices and adjustments in the innovation process necessary to sustain and support it.

The requisite of failure is that it be used objectively as a tool. Failure must constantly be identified as a part of the metrics that assess the trajectory of an innovation and help determine choices and actions that need to be taken as a result of the information that a failure provides to leaders of the innovation process. As outlined previously in this chapter, if failure is engaged as a productive and positive tool set for enumerating the success of a particular innovation trajectory, the emotional and personal content often affiliated with it can be minimized and potentially eliminated. In this case, it is the obligation of leaders to create that objective and safe approach to the utility of failure as an objective and meaningful tool along the continuum of innovation work. Leaders who do not create this safe and productive capacity for the use of failure metrics actually contribute to the emotional trauma and debilitation. Negative feelings and responses to failure in the organization should come as no surprise to leaders if their organizational members are failure sensitive and risk averse. If the leadership climate generates and supports those negative sentiments and punishes or creates an adverse response to notions, mechanisms, processes, and outcomes that result from the aversion to risking and failing, then debilitating failure is guaranteed. Failure is good only if it is perceived as good and only if it produces values that result in better decisions, more effective action, and exciting processes and products that demonstrate the positive use of failure analytics as a part of the process of producing a dynamic outcome (**Figure 11-7**).

Discussion

When considering the leadership of innovation, what particular personal skill sets do you bring to the engagement of innovation? As this chapter closes, what specific skills do you need to focus on developing in your capacity to embrace failure as an objective tool for managing innovation? How will you test your new and developing skills in your leadership role?

Figure 11-7   A failure of leadership

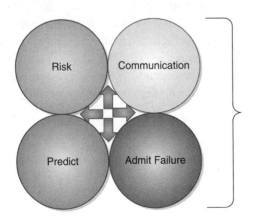

Risk

Communication

Predict

Admit Failure

Impact

- Position for Success
- Predict the Trajectory
- Engage the Stakeholders
- Move Innovation Forward
- Assure Organizational Thriving
- Sustain Future Orientation

Case Example: Leadership

Leticia Morgan, RN, BSN, had been approached by one of her staff members with a new digital device and software that would help monitor the movement of geriatric patients in their homes and inform the geriatric continuum of care nurse coordinator if the patient was involved in a safety risk activity. The nurse had been working on this idea for the last couple of years, and now she was ready to move her idea into a useful product. The nurse inventor had kept Leticia informed during every stage of her idea creation, but Leticia had paid only cursory attention to the progress. Now this nurse was approaching her to determine if there were any formal steps or processes she needed to go through in the organization to access supports and systems that might help take her invention to production.

Leticia had heard about her health agency's interest in facilitating monitoring the care of homebound patients but was not sure how it worked. When she heard about the innovation development process, Leticia thought it was very complicated and detailed and was directed mostly to helping physicians develop practice innovations within their own specialties to advance their technology and financial partnership with the health organization. Leticia was pretty sure they would not be interested in any nursing idea that did not appear to make much difference in nurses' work. Leticia informed the nurse inventor that it might be wiser for her to find a patent or invention organization outside the health agency that might be interested in an invention like hers because the organization's resources were tight and there would not be much support inside the system. The nurse inventor was discouraged, leaving the conversation with Leticia believing that her potential innovation was not significant enough to pursue and feeling that perhaps she should simply let it go.

Discussion

Leticia and the nurse inventor practiced in an organization that did have an organized and structured innovation process. Leticia assumed that from what she had understood about process, it was directed more to position inventors who had a larger stake in the financial impact for themselves and the organization. Leticia further assumed that the invention was not significant enough for further consideration and directed the nurse inventor elsewhere. This scenario can be replicated in a number of health organizations across the country and create some real challenges for inventors and a potential limitation on the possibilities and implications for an innovation that never gets to see the light of day.

Questions

1. What do you think of Leticia's original relationship with the nurse inventor during the idea stage over the past 2 years?
2. How thorough do you think Leticia's understanding of the agency's innovation process was, and how did that influence her advice to the nurse inventor?

3. If you were the nurse leader in Leticia's place, what series of activities and interactions would you have with the nurse inventor? What stages or phases of the innovation process might you facilitate for the nurse inventor's efforts?

4. How many levels of failure are you able to identify in this scenario? (Keep in mind that there is evidence in this scenario of failure at the systemic, departmental, leadership, and individual levels.)

5. What steps would you take to address the failures you identified in question 4 to keep these kinds of failures from occurring again and, instead, facilitate an environment of innovation supportive of invention?

SUMMARY

From an objective perspective, the only role that failure plays is in the evaluation and assessment of organizations' and individuals' movement to success and thriving. The incongruent fear of failure generally expressed by leaders and others does not come near representing the significance of the value of failure as a metric along the trajectory of the journey to successful innovation. Instead, engaging and embracing failure as a viable and useful measure of progress is a much more realistic and valuable perspective of the role of failure and one that provides great utility in the innovation process. Leaders must confront individual and organizational apprehensions regarding the role of failure and make issues related to the management of failure a fundamental part of the leadership development process. If the mechanisms and characteristics of failure are utilized as positive tools in evaluating the mechanisms and processes of innovation, a more disciplined, appropriate, and meaningful experience of innovation development can be generated in individuals and in the organization. Failure is a tool, not a condition.

REFERENCES

Akintoye, A., Goulding, J., & Zawdie, G. (2012). *Construction innovation and process improvement*. Ames, IA: Wiley-Blackwell.

Anderson, N., & Costa, A. C. (2010). *Innovation and knowledge management*. Los Angeles, CA: Sage.

Bennis, W. G., Sample, S. B., & Asghar, R. (2015). *The art and adventure of leadership : Understanding failure, resilience and success*. Hoboken, NJ: Wiley.

Bolman, L. G., & Deal, T. E. (2013). *Reframing organizations : Artistry, choice, and leadership* (5th ed.). San Francisco, CA: Jossey-Bass.

Cleary, J. (2014). *The Cambridge companion to Irish modernism*. New York, NY: Cambridge University Press.

Davila, T., & Epstein, M. (2014). *The innovation paradox: Why good businesses kill breakthroughs and how they can change*. San Francisco, CA: Berrett-Koehler.

Erickson, J. I. (2013). Reflections on leadership talent: A void or an opportunity? *Nursing Administration Quarterly, 37*(1), 44–51. doi:10.1097/NAQ.0b013e3182751610

Harford, T. (2012). *Adapt: Why success always starts with failure.* New York, NY: Farrar, Straus & Giroux.

Hoque, F., & Baer, D. (2014). *Everything connects: How to transform and lead in the age of creativity, innovation, and sustainability.* New York, NY: McGraw-Hill Education.

Kale, V. (2015). *Inverting the paradox of excellence: How companies use variations for business excellence and how enterprise variations are enabled by SAP.* Boca Raton, FL: CRC Press.

LaRusso, N., Spurrier, B., & Farrugia, G. (2015). *Think big, start small, move fast: A blueprint for transformation from the Mayo Clinic Center for Innovation.* New York, NY: McGraw-Hill Education.

Ormerod, P. (2010). *Why most things fail and how to avoid it.* New York, NY: Wiley.

Owens, T., & Fernandez, O. (2014). *The lean enterprise: How corporations can innovate like startups.* Hoboken, NJ: Wiley.

Porter-O'Grady, T., & Malloch, K. (2016). *Quantum leadership: Building better partnerships for sustainable health* (4th ed.). Burlington, MA: Jones & Bartlett Learning.

Shaw, R. (2014). *Leadership blindspots: How successful leaders identify and overcome the weaknesses that matter.* San Francisco, CA: Jossey-Bass.

Sills, D. L., Wolf, C. P., & Shelanski, V. B. (1982). *Accident at Three Mile Island: The human dimensions.* Boulder, CO: Westview Press.

Sundheim, D. (2013). *Taking smart risks: How sharp leaders win when stakes are high.* New York, NY: McGraw-Hill.

Talukder, M. (2014). *Managing innovation: Adoption from innovation to implementation.* Surrey, UK: Gower.

U.S. Congress, Senate Committee on Commerce, Science, and Transportation, Subcommittee on Science, Technology, and Space. (1986). *Space shuttle accident: Hearing before the Subcommittee on Science, Technology, and Space of the Committee on Commerce, Science, and Transportation, United States Senate, Ninety-ninth Congress, second session, on space shuttle accident and the Rogers Commission report, February 18, June 10, and 17, 1986.* Washington, DC: US Government Printing Office.

von Held, F. (2012). *Collective creativity: Exploring creativity in social network development as part of organizational learning.* Wiesbaden, Germany: Springer.

Innovation and Evidence as an Integrated, Iterative Process

Shifting Workforce Paradigms: From Quantity to Value-Driven Staffing Using Evidence and Innovation

Kathy Malloch and Tim Porter-O'Grady

The enterprise that does not innovate ages and declines. And in a period of rapid change such as the present, the decline will be fast.

—PETER DRUCKER

CHAPTER OBJECTIVES

Upon completion of this chapter, the reader will be able to:

1. Examine the driving forces and current challenges requiring change in health care.
2. Develop insights into an innovative healthcare value model as the infrastructure to improve nurse staffing adequacy.
3. Assess the clinical productivity model as a strategy to integrate disciplines across the continuum.

INTRODUCTION

Providing adequate caregivers and staff support for patient needs is foundational for effective healthcare organizations, clinics, and home care settings to be able to achieve valued outcomes. This work is complex and clearly impacted by emerging evidence, new technology, innovative ideas, and the existing organizational culture in which care

369

is provided. In this chapter the driving forces requiring change, the new opportunities that support innovations in healthcare delivery, challenges and obstacles to progress, and a value-based approach for more effective care from an evidentiary perspective, as well as the anticipated outcomes from this value-driven model, are presented. The content of this chapter focuses on available evidence as the foundational content for effective work and identifies gaps in knowledge or absence of evidence as opportunities for innovation and innovative strategies. Challenges in advancing this work should be viewed not as obstacles but rather as opportunities to tap into the infinite wisdom of healthcare colleagues and move forward with energy and enthusiasm in changing health care for the better. The interactive dynamic of evidence and innovation provides a purposeful framework from which to view this work.

> *The key to success is for you to make a habit throughout your life of doing the things you fear.*
>
> —VINCENT VAN GOGH

DRIVING FORCES FOR CHANGE AND INNOVATION IN STAFFING

There are numerous drivers and incentives to improve not only the management of nurse staffing, but also the overall quality of the healthcare experiences that are nearly always impacted by the quality of nurse staffing. Several regulatory and accrediting agency drivers that are facilitating significant change in the way health care is delivered include the Centers for Medicare and Medicaid Services (CMS), the Institute of Medicine (IOM), and the Institute for Healthcare Improvement (IHI).

The CMS road map for value-based purchasing (Centers for Medicare and Medicaid Services [CMS], n.d.) and the Medicare Modernization Act and the Deficit Reduction Act have shifted the government from a passive payer of services to an active purchaser of higher-quality, affordable care. The overall intent of these regulations is to promote efficiency in resource use while providing high-quality care in settings such as hospitals, home health, nursing homes, and medical homes. Nursing is a significant part of resource allocations and necessarily must embrace more effective, evidence-driven ways of providing care.

CMS has also advocated for and legislated improvements in care coordination, alignment of financial incentives with outcomes, adoption of electronic health records, e-prescribing, increases in the percentage of population-based payment, and joint team accountability for outcomes (CMS, 2015; Welton, 2010). The meaningful use initiative now requires increasing levels of electronic documentation.

The IHI identified the Triple Aim of simultaneously improving population health, improving the patient experience of care, and reducing costs per capita as the expectation for transformed healthcare systems (2012). The Triple Aim has become an organizing framework for the U.S. National Quality Strategy. Necessarily, improvements in nurse staffing and resource use are essential in supporting the Triple Aim.

NEW OPPORTUNITIES

In addition to the driving forces, there are several advances that provide opportunities to improve the healthcare system. These include an increased evidentiary focus, technology advances, and increasing consumerism focusing on value.

Evidentiary Focus

Much attention has been given to staffing based on evidence or research that has tested and validated practices. A critical mass of research supporting the presence of registered nurses in hospitals is now recognized. Nurses educated at the baccalaureate level also positively impact or decrease patient mortality (Aiken, Clark, Cheung, Sloane, & Silber, 2003; Aiken, Clark, Sloane, Sochalski, & Silber, 2002; Buerhaus, Donelan, Ulrich, Norman, DesRoches, & Dittus 2007; Kane, Shamliyan, Mueller, Duval, & Wilt, 2007; Lang, Hodge, & Olson, 2004; Needleman et al., 2002; Needleman, Buerhaus, Pankratz, Leibson, Stevens & Harris, 2011; Savitz, Jones, & Bernard, 2005; Tourangeau, Cranley, & Jeffs, 2006; Upenieks, Akhavan, Kotlerman, Esser, & Ngo, 2007; White, 2006). Further, new science specific to healthcare organizations in the Magnet Recognition Program shows better patient outcomes on mortality measures and significantly better outcomes compared to non-Magnet hospitals (Friese, Xia, Chaferi, Birkmeyer & Banerjee, 2015).

New science for staffing specific to clinical specialties, skill mix, environmental influences, and the linkage of staffing models to clinical outcomes is being developed and published regularly (Malloch, 2015; Needleman et al., 2011). In addition to new staffing science is evidence for IOM interprofessional practice (IPP). IPP has an impact on patient safety, provider and patient satisfaction, quality of care, community health outcomes, and cost savings, as well as a direct impact on the relationship among interprofessional education (IPE) and patient, population, and system outcomes (Institute of Medicine, 2015).

Value research is also emerging. The Agency for Healthcare Research and Quality (AHRQ) has advanced value research, which focuses on finding a way to achieve greater value in health care with cost and waste reductions while maintaining or improving quality (AHRQ, 2015)

Technology Advancements

Advances in technology continue to emerge for both patient care delivery and the management of information. With the introduction of the electronic health record, platforms for the management of large data sets are now available as well as the introduction of standardized clinical language. The standardized language further supports data comparisons across settings and enables providers to coordinate and collaborate more easily on patient care, which can improve healthcare outcomes and enable providers to achieve performance standards (CMS, n.d.).

Consumerism

Finally, users of the healthcare system are more involved than ever. Person and family-centered care is now the expectation (Barnsteiner, Disch, & Walton, 2014), whereby persons are empowered, actively participate, and are informed of all costs and the anticipated value of services. Both provider and healthcare organization performance metrics, as well as Hospital Consumer Assessment of Healthcare Providers and Systems (HCAHPS) scores, are published regularly. Consumers also access staffing data for healthcare facilities on a routine basis. The importance and utility of a personal health record continues to increase. Users of the healthcare system want their information consolidated into one file and readily accessible when needed. User ownership and management of one's personal health record is now an expectation of increasing numbers of patients. These opportunities, along with other driving forces, continue to support the case for value-based health care, of which staffing is an integral part.

Embedded within each of these initiatives are issues and concerns about the availability and productivity of nursing resources. As previously noted, the work of changing current systems and practices is complex and requires courage, persistence, and evidence to shift the current trajectory. While there is supporting evidence for this journey, there are also obstacles and challenges that must be reckoned with. The obstacles or challenges to this work are discussed in the next section.

CHALLENGES AND OBSTACLES TO CHANGE

There are many challenges and obstacles within the healthcare system that make it difficult to move forward with improvements to the healthcare system. Despite the clear and convincing theoretical rationale for system change, it is often ignored. These obstacles to making the needed transformation happen cannot be dismissed or taken lightly. Creating a new healthcare model requires support, passion, evidence, and resources. For many healthcare leaders, the process involved in making a significant system change is far too complex to embrace. Many leaders will struggle with any modification of the current system under the misguided notion that the system is functional and provides the appropriate information to make decisions supportive of quality patient care outcomes. In this section, several of these challenges will be discussed. The control and influence of the existing powerful organizational infrastructures over nursing resource allocation, coupled with the inability of nursing to articulate its specific work and outcomes achieved within the existing productivity framework, the environment of health care, and the determination of productivity using a single metric are imposing obstacles that many may find difficult to challenge.

Historically, services are provided and documented by siloed or individual disciplines and then pasted together into a summative document without identified connections among the individuals contributing to patient care. Most healthcare organizational cultures are steeped in traditions that support the silo mentality and stability of operations.

The historical adequacy of the overarching position of medicine and its specific measures of procedural-based coding and billing have precluded the need for more accurate clinical productivity measures for nursing that are quantifiable, credible, and useful. Unfortunately, the development of appropriate measures for nursing work tend to garner attention only during times of nursing shortage and nursing dissatisfaction.

Organizations today may struggle to control costs through cost reductions associated with the poorly defined work of nursing, yet the need for competently educated practitioners remains significant. Despite the increases in nursing education and the increasing complexity of nursing work, clarity in the work of nursing and appropriate workforce measures have not emerged to achieve the desired recognition of the value of nursing work in the marketplace. Because it is poorly defined and described, nursing work is difficult to measure and evaluate, which too often results in uncertain patient outcomes. When attempts are made to decrease or increase nursing resources for work that is poorly defined, the effects of these measures on patient outcomes is uncertain as well. While it is believed that less nursing care results in poor patient outcomes, such conclusions are not universally supported. The lack of evidence identifying the specific interventions of nursing and their implications for patient outcomes must be addressed. Tallying simple hours of care, without delineating the actual work performed, will not produce data that can be confidently correlated to patient outcomes, whether those outcomes are positive or negative. Describing the work of nursing from an evidence-based perspective is the first step in the process; the second step, integrating these principles into practice, is evolutionary and ongoing.

Inconsistent Identification of the Work of Nursing

Not all work of nursing is visible and measurable; intuition, caring behaviors, and trust are essential in the provision of care and yet are not readily captured in traditional knowledge worker models or productivity systems. The tangible work of nursing is more easily measured than intangible work. While the work of nursing is defined in each state's nurse practice act and professional standards of the American Nurses Association (ANA), each organization has created unique models and frameworks to guide the practice of nursing. Most frequently, the frameworks are based on body system checklists and assessments. Few organizations focus on nursing care interventions on the basis of practice acts or professional standards.

Another challenge is the work that nurses actually do during their work time. A high percentage of time is spent on activities not related to direct patient care. In a Hill-Rom study of acute care organizations, approximately 85% of nurses' time was spent on direct and indirect activities that did not move the patient along the care path (Lanser, 2001). Murphy (2003) reported that wasteful work—including excessive documentation requirements; inefficient shift-to-shift or departmental reports; and searching for colleagues, supplies, and equipment—consumed 35% of hospital employees' time. More recently, the Advisory Board Company identified that nurses spend 25% of their time on indirect patient care (2012).

Another aspect of this challenge is that nurses find it quite difficult to give up any of their current nursing work because all work is believed to be valuable and appropriate. Non-value-added work includes both direct and indirect nursing work and work resulting from system inefficiencies. The following examples identify tasks that do not provide value to patient outcomes:

- Provision of patient education to patients who are historically noncompliant: It is unrealistic to expect that an 80-year-old diabetic patient will become enlightened and change his or her behaviors in an acute care setting. Extensive reviews and presentation of information in these situations serve only to complete checklists and provide inappropriate feelings of accomplishment. Brief, meaningful encounters with known noncompliant patients are necessary to check for new interest; however, this is more effective in post-acute-care settings. In the value equation, unrealistic interventions render the equation out of balance given the lack of outcomes and overuse of scarce resources associated with these efforts.
- Frequency of vital signs: When a patient has consistent and stable vital signs, is it necessary to repeat these measures every 4 hours, especially when caregivers are present who can monitor the patient?
- Telemetry monitoring: Is all telemetry monitoring value based? Is the intervention of telemetry monitoring linked to improvements in the patient's status, and is it an effective use of available resources? Or is telemetry monitoring used for routine patient oversight?

- Searching for equipment and supplies: Does this task promote the patient's movement along the healing continuum?
- Passing out meal trays: Is this the best use of a nurse's time? Should someone from another division or support staff handle this task?
- Searching for other providers and colleagues: Is this an appropriate task for nurses?
- Replenishing procedure carts and monitoring levels in supply rooms: Do these activities directly affect the patient?
- Searching for information and reference manuals: Can this task be managed differently?

Lack of Linkage between Nurse Actions and Patient Outcomes

The next challenge is not only the lack of linkage between nurse work and patient outcomes, but also the inconsistent use of linkage evidence that is available. The evidence supporting a relationship among caregiver performance, patient outcomes, and financial performance is strong (Aiken et al., 2003; Aiken, Smith, & Lake, 1994; Blegen & Vaughn, 1998; Cho, Ketefian, Barkauskas, & Smith, 2003; McCue, Mark, & Harless, 2003). Evidence supporting the relationships among variables in the organizational structure and patient outcomes has also been identified. Unfortunately, the intervening specific work processes that produce those outcomes have not been clearly articulated, nor are they embedded in the analysis of these relationships.

The challenge in identifying truly valued work is coupled with the reality that evidence is lacking to support some interventions that may, indeed, positively affect patient outcomes. The historic lack of connection between the economic viability of the organization and its effects on the satisfaction and performance of its nursing resource is an untenable factor in the future consideration of the viability of healthcare organizations. The failure to clearly tie practice elements and activities to specifically defined outcomes makes it exceptionally difficult to identify any unique and specified value for nursing practice. Nurses cannot claim value on one hand and provide little definitive evidence of that value on the other hand.

Too many nurses ignore the need to balance clinical performance against resource availability and quality outcomes. Because of the history of nursing and its predominant focus on clinical process, rather than specific identification with clinical outcome, many nurses have become addicted to process (Hughes & American Nurses Association, 1958). In fact, for many nurses, the process has become ritual, routine, and intellectually mindless. Further, experience itself has become a mantra, even though in most cases experience tends to be a limitation; the more experience one has, the more one is inculcated in the values that experience provides (Smith, 2002). *Competent* practice is *changing* practice. As technology enhancements and innovations continually challenge the foundations of clinical practice, it is the very fluidity, flexibility, and mobility of clinical practice that ensures its continuing viability and efficacy. This blind dependence and valuing of experience over innovation and education must be overcome if meaningful value is to be found and defined (Corey, 2001).

Inconsistent Time Allocations for Nursing Work

There is precious little data about how much time is required for nursing interventions and the recognition of the optimal provider to do this work. The greatest stumbling block for quantification of nursing work is the lack of consensus about the appropriate measurement technique, such as motion and time studies, historical use of nurses' time, and comprehensive assignment analysis methods (Malloch, 2015).

Calculation of time requirements for patient care needs requires more granularity than previously considered. Time considerations for the additional handoff requirements of admissions, discharges, and transfers has been identified and continues to be studied using electronic records. Time for nurse surveillance and nursing care that encompasses oversight of the patient without a specific intervention has also been calculated and linked to adverse patient outcomes when not provided.

Limited Productivity Measurement and Evaluation

The current metric of hours per patient day identifies how long it took for the care to be delivered but not what was done; it is an incomplete representation of the work of nursing that does not incorporate structural and environmental considerations in productivity measures. Relative value unit (RVU) measures attempt to recognize the degree of patient care variation based on a median unit, but they are limited by the description of the value of 1.0 unit. The limited accuracy and completeness of describing 1.0 RVU continues to be problematic because descriptors for all categories of the core work of nursing are not included in this system.

Measurements that are limited to comparisons of total hours worked per patient day and projected budgeted hours can only provide a limited perspective of value. Such comparisons provide no information specific to the level of patient acuity, provision of appropriate interventions, achievement of clinical outcomes, and absence of adverse outcomes—all of which require a framework for productivity measurement based on principles that integrate values of effectiveness, utility, and cost.

Knowing which outcomes resulted from which work performed by which category of caregiver is critical if the profession is to effectively articulate its value and contribution to the health of individuals. Understanding the important relationships among specific work processes and integrating them into the productivity measurement systems of organizations will require new knowledge, new mental models, and commitment to staffing on the basis of evidence or trend data created from best practices.

Unfortunately, this approach and limited analysis have been used in most organizations to measure nurse productivity and to make decisions specific to the allocation of staffing resources. The hours used are typically compared to patient units of service without considering the actual output, which is an essential component of a productivity measure. These traditional productivity measures of hours used per patient day represent a limited analysis and do not reflect the notion of theoretical productivity, which calls for the greatest output for the least input (Drucker, 1990).

Nonsupportive Physical Environment

Pinkerton and Rivers (2001) identified 64 variables that affect nurse staffing needs, including variables specific to interdepartmental interactions, intradepartmental interactions, the care environment, professional competency, physicians, and the external environment. Physical environments are a critical element of the care dynamic itself, not only for patients, but also for providers. Unfortunately, there is wide variability in the use of evidence in the creation and sustaining of current healthcare environments. The building, structural format, color, inclusion of nature, and peaceful aesthetics help create a viable milieu to work within (Ulrich, Quan, Zimring, Joseph, & Choudhary, 2004).

Poorly designed work spaces, heavy equipment, the absence of patient lift equipment, and the lack of noise control have negatively impacted both patients and caregivers. Further, the conditions of stress embedded in clinical work have a tremendous impact on retention and turnover in clinical practice. Nurse fatigue and burnout have been identified as major stressors for both nurses and patients (Geiger-Brown et al., 2012; Martin, 2014; Stimpfel, Lake, Barton, Gorman, & Aiken, 2013).

Mixture of Technology and Minimal Interoperability/Lack of Actionable Data

The use of multiple applications for clinical documentation and management information requires users to sign in and sign out of multiple applications during their work time. The inefficiencies of isolated applications render the information fragmented and leaves the aggregation of data to the user to obtain meaningful information for clinical decisions. Further, within applications, caregivers are required to review multiple other areas of documentation to determine the status of the patient condition.

Evidence Lacking in Staffing and Assignment Processes

The nurse–patient assignment process has also lacked an evidentiary foundation; namely, matching required hours of patient care to the appropriately competent caregiver. The simplicity of ratio calculations for nurse–patient assignments has overshadowed the benefits (including greater accuracy) that might be realized with the use of multiple data values. Overcoming the deeply entrenched tradition of ratio or grid-based staffing models to create evidence-based processes that recognize and address the daily variations of patient care needs and staff availability requires courage and commitment to the creation of a better system. The obvious simplicity of these historical calculations is antithetical to the real goal of quality patient care. To overcome this resistance, increasing numbers of organizations are selecting computerized database management systems to provide more sophisticated, more complex, and timely data that can be used to develop the next generation of productivity measurements. The reality is that it is difficult to use resources effectively without such systems and evaluations.

Lack of Standardized Language

In attempting to arrive at the truth, I have applied everywhere
for information, but in scarcely an instance have I been able
to obtain hospital records fit for any purposes of comparisons.

—FLORENCE NIGHTINGALE

At one point, the ANA approved 13 standardized languages that support nursing practice, 10 of which are considered languages specific to nursing care (Rutherford, 2008). The use of multiple descriptions for similar concepts is confusing and difficult to automate. Information in healthcare records must be searchable, shared, and synthesized as needed (Warren, 2012). The use of standardized healthcare language requires that the interventions of nursing must be specified and described with sufficient clarity so another researcher or practitioner can replicate the action. Standardized language comprises terminology and communication styles that can be used in all settings by all clinicians, is grounded in clinical practice and research, is functionally appropriate for computerized clinical documentation systems that need to simplify the exchange, and makes it easier to manage and integrate clinical data into the electronic health record. The language must allow for the measurement of patient, family, and community healthcare interventions and outcomes (Moorhead, Johnson, & Maas, 2004).

Although this next section focuses on the work of nursing, it is imperative for all professional and support providers to recognize the current limitations in determining their value and create similar linkages among services and valued outcomes. The proposed innovative model is designed to serve as a framework for the conceptualization of the interrelationships of organizational elements.

A pile of rocks ceases to be a rock pile when somebody contemplates it with the idea of a cathedral in mind.

—Antoine de Saint-Exupéry

THE VALUE APPROACH: AN INNOVATIVE MODEL TO ADVANCE STAFFING ADEQUACY

At long last, the rules are changing! Value is now the driver for healthcare work as identified earlier in this chapter. It is now back to the future as healthcare leaders work to achieve the expected value outcomes from an evidentiary paradigm. Considering both the challenges and the opportunities in health care, leaders are well positioned to advance the value model. In this section, the basic components of a healthcare staffing value model are presented (**Figure 12-1**). These components include principles for an evidentiary value

---

Figure 12-1   Healthcare value model mind map: Basic components

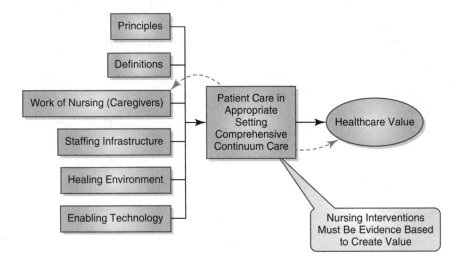

model, a description of healthcare value, description and measurement of nursing work using a clinical productivity model, and anticipated outcomes from a value-driven system.

Principles in a Value Model

Foundational principles to guide the development of this innovative model are presented. Principles for designing this model are more effective in a complex and ever-changing world than specific procedures and algorithms. Principles should be longer lasting, and procedures and algorithms change rapidly. The principles include the following:

- Person and family-focused care is provided within the context of each patient's life position
- Coordinated team efforts are essential for and by providers and patients
- Objective and measurable outcomes are associated with each intervention or strategy
- Providers are selected based on cost and outcomes; the goal is the highest quality and the lowest cost optimizing the full scope of practice for each role
- The environment is supportive of patients and caregivers
- The most current evidence is integrated into this work

Value Definitions

Although there are many definitions of value and value-based health care, the following are simple and reflective of the desired outcome:

- Value is considered as patient health outcomes per dollar spent; value is the only goal that can unite the interests of all system participants. It will require fundamental restructuring of healthcare delivery, not incremental improvements (Porter, 2012).
- Value-based care means safe, appropriate, and effective care with enduring results at a reasonable cost; it means using evidence-based medicine and proven treatments and techniques that take into account the patient's wishes and preferences (Dartmouth-Hitchcock, 2015).

CLARIFYING THE WORK OF NURSING

The challenge is to create a value-driven model based on evidence for nursing work that includes all valued nursing care, its economic component, and the intangible work that nurses bring to the bedside (Welton, 2011). There are three types of nursing work: objective and observable interventions, intangible interventions or absence factors, and overlapping interventions. All must be included in a staffing productivity model.

The work of nursing is about providing appropriate goal-oriented services rather than providing as many services as possible irrespective of the cost and outcomes. Value choices for care, rather than rich choices (choices for care that are nice but not linked to the outcome, such as back rubs twice a day or bed baths for ambulatory patients), that take into account fiscal implications, appropriateness of nursing care specific to outcomes, and goodness of fit, service quality, and patient impact are needed. The process of quantifying and enumerating the work of nursing must be embraced if we are to develop valid and reliable information and systems to guide nurse staffing. This effort will, in turn, provide credibility within the financial sectors of health care.

To identify value, there also needs to be objective and measurable elements that can be related to outcomes using standardized language to embed in current measurement structures and electronic databases. The description also requires recognition and integration of a societal mandate for nursing, the professional scope of practice, and the economic realities of the marketplace (American Nurses Association [ANA], 2003). A qualitative, descriptive overview of the work of nursing must include more than just tasks that are easily observed and quantified, such as procedures and administration of medications.

Quantifying the work of nursing using a standardized approach to patient intensity is the foundation for a valid and reliable patient intensity needs system, another important element of an evidence-based workforce management system (ANA, 2008). The patient intensity level used by an organization must reflect the major clinical intervention categories applicable to all clinical specialties. At a minimum, categories specific to the technical work of nursing, monitoring activities, interdisciplinary coordination, communication, and leadership must be represented. Examples of interventions within those categories include patient assessment, medication administration, intravenous access and line management, pain management, safety or restraint management, and interpretation of vital signs.

In addition to these categories, the following must be included:

- Monitoring progress and oversight of patient conditions
- Management of information, namely, knowing not only what to communicate, but also to whom and when to communicate
- Patient and family education as well as information management among members of the caregiver team

- Creating and modifying plans of care in a timely manner based on patient conditions
- Leadership behaviors specific to the delegation and supervision of work processes of other staff and precepting new nurses
- Continuum care coordination, namely coordination of the work of all disciplines caring for the patient

It is clear that to ensure effective resource management, workforce systems must be transformed into evidence-based systems and reflect a prevailing and sustaining reality (ANA, 2012). Optimum nursing care, according to Welton (2011), represents a balance between the intensity and quality of the delivered nursing care, including costs, safety, and outcomes of that care.

Continuum Care Coordination

The work of care coordination has been moved among clinical roles and typically focuses on utilization management or the amount of resources or dollars that are available for a patient. Historical goals have been to avoid overuse of resources at the expense of patient achievement of desired goals. The proposed value model requires the registered nurse to assume the care coordination role across the continuum for several reasons. The nurse is located at the intersection of the provision of all healthcare services. It is the nurse's role to coordinate, integrate, and facilitate all of the clinical functions related to the delivery of patient care. Nurses are deeply entrenched in daily processes of relationship management with all patient care team members (e.g., physicians, nurses, managers, allied health personnel, and unlicensed assistive personnel). Experience and collective wisdom emerge from team members who work together effectively. It is vital to recognize nursing's central role, however, as nurses integrate all of the work of other disciplines with regard to a patient's progress along the healing continuum. This realization is the key to the clinical success of the entire health organization (While et al., 2004). However, empirical evidence of the critical value of *intersection management—* that is, interdisciplinary coordination—is needed.

Continuum care coordination is a much-needed service for patients within the value model. As previously noted, it has been difficult to determine and quantify the value of those activities that are predominantly focused on coordinating and integrating processes. Because this type of coordination and integration account for the majority of professional nursing activity (in terms of value), it is clearly important to provide a financial definition for it (Rubin, Plovnick, & Fry, 1975). Although nursing must clearly delineate its own specific functions and activities, the importance attached to those functions and activities is not gained unilaterally.

Fulfilling the role of care coordination clearly places the nurse in a critical position with regard to the financial and service viability of the organization. In addition, elements of high levels of quality in the delivery of clinical service are influenced and often coordinated by nursing professionals. Nurses are the eyes of all other providers; in this eyes-and-ears role, nurses evaluate the patient's condition, response, and progress in a timely fashion. Therefore, in a high-level interface, nurses have a direct and powerful impact on the clinical and service viability of the organization. Through this direct relationship, nurses control the financial variables that ultimately affect the economic viability of the organization as a whole (Finkler & Graf, 2001).

Missed Nursing Care

Missed nursing care must also be considered. Examination of nursing from the opposite side of the outcome—namely, from the time before nursing occurred or in the absence of nursing as it is now known—is both illustrative and enlightening to assist in the description of nursing. When nursing is absent, it is not merely medications that are not administered and dressings that are not changed; much more occurs. What is lost is subtle at first and then overwhelmingly thunderous. Patients are not monitored regularly for condition changes; failure to rescue is common, and emergency codes occur; condition changes are not communicated to physicians; care is not coordinated; patient knowledge is not improved; and measures of preventable conditions, such as pressure ulcers, urinary tract infections, pneumonia, and length of stay, all increase—these are the intangible interventions that need to be described and included as nurse work. Kalish (2014) has recently identified nine elements of regularly missed care: ambulation, turning, delayed or missed feedings, patient teaching, discharge planning, emotional support, hygiene, intake and output documentation, and surveillance. Failing to fully account for the work of nursing and to be sure that there is not missed care will compromise the integrity of the value model.

Discussion

Nurses in your department believe there is much nursing care that is missed. What is available in your current systems to determine what has not been done? How would you propose to determine if discharge planning has been missed? Or if hygiene has been missed and how often it has been missed? After you quantify this information, how can you use the clinical productivity model to assure that the care will not be missed in the future? Finally, how were patient outcomes impacted in light of missed care?

Overlapping Patient Care

The nature of nursing practice should be closely examined to better understand the boundaries of nursing; that is, boundaries that overlap with other disciplines and boundaries that are unique to the nursing profession. The work of care coordination, assessment, planning, and identified procedures should be retained by nurses, and activities of daily living, vital sign monitoring in many situations, and administration of routine medications should be delegated and shared with appropriate disciplines, such as paramedics, nursing assistants, and licensed practical nurses (Pittman & Forrest, 2015; Rheaume & Belliveau, 2015).

Some of the work performed by nurses can be performed by other disciplines or support staff. Nursing will have an especially difficult time in meeting the obligations of discipline-specific definitions if it continues to perform these tasks without further evaluation and efforts to assure the highest quality of care at the lowest cost. Examples of overlapping interventions include vital sign monitoring, activities of daily living, and medication administration in selected settings. The challenges for nursing derive from its historical commitment to the process and its lack of a clearly defined relationship to clinical outcomes. The more valuable activity for nursing in undertaking this process will be to assess the time commitments related to coordinating, integrating, and facilitating the clinical work of all the disciplines, then assign a specific value to that time and effort. Important to this process, which will put nursing farther along the road to adoption of an evidence-based format, is attention to the following factors:

- Establishing a clear value for the support functions of managing supplies and equipment for nurse work.
- Enumerating the type and character of coordinative and integrative activities that are fundamental to the role of the nurse.
- Specifically identifying particular clinical practice standards and professional performance characteristics against which value can be established so the outcomes indicated by them can be more clearly defined.
- Creating a method (formula) for determining costs and value related specifically to the clinical and coordinative activities undertaken at the point of service that reflect the standard of practice identified there.

The elimination of non-value-added work also provides more time for nurses to give comfort to and talk with patients, develop and update plans of care, and provide patient and family education—all types of work that are typically foregone when time is scarce.

Creating Linkages between Work and Value for the Patient

After the work of nursing is described, its linkage to patient outcomes and available resources must be established. A specifically defined tie among clinical tasks, best practices, and the payment formats within which they are financed is an essential element of the value model. The value equation in which clinical practice, performance outcomes, and the available payment structure are examined serves as a template to assess the overall value of the nursing work (Malloch & Porter-O'Grady, 1999). Desirable outcomes of nursing interventions include achievement of clinical goals, improvement in the ability to manage one's own health, and a safe environment as measured by the absence of adverse outcomes. Examples of outcomes specific to nursing that affect not only the patient, but also the conditions that influence a patient's health, include the following:

- Increased ability to provide self-care
- Improved mobility
- Improved stress management and coping skills
- Improved knowledge of clinical condition
- Improved knowledge of healthy behaviors specific to nutrition and mobility
- Improved parenting skills
- Community health and well-being
- Improved knowledge of behaviors for safety specific to health care

The purpose of quantification of caregiver work is to develop information to extend the current productivity system that identifies the direct link among the evidence-based work of caregivers, value-based outcomes, and payment. Necessarily, this effort requires quantification of the specific work and the link or relationship of the work to the achievement of desired value-based outcomes. The health status of the patient must be affected positively to justify the resource expenditure.

Discussion

Achieving value in healthcare organizations begins at the unit or shift level. Using the value equation, namely resources will result in the desired clinical outcome for the patient, a group of nurses in a Magnet organization decided to see if their pain management service resulted in value for the patients. Nurses were aware that the revenue for this unit exceeded budget targets, and the hours for nurse staffing were within the budgeted allocation. As the team discussed this process of value analysis, they realized that patient feedback specific to sustainable pain relief was not a metric considered in evaluating the program.

- What is your reaction to this scenario?
- What changes do you think are necessary to determine the value of this program to patients?
- If the revenue and hours of nursing care were over budget and the patients experience significant relief from their pain, what would be the next steps in your assessment of the pain clinic?
- Are there other areas of patient care in which this analysis would be similar?

To clearly delineate nursing value, it is crucial to utilize the prevailing methodology, which uses payment factors as a part of value determination. The most obvious unit of value is the Diagnosis-Related Group (DRG), the predominant value unit that is used for payment in healthcare organizations. No matter which approach is ultimately identified and used, it must be consistent, be reducible to financial value, integrate and link the contributions of the healthcare disciplines, and be useful as an evaluative and comparative mechanism. In addition, it should provide an opportunity to evaluate the criteria, performance, and impact of medical practice.

Finally, there are several tools to examine the value of nursing in addition to clinical outcomes. These analyses can further document the value of nursing care. Each method is based on specific goals (Stone, Curran, & Bakken, 2002) and includes the following:

- Financial metric of cost minimization: Costs are compared among alternatives only; equal effects are assumed; no outcomes are measured
- Value metric of cost effectiveness: Consequences are measured in the same units among alternatives; outcomes are measured using ratios such as expenditures/outcome or dollars/life years gained
- Value metric of cost utility: Effects include both quantity and quality measures; measures are dollars or quality of life years gained
- Financial metric of cost benefit: Effects are measured as a single dollar measure; measures are in dollars gained
- Value metric of cost consequences: Costs and effects are listed separately; effects among alternatives may have different measures; expenditures and a separate list of outcomes are measured

Each of these evaluation methods offers a different lens through which to view the work of nursing. Ultimately, a combination of several methods is likely to better represent nursing work based on the intended goals and resources.

Supporting Effective Staffing Infrastructure Elements

To achieve staffing adequacy, specific organizational infrastructure elements are needed. The first is appropriate caregiver resources; that is, competent caregivers and support staff to meet identified patient care needs. The staffing infrastructure also includes a scheduling system, patient needs system, and time and attendance systems that are preferably interconnected and interoperative so that staffing adequacy can be obtained. The following elements are essential components within an effective staffing system:

- Nursing time required to perform identified care (Malloch, 2015)
- Appropriate skill and competence of each caregiver, addressing the overlapping of selected interventions by different disciplines

- Performance standards, including levels of expectations for clinical competence, differentiation among provider levels, and clearly delineated performance expectations for specific patient populations or DRGs
- Nurse–patient assignment criteria and a staffing adjustment process that addresses changes in patient conditions and needs
- Understanding of environmental factors impacting staffing and the cost factors associated with delivery of care
- Available resources (supplies, equipment, medication, etc.) for each patient

Supportive Environment

There are several considerations for the environment of care. First is a culture with supportive leadership embracing engagement, openness, and valuing of the clinical provider as a key aspect of creating an appropriate supporting structure. A host of considerations must be taken into account in regard to the physical work environment and its impact on risk and safety from both providers' and patients' perspectives. These issues also exert a powerful effect on the cost of providing service and the ability to create an environment that establishes a marketable relationship between the organization and those whom it serves. Much evidence supports the existence of a close relationship between environmental issues of safety and clinical error rates. As a consequence, fiscal and service leaders should be able to make a clear distinction of the costs associated with these environmental and structural factors. Also, these factors should be incorporated into any data analysis related to productivity and work value determinations.

The Center for Health Design's Pebble Project model addresses issues including the desirability of the environment for the patient, the market value of a healing environment to the community, and the fiscal impact of reducing length of stay, care intensity, and patient need. According to this model, creating a physical environment that facilitates healing is as important as other influences on cost (Berry et al., 2004).

Environmental considerations are critical to establish evidence of the environment's influence on clinical practice as well as economics and health service costs. In building an evidentiary value model, the following issues and relationships should be considered:

- Identification of specific healing, comfort, and patient satisfaction considerations related to the physical environment and structural context for care
- Delineation of the structural and organizational (delivery system) considerations affecting clinical practice and specific elements of work flow
- Enumeration of the impact of physical plant, environment, and structures on provider attitudes, satisfaction, and turnover rates
- Determination of the impact of environment and structure on issues of clinical error, patient safety, and circumstances of care

- Incorporation of structural and environmental considerations in productivity measures and formulas associated with appropriate resource use and service time values

Enabling Information Technology Platform for Data Management

The development of a data management system that collects, sorts and provides reports in an easy-to-access format is essential in an evidentiary model. Using an evidence-based framework to determine optimal productivity, patient–staff ratios, clinical assignments, provider categories, and relationships to patient outcomes is now fundamental in efforts to accurately determine value and its effects on quality and cost (Harrington & Estes, 2004). Indeed, the accuracy of the financial data pertaining to the clinical relationship between patient and provider is now an essential construct of appropriate, meaningful, and sustainable delivery of clinical services. Failing to include these environmental and structural considerations in the determination of productivity and clinical care not only contributes to a lack of cost control, but also facilitates the inappropriate and possibly expensive use of unevaluated human resources.

A new productivity metric is needed that reflects the complex work involved in the practice of nursing. This new metric would replace the traditional comparison of hours worked to hours budgeted. Metrics that reflect the output of care as compared to the input of providers and is adjusted for environmental factors provides a more accurate representation of nursing productivity.

An integrated data infrastructure in which nursing practice is included according to the context of both clinical quality and financial enumerators is necessary for monitoring and evaluating the value model. Integrated data systems that link services, costs, and outcomes add the nurse–patient assignment to electronic operational databases to allow specific identification of which nurse cared for which patients. Moving in this direction will significantly change how we view nursing performance (Welton, 2010). The financial success of system participants does not equal patient success, rather it is the aggregated cost the patient is responsible for, such as deductibles and non-covered items. It is important to be transparent and identify costs around the full cycle of care for the patient's medical condition rather than charges billed or collected (Porter, 2012).

The purpose of creating a new clinical productivity model is not to more accurately represent the work of nursing as we now know it, but rather to create a new mindset that moves leaders from expecting adequate numbers of nurses to focusing on achieving adequate patient care outcomes within the existing healthcare structure and resources. Three strategies are essential in the creation of a more contemporary model:

- Embedding the new measures within existing systems
- Evaluating performance in an aggregated model
- Managing the variance or system feedback to ensure system sustainability

From an evidence-based practice perspective, it may be more helpful to clearly articulate nursing's value within an economic framework to join all interdisciplinary activities under the rubric of an integrated clinical standard of practice. It is this linkage and integration among the disciplines that will create the composite framework for value determination. The evidence of impact on patient outcome, the viability of clinical processes, and the cost framework that supports clinical practice can be more clearly elucidated when the disciplines speak the same language and use a common framework. Until that time, however, focusing on effective nursing workforce management and creating an integrated structure for valuing that work will be critical first steps toward valuing nursing practice, establishing its relationship to financial and payment concerns, and providing a baseline with which nursing resource value can be connected across the interdisciplinary healthcare network.

An integrated data set connects the financial, accounting, and budgeting processes of the organization to workforce management and resource allocation within the context of specific clinical protocols or DRGs. Developing, refining, and maintaining a clinical resource information infrastructure for real-time data related to acuity, patient demand, resource allocation, clinical standards or protocols, structural and environmental considerations, and a continuous and effective reporting mechanism requires an evolutionary process in which long-time disparate processes can be strategically linked.

An integrated data management system also supports the work of addressing the challenges of change and innovation. Improvements that focus on the elimination of non-value-added work and increasing productivity include computerized electronic health records, technology for communication, pocket reference guides, personal digital assistants, and pocket-sized hand sanitizer packets.

Variance Management: A Daily Dynamic

Daily data assessments of critical variables specific to clinical and financial targets are important not only to understand the current state, but also to make course corrections if needed.

The most significant information produced from any system relates to variances; that is, the differences between the desired outcome and the actual outcome. Seldom is there a perfect match between what is desired and what actually results. The resulting variance between time for patient care needs and time provided by staffing resources reflects the reality of balancing the workforce processes with the inherent expectations for reducing, eliminating, or managing these differences. It is this variance that provides the data from which to manage, monitor, and improve system performance. Merely counting and documenting the desired and actual outcomes does not provide any value for the system in outcome management. Instead, ensuring the accountability of the articulation and reporting of variance management are essential unifying links in the process. Efforts to produce high levels of quality without devoting adequate human or financial resources to support those efforts is irrational and doomed to eliminate (destroy) the system. Effective evaluation processes lay the foundation for safe and timely management of the variance between what is desired and what actually occurs.

Discussion

As nurse manager on a unit, you would like staff nurses to become familiar with variance management for their own shift. What guidelines would you establish for determining when a variance is over or under target? How would you assist the nurses in determining if patient care is or will be negatively impacted? Is this about using evidence that is available, or being innovative and creating a new strategy for variance management?

Leaders are continually challenged to consider variations in the known natural clinical variances of disease, levels of severity, patients' responses to treatment, variability in work flow due to random arrivals of patients, and inherent variability of clinicians in regard to their knowledge, critical thinking, prioritizing, and communication skills. According to Long (2002), the goal is to eliminate artificial variance—that is, clinical errors, medication errors, lack of knowledge, inappropriate scheduling, and scheduling based on staff needs rather than patient needs. Leaders should focus on further managing the natural variation or the uncertain occurrence of care needs by patients, both predicted and unpredicted, and the inherent professional differences in ability that will always exist.

System variances result in high and low levels of workload, characterized by frequent internal diversions of patients to other units, backups in the postanesthesia care unit, external diversions from the emergency department, staff overload, and increased length of stay as a consequence of system gridlock. When a system variance is identified, the following management practices are indicated:

- Delineate protocols and link their required interventions to desired outcomes.
- Create a framework to examine performance standards.

- Define the linkage among interventions, best practice, and payment formats.
- Continue to monitor, evaluate, and adjust for gaps in desired linkages needed for value (cost–service–quality).

A staffing variance occurs when there is a difference between the identified patient care needs and the resources available to meet those needs. Given that there will always be discrepancies between needs and available staff, and given that nurses will continue to accept responsibility for providing safe, competent care, the development of strategies to manage this type of variance is essential. When a staffing variance is identified and efforts to obtain additional staff are exhausted, consider the following 10 strategies:

- Take a teamwork approach: Commit to working as a team to address the gap. Planned variance management from a team perspective is proactive and minimizes stress. In contrast, individual variance management is impulsive, reactive, and highly stressful.
- Prioritize: Identify specific patient care issues that require immediate attention and those that can be safely left until later in the shift or for the next shift.
- Manage decision making: As a team, determine how work will be organized or reorganized, then assign work for the shift based on the type of staff available and patient needs. Decide which aspects of care can be eliminated or safely assigned to others.
- Delegate and supervise: Delegate work to the appropriate caregivers and supervise accordingly to ensure that the work is being performed as required.
- Control work flow to the unit: Reroute admissions if possible and appropriate.
- Communicate: Arrange for a short midshift report to assess how well all team members are managing the workforce and reassign and reprioritize tasks as needed. Communicate how breaks and lunches will be organized.
- Plan: After the team is organized, have each team member do a quick walkabout to assess those clients identified as high priority.
- Evaluate: If circumstances require modification of a patient's plan of care, inform the patient about these changes and provide clear, factual information about the care the patient can expect.
- Document: Complete a variance report that identifies the specific patient care concerns. Clearly describe the safety concerns. Provide examples of care that could not be completed or situations in which the timing of prescribed interventions was delayed.
- Communicate: Share the variance management data with stakeholders and develop plans to minimize future gaps.

Box 12-1 Key Variance Assessment Questions

1. How many shifts are within, under, or over targeted staffing?
2. How many nurse–patient assignments were within capacity? Over? Under?
3. How do these results compare with target performance goals?
4. How many adverse patient outcomes occurred when targets were not met?

Variations from target staffing can also be calculated on a shift-by-shift basis. These data provide an overview of staffing patterns and opportunities to sustain or adjust current practices. In a large study by Needleman and colleagues, 15.9% of all shifts were 8 hours or more (8-hour shifts) below targeted staffing requirements. Both below targeted staffing and high turnover were associated with increased levels of mortality (Malloch, 2015; Needleman et al., 2011). Organizations will necessarily establish target performance levels and determine if 15.9% is acceptable.

New Units of Service: Comprehensive Continuum Approach

The historical inadequacy of summative task workforce calculations can be improved upon by using an aggregated or comprehensive workforce unit approach to measure patient care; the latter approach better represents the essence of the work of not only nursing, but also all other caregiver work.

New models that embrace and reflect the reality of nursing patient care services, focusing on the holistic and dynamic human condition with associated scientific, societal, and economic factors, will improve the ability of leaders to manage resources from an evidence-based perspective. A model that views and measures the work of patient care as an aggregated whole, rather than as a series of disconnected tasks, better represents the work of caregivers in a much simpler way. An extension of the nursing patient classification system to include all disciplines providing care further enhances the robustness of a clinical productivity system. The ideal workforce management system is one in which the unit of service is multidisciplinary and patient specific for a defined period of time. All disciplines providing services are integrated and considered as a multidisciplinary comprehensive unit of care. The work of each discipline can be identified on the basis of interventions and associated contributions to patient outcomes. This unit of care represents the integrated, interwoven contributions of associated disciplines, such as hospitalists, physical therapy, respiratory therapy, and social services.

This new model also must integrate the achievement of clinical outcomes resulting from the services provided, the number of hours of care for the service, and the level of provider required to achieve these outcomes. Further, the effects of this integration are reflected in the patient care value equation in which resources, outcomes, and value are examined and evaluated, forming the philosophical foundation for a new, aggregated productivity model.

The purpose of modifying current processes and measures is not to devalue the historical clinical productivity measurement, but rather to extend the existing productivity system to quantify the relationship among patient care services, value, and payment, and to adjust for those variables that influence the work of nursing. To be sure, this work may prove challenging. Reengineering anything is a risk that requires knowledge of not only the desired state of improvement, but also the failures that one desires to correct. Successes provide confidence that something right is occurring but not necessarily *why* it is right. Failures provide unquestionable proof that we have done something wrong. Creating new measurement models for healthcare clinical labor productivity requires knowledge of the best features of effective existing processes and failures that have negatively influenced outcomes.

As we move though the productivity enhancement journey, it is important to remember that 100% productivity requires homogeneity—namely, patients with the same disease, patients arriving at the same rate, providers equal in their ability to provide patient care, and families with the same level of knowledge and understanding. In other words, 100% productivity is a mythical, ideal state that does not exist in clinical settings. The most reasonable approach for operational decision making is longitudinal monitoring of productivity by organizational units combined with indicators of quality of patient care (Advisory Board Company, 2014; O'BrienPallas, Thomson, Hall, Pink, Kerr, Wang, et al., 2004). This care must be described, documented, and measured using a standardized patient classification system to support decisions that will support safe patient care. O'BrienPallas and colleagues (2004) identified 85% as the optimal nursing unit productivity, with 93% as the maximum productivity because 7% of the shift is made up of mandatory breaks.

ANTICIPATED OUTCOMES FROM A VALUE-DRIVEN SYSTEM

Making changes and improvements in healthcare staffing to create an optimal value model will evolve over time. Using an evidentiary approach strengthens the quality and reliability of decisions and further illuminates opportunities for innovation. Using a value model framework is intended to improve not only allocation and matching of staff resources to patient needs, but also improved clinical outcomes through coordinated care, more affordable care, the availability of actionable data, and data to identify gaps in processes and opportunities to reduce those gaps. **Figure 12-2** provides an overview of the component details of the value model.

Figure 12-2 Healthcare value model mind map: Component details

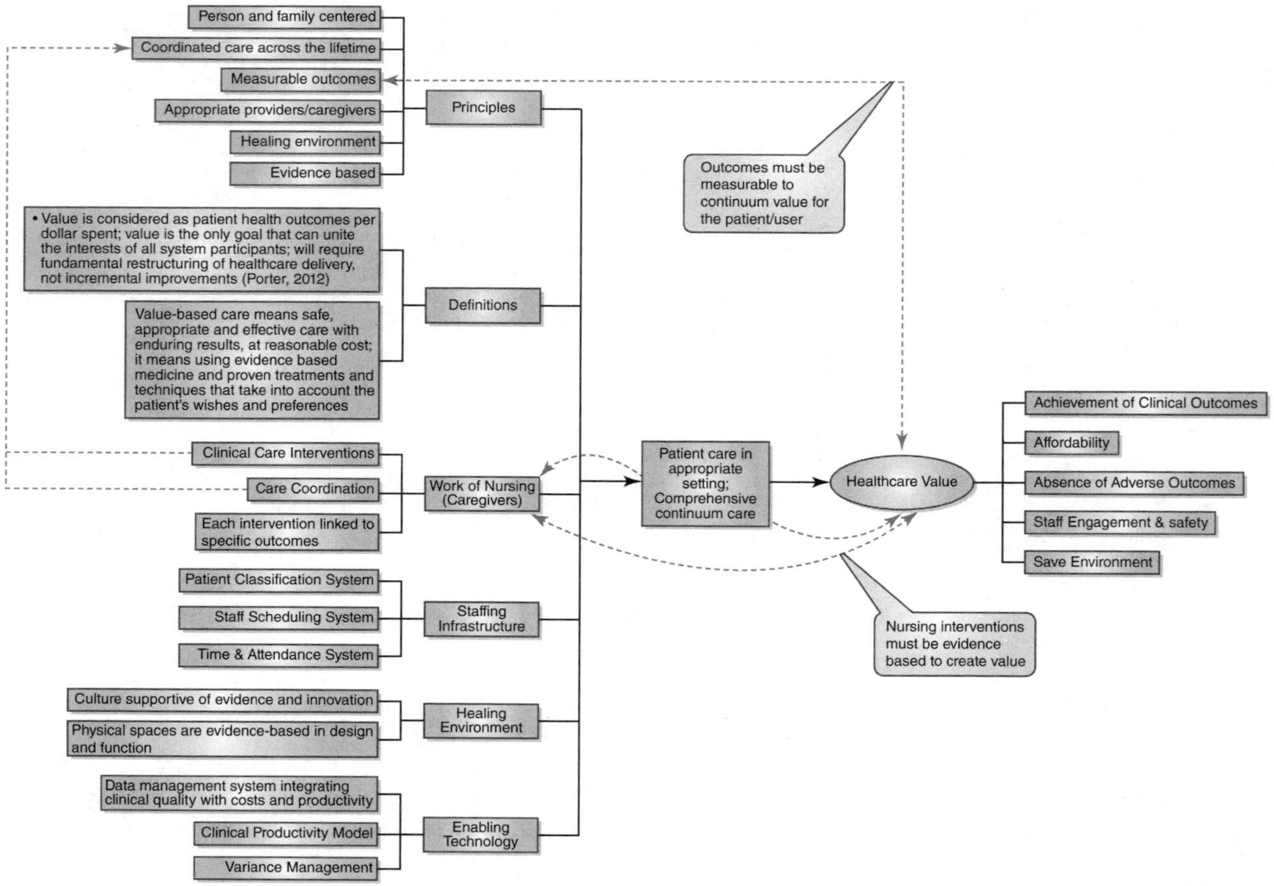

Principles
- Person and family centered
- Coordinated care across the lifetime
- Measurable outcomes
- Appropriate providers/caregivers
- Healing environment
- Evidence based

Definitions
- Value is considered as patient health outcomes per dollar spent; value is the only goal that can unite the interests of all system participants; will require fundamental restructuring of healthcare delivery, not incremental improvements (Porter, 2012)
- Value-based care means safe, appropriate and effective care with enduring results, at reasonable cost; it means using evidence based medicine and proven treatments and techniques that take into account the patient's wishes and preferences

Work of Nursing (Caregivers)
- Clinical Care Interventions
- Care Coordination
  - Each intervention linked to specific outcomes

Staffing Infrastructure
- Patient Classification System
- Staff Scheduling System
- Time & Attendance System

Healing Environment
- Culture supportive of evidence and innovation
- Physical spaces are evidence-based in design and function

Enabling Technology
- Data management system integrating clinical quality with costs and productivity
- Clinical Productivity Model
- Variance Management

Outcomes must be measurable to continuum value for the patient/user

Patient care in appropriate setting; Comprehensive continuum care

Healthcare Value

Nursing interventions must be evidence based to create value

- Achievement of Clinical Outcomes
- Affordability
- Absence of Adverse Outcomes
- Staff Engagement & safety
- Save Environment

All care providers must now be cognizant of the relationship among what they do, what it costs, and what is achieved as a result of having done it. In an evidence-based value format, managerial decisions must reflect a balancing of the value equation—namely, the tension among service, resources, and outcomes (Malloch & Porter-O'Grady, 1999). This three-legged stool upon which clinical and performance viabilities are based becomes unbalanced when any one of the value factors is emphasized in a way that sacrifices its relationship to the other factors. Untenable and uncontrolled emphasis on providing service without consideration to issues of resource utilization creates an imbalance that ultimately diminishes service sustainability. Equally importantly, a focus on producing high levels of quality without efforts to develop the human or financial resources necessary to obtain and sustain that quality creates an imbalance. An uncontrolled and overriding focus on managing costs ultimately limits and threatens the organization's ability to provide adequate service or to ensure the high quality of that service. Again, the imbalance inherent in these situations is obvious.

The economic and financial sustainability of the organization depends on finding a continuous and dynamic balance among the three elements of the value equation and keeping them in accord. To achieve this goal, productivity measurement must transcend its current constraints and evolve into a multifaceted model that reflects the complexity of the work of nursing. This level of understanding is much different from the simple and limited cost–benefit evaluation that compares work hours to budgeted units of service. Imagine the long-term impact that reactive cuts to the nursing resource create during an economic downturn and the turnaround toll that is later exacted when these reduced numbers increase both risks and costs, alter the organization's market position, and raise recruitment and salary costs to untenable levels. Cutting out the core of a business does more than just alter the current balance sheet; it ultimately damages the sustainability of the business itself and positions it on a negative trajectory from which it may never fully recover.

Case Example: Care coordination assessment

Cynthia Walker, RN, MSN, has recently been promoted to chief operating officer. One of her executive responsibilities is to assure there is an appropriate infrastructure for care coordination across the patient lifespan. She has a good understanding of the work and intended outcomes of this initiative; however, she is not certain how to assess current staffing for care coordination across the continuum life span. She would like to know the current status of care coordination. She believes the following information is needed:

- Identify those involved in handoffs, care planning, discharge planning, home health, and nonacute care placements.

- Identify and review existing policies and protocols for handoffs, care coordination, case management, and discharge planning processes. Identify the level of available evidence to support these policies and protocols.
- Interviews with 10 patients who use the organization's services and have chronic disease conditions, asking about their perceptions of care coordination across their life span.
- Interviews with 10 wellness users who access organizational services for regular health support and wellness maintenance about their perceptions.
- Review available metrics specific to care coordination processes.

Questions
1. Will this information be adequate to achieve Cynthia's desired goals?
2. Is additional information needed?
3. Is some of the information not necessary?
4. What would be the next steps in this process after the assessment is completed?
5. What innovations are needed to facilitate the required changes?

Case Example: Staffing adequacy

Sheila Baumgarten, PhD, RN, has been the director of the medical product line for 20 years. She is also a nurse informaticist and would like to see more use of software for clinical and management analyses. She is responsible for both acute care and postacute care services, including clinical, diagnostic facilities, and home health services. She has long been challenged with the limited utility of the financial productivity model. She recognizes that some of the resistance of executives has been due to the lack of software applications to collect and sort essential data elements for more comprehensive analysis of multiple data points.

The organization recently purchased the ideal software to create a comprehensive clinical productivity system. The nurse executive of the system asked Sheila to lead a team to develop the optimal clinical productivity system. She is excited and also cautious about how to do this work effectively using the current evidence for practice and outcomes and to be innovative in designing a robust model to address the current challenges. She has decided to start small and selected DRG 89, simple pneumonia and pleurisy, to begin this work.

Sheila identified key stakeholders to collaborate with and create the desired model. The following information has been identified by the group as necessary to create a clinical productivity system:

- Inputs:
  - Number of patients with DRG 89 for the past 12 months
  - Hours of care provided to each patient by registered nurses (RNs) and nursing assistants (NA)

- Intensity projected needs for patient care (patient acuity) in hours
- Budgeted hours of care for each patient
- Outcomes:
  - Actual length of stay (average)
  - Target length of stay (average)
  - Cost of care (average per patient)
  - Hospital Consumer Assessment of Healthcare Providers and Systems (HCAHPS) scores for patients (average)
  - Patient satisfaction with clinical outcomes
  - Number of falls, medication errors, and pressure ulcers

The following information was readily available:

- 200 patients with diagnosis DRG 89
- RNs provided an average of 47 hours to each patient (data extracted from patient acuity system and staffing information)
- NAs provided an average of 14 hours to each patient
- Patient intensity hours from the acuity system averaged 65 hours for each patient
- Budgeted RN and NA hours for each patient averaged a total of 68 hours for the RN and NA
- Patient satisfaction is 10% lower than the target performance goal
- Patient falls with injury increased by 10%
- No change in pressure ulcers or medication errors

Questions

1. As a team, consider these data and what they mean.
2. Is this data adequate for a new clinical productivity system?
3. What actions would you take, knowing that the hours used were below both the acuity and budgeted hours?

REFERENCES

Advisory Board Company. (2012). Survey: Nurses spend 25% of shift on indirect patient care. Retrieved from https://www.advisory.com/daily-briefing/2012/02/02/nurses

Advisory Board Company. (2014). Nursing productivity benchmark generator. Retrieved from https://www.advisory.com/technology/workforce-compass/members/tools/nursing-productivity-benchmark-generator http://www.ahrq.gov/cpi/portfolios/value/index.html

Aiken, L. H., Clark, S. P., Cheung, R. B., Sloane, D. M., & Silber, J. H. (2003). Education levels of hospital nurses and patient mortality. *Journal of the American Medical Association, 290*(12), 1–8.

Aiken, L. H., Clark, S. P., Sloane, D. M., Sochalski, J., & Silber, J. H. (2002). Hospital nurse staffing and patient mortality, nurse burnout, and job dissatisfaction. *Journal of the American Medical Association, 288*(16), 1987–1993.

Aiken, L. H., Smith, H. L., & Lake, E. T. (1994). Lower Medicare mortality among a set of hospitals known for good nursing care. *Medical Care, 32*(8), 771–787.

American Nurses Association. (2003). *Nursing's social policy statement* (2nd ed.). Washington, DC: Author.

American Nurses Association. (2008). Safe staffing saves lives. Retrieved from http://www.nursingworld .org/HomepageCategory/Announcements/Safe-Staffing-Saves-Lives.html http://www.safestaffingsaveslives.org/default.aspx

American Nurses Association. (2012). *Principles of nurse staffing* (2nd ed.). Silver Spring, MD: Author. Retrieved from http://www.nursingworld.org/MainMenuCategories/ThePracticeofProfessionalNursing /NursingStandards/ANAPrinciples/ANAsPrinciplesofNurseStaffing.pdf

Barnsteiner, J., Disch, J., & Walton, M. K. (2014). *Person and family centered care.* Indianapolis, IN: Sigma Theta Tau International.

Berry, L., Parker, D., Coile, R., Hamilton, D. K., O'Neill, D., & Sadler, B. (2004). *Can better buildings improve care and increase your financial returns?* Chicago, IL: Frontiers of Health Services Management.

Blegen, M. A., & Vaughn, T. (1998). A multisite study of nurse staffing and patient occurrences. *Nursing Economic$, 16*(4), 196–203.

Buerhaus, P. I., Donelan, K., Ulrich, B. T., Norman, L., DesRoches, C., & Dittus, R. (2007). Impact of the nurse shortage on hospital patient care: Comparative perspectives. *Health Affairs, 26*(3), 853–862.

Centers for Medicare and Medicaid Services. (n.d.). Roadmap for implementing value driven healthcare in the traditional Medicare fee-for-service program. Retrieved from http://www.cms.gov/Medicare/Quality-Initiatives-Patient-Assessment-Instruments/QualityInitiativesGenInfo/downloads/vbproadmap_oea_1-16_508.pdf

Centers for Medicare and Medicaid Services. (2015). Better care, smarter spending, healthier people: Improving our health care delivery system. Retrieved from http://www.cms.gov/Newsroom/MediaReleaseDatabase /Fact-sheets/2015-Fact-sheets-items/2015-01-26.html

Cho, S. H., Ketefian, S., Barkauskas, V. H., & Smith, D. G. (2003). The effect of nurse staffing on adverse events, morbidity, mortality, and medical costs. *Nursing Research, 52*(2), 71–79.

Corey, M. (2001). *Groups: Process and practice.* London, U.K.: Wadsworth.

Dartmouth-Hitchcock. (2015). What is value-based care? Retrieved from http://www.dartmouth-hitchcock. org/about_dh/what_is_value_based_care.html

Drucker, P. (1990). *Managing the nonprofit organization.* New York, NY: Harper Collins.

Finkler, S., & Graf, C. (2001). *Budgeting concepts for nurse managers.* New York, NY: W. B. Saunders.

Friese, C. R., Xia, R., Chaferi, A., Birkmeyer, J. D. & Banerjee, M. (2015). Hospitals in 'Magnet' program show better patient outcomes on mortality measures compared to non 'Magnet' hospitals. *Health Affairs, 34*(6), 986–992.

Geiger-Brown, J., Rogers, V. E., Trinkoff, A. M., Kane, R. L., Bausell, R. B., & Scharf, S. M. (2012). Sleep, sleepiness, fatigue, and performance of 12-hour-shift nurses. *Chronobiology International, 29*(2), 211–219.

Harrington, C., & Estes, C. L. (2004). *Health policy: Crisis and reform in the U.S. health care delivery system* (4th ed.). Sudbury, MA: Jones and Bartlett Publishers.

Hughes, E. C., & American Nurses Association. (1958). *Twenty thousand nurses tell their story: A report on studies of nursing functions sponsored by the American Nurses Association.* Philadelphia, PA: Lippincott.

Institute for Healthcare Improvement. (2012). A guide to measuring the Triple Aim: Population health, experience of care, and per capita cost. Retrieved from http://www.ihi.org/resources/Pages/IHIWhitePapers /AGuidetoMeasuringTripleAim.aspx

Institute of Medicine. (2015). Measuring the impact of interprofessional education (IPE) on collaborative practice and patient outcomes. Retrieved from https://www.iom.edu/Reports/2015/Impact-of-IPE.aspx

Kalisch, B. J. (2014). Missed nursing care: A qualitative study. *Journal of Nursing Care Quality, 21*(4), 306–313.

Kane, R. L., Shamliyan, T. A., Mueller, C., Duval, S., & Wilt, T. J. (2007). The association of registered nurse staffing levels and patient outcomes: Systematic review and meta-analysis. *Medical Care, 45*(12), 1195–1204.

Lang, T. A., Hodge, M., & Olson, V. (2004). Nurse–patient ratios: A systematic review on the effects of nurse staffing on patient, nurse employee and hospital outcomes. *Journal of Nursing Administration, 34*(7–8), 326–337.

Lanser, E. G. (2001). Leveraging your nursing resources. *Healthcare Executive, 80*(10), 50–51.

Long, M. C. (2002). *Translating the principles of variability management into reality: One physician's perspective.* Boston, MA: Boston University, School of Management, Executive Learning.

Malloch, K. (2015). Measurement of nursing's complex health care work: Evolution of the science for determining the required staffing for safe and effective patient care. *Nursing Economic$, 33*(1), 20–25.

Malloch, K., & Porter-O'Grady, T. (1999). Partnership economics: Nursing's challenge in a quantum age. *Nursing Economic$, 17*(6), 299–307.

Martin, D. (2014). Literature review: Nurse fatigue related to shift length. *Arizona State Board of Nursing Regulatory Journal, 9*(3), 4–5.

McCue, M., Mark, B. A., & Harless, D. W. (2003). Nurse staffing, quality, and financial performance. *Journal of Health Care Finance, 29*(4), 54–76.

Moorhead, S., Johnson, M., & Maas, M. (2004). *Nursing outcomes classification (NOC)* (3rd ed.). St. Louis, MO: C. V. Mosby.

Murphy, M. (2003). *Research brief: Eliminating wasteful work in hospitals improves margin, quality, and culture.* Washington, DC: Murphy Leadership Institute.

Needleman, J., Buerhaus, P., Mattke, S., Stewart, M & Zelevinsky, K. (2002). Nurse staffing levels and the quality of care in hospitals. *New England Journal of Medicine, 346*(22), 1715–1722.

Needleman, J., Buerhaus, P., Pankratz, S., Leibson, C. L., Stevens, M. S., & Harris, M. (2011). Nurse staffing and inpatient hospital mortality. *New England Journal of Medicine, 364*, 1037–1045.

O'BrienPallas, L., Thomson, D., Hall, L. M., Pink, G., Kerr, M., Wang, S., et al. (2004). Evidence based standards for measuring nurse staffing and performance. Retrieved from http://www.researchgate.net/publication/228738285_Evidence-based_Standards_for_Measuring_Nurse_Staffing_and_Performance.

Pinkerton, S., & Rivers, R. (2001). Factors influencing staffing needs. *Nursing Economic$, 19*(5), 236–237.

Pittman, P., & Forrest, E. (2015). The changing roles of registered nurses in Pioneer ACOs. *Nursing Outlook, 63*(5), 554–565. Retrieved from http://www.nursingoutlook.org/article/S0029-6554(15)00179-7/references

Porter, M. E. (2012). *Value-based health care delivery.* Presentation at HBS Healthcare Initiative & Healthcare Club, March 7, 2012.

Rheaume, A., & Belliveau, E. (2015). The changing boundaries of nursing: A qualitative study of the transition to a new nursing care delivery model. *Journal of Clinical Nursing. 24*(17–18); 229–2537.

Rubin, I. M., Plovnick, M. S., & Fry, R. E. (1975). *Improving the coordination of care: A program for health team development.* Cambridge, MA: Ballinger.

Rutherford, M. (2008). Standardized nursing language: What does it mean for nursing practice? *OJIN: The Online Journal of Issues in Nursing,* Retrieved from: http://www.nursingworld.org/MainMenuCategories/ThePracticeofProfessionalNursing/Health-IT/StandardizedNursingLanguage.html

Savitz, L. A., Jones, C. B., & Bernard, S. (2005). Quality indicators sensitive to nurse staffing in acute care settings. In K. Henriksen, J. B. Battles, E. S. Marks, & D. Lewin (Eds.), *Advances in patient safety: From research to implementation* (pp. 375–385). Rockville, MD: Agency for Healthcare Research and Quality.

Smith, J. (2002). Analysis of differences in entry level or and practice by educational preparation. *Journal of Nursing Education, 41*(11), 491–495.

Stimpfel, A. W., Lake, E. T., Barton, S. Gorman, K. C., & Aiken, L. H. (2013). How differing shift lengths relate to quality outcomes in pediatrics. *Journal of Nursing Administration, 43*(2), 95–100.

Stone, P. W., Curran, C. R., & Bakken, S. (2002). Economic evidence for evidence based practice. *Journal of Nursing Scholarship, 34*(3), 277–282.

Tourangeau, A. E., Cranley, L. A., & Jeffs, L. (2006). Impact of nursing on hospital patient mortality: A focused review and related policy implications. *Quality and Safety in Health Care, 15*(1), 4–8.

Ulrich, R., Quan, X., Zimring, C., Joseph, A., & Choudhary, R. (2004). *The role of the physical environment in the hospital of the 21st century: A once in a lifetime opportunity.* Concord, CA: Center for Health Design.

Upenieks, V. V., Akhavan, J., Kotlerman, J., Esser, J., & Ngo, M. J. (2007). Value added care: A new way of assessing nursing staffing ratios and workload variability. *Journal of Nursing Administration, 37*(5), 243–252.

Warren, J. (2012). Importance of standardized terminology in healthcare information systems. Retrieved from http://www.aacn.nche.edu/qsen-informatics/2012-workshop/presentations/warren/Importance-of-Standardized-Terminology-Warren.pdf

Welton, J. M. (2010) Response to nurse staffing and quality of care with direct measurement of inpatient staffing. *Medical Care;* 48(100; 940.

Welton, J. M. (2011). Value based nursing care. *Journal of Nursing Administration, 40*(10), 399–401.

While, A., Forbes, A., Ullman, R., Lewis, S., Mathes, L., & Grifiths, P. (2004). Good practices that address continuity during transition from child to adult care: Synthesis of the evidence. *Childcare Health and Development, 30*(5), 439–452.

White, K. M. (2006). Policy spotlight: Staffing plans and ratios. *Nursing Management, 37*(4), 18–22, 24.

CHAPTER 13

Shared Governance: The Infrastructure for Innovation

Gregory L. Crow and Gregory A. DeBourgh

> *I am on the edge of mysteries and the veil is getting thinner and thinner.*
>
> —LOUIS PASTEUR

CHAPTER OBJECTIVES

Upon completion of this chapter, the reader will be able to:

1. Analyze the relationship among shared governance, innovation, and the change agent's role in leading change.
2. Analyze the change agent's role in relation to each phase of the diffusion of innovation process.
3. Compare and contrast your organization's operations with the distinctive characteristics of rigid and frozen organizations.
4. Analyze the potential benefits of using a think tank approach to problem identification and resolution within healthcare organizations.

INTRODUCTION

This chapter is about using the time-tested organizational arrangement of nursing shared governance and evolving it to whole-systems shared governance, with an important functional addition. Whole-systems shared governance can be the think tank that then becomes the engine of creativity and innovation in a healthcare organization. Caliva and Scheier define *think tank* as a "process for in-depth consideration of issues and challenges whose relevance reaches beyond the individual person or program and the immediate time frame" (1992, p. 2). Think tanks endeavor to step beyond everyday needs, provide a powerful tool for dealing with deeper and longer-range issues, help to develop whole-systems thinking patterns (seeing the big picture), and can stimulate creativity in an industry that today seems more concerned with standardization rather than innovation. Every healthcare organization needs a leader who can balance the need for standardization (in an effort to prevent mistakes) against the organization's long-term need to challenge the many orthodoxies of what is currently defined as good patient care.

Burton and Moran (1995) note that a successful organization is one that is constantly changing by continuously focusing on its primary purpose and ways to keep that purpose aligned with its environment as that environment evolves. Discovery, which is a primary function of think tanks, is one part of the process that allows the organization to blend new discoveries into its strategic direction with tactical support to see that it occurs. Drucker (1995) informs us that for an organization to be well organized to deal with change, it must be decentralized. Shared governance, be it nursing shared governance or whole-systems shared governance, is the right decentralized structure and process to propel an organization forward into its preferred future.

A high-functioning whole-systems shared governance model working in conjunction with senior leadership (the C-suite, as in chief operating officer, chief nursing officer, etc.) and the board of directors can create a future-focused think tank. This arrangement has the potential to be the stimulus to constantly evolve the healthcare organization in an effort to meet the ever-changing and complex healthcare needs of those it serves, and to manage the ever-changing and complex workplace needs of its employees. The healthcare organization that fails to satisfy its employees will soon find itself not meeting the needs of its patients, families, and community.

Drucker (1995), and Martins and Martins (2002) note that as an organization finds itself in the midst of great change, effective leaders try to create an institutional framework in which creativity and innovation are accepted as a basic cultural norm. Whole-systems shared governance can be that healthcare organization's institutional framework to stimulate innovation, constantly adjust the internal culture to acknowledge the need for change, and inspire the organization to meet the challenges of today and tomorrow.

To be an effective resource to the healthcare organization, whole-systems shared governance must evolve from mostly solving past, present, and known near-future issues to becoming an integral part of the healthcare organization's systems that continuously scan the local, state, and national healthcare environments to identify long-term, future-focused challenges that impact the viability of the healthcare organization and its ability to respond to both known and unknown challenges as they arise. Whole-systems shared governance councils, and the members who serve on them, must become adept at piercing the external boundaries of the healthcare organization in a constant search of what is on the horizon that will impact the healthcare organization.

Boundary spanners are vital to organizational success; they are the employees (both management and staff) who see and understand where the healthcare world is going, translate that direction into action, and disseminate it throughout the organization. Working with the C-suite, councils must then take the necessary steps for the healthcare organization to flourish in any given environment. Goodness of fit between the healthcare organization and the healthcare organization's environment is the only successful path to sustainability.

Challenges, both big and small, continuously confront healthcare organizations. Those healthcare organizations that accurately identify various threats and opportunities on near and far horizons and then take the necessary steps to meet those challenges will flourish. Perhaps more importantly, those organizations can create their preferred futures rather than be passive recipients of their tomorrows. The preferred future of any healthcare organization is not given—it must be earned.

SYSTEMS

The origin of much of our current frustrations in healthcare organizations is because, in the past century, the American healthcare system shifted from being a complicated system to a complex system. However, many of our healthcare organizations did not make the same shift. They are basically organized, structured, and operated much like hospitals in the mid-20th century. Minus our technology, decor, medications, and dress, a nurse from the mid-20th century would be able to not only recognize, but also feel comfortable in, many of our healthcare organizations today. Our problems are in the 21st century, yet our tools and strategies for solving current problems are of the 20th century.

Complexity science teaches us that the complex healthcare problems we face today cannot be adequately resolved by healthcare organizations that are trapped in the traditional mechanistic hierarchical systems of yesteryear. The tools we use to solve today's problems must be equal to the task. We need many tools in our toolboxes to manage and lead in contemporary, complex healthcare environments. When the only tool you have is a hammer, everything looks like a nail. One cannot build a system with a single tool.

The basic elements of an open system are inputs, throughputs, outputs, feedback, negative entropy, and homeostasis. Open systems are systems that communicate with, and are dependent on, their environments for the energy they require (inputs) to produce useable outputs for their environment. Throughput is the process by which a system transforms environmental inputs into useable outputs. To do this, the system must be organized so it is able to anticipate environmental demands and produce exactly, or approximately, what the environment needs. Open systems are linear and use processes in which small inputs produce small outputs, and large inputs produce large outputs. The system is dedicated to maintaining homeostasis (a steady state), where the goal is to preserve the system as is. The as-is state is the goal, not adaptation.

Systems must be alert to continuous feedback. Feedback is used to keep the system on a steady and unchanging course. To maintain this steady course, open systems do not tolerate or encourage emergent properties to surface (Schneider & Somers, 2006). The system, in our case the healthcare organization, uses Herculean efforts to keep emergence from occurring. Emergence means that the machine is producing variance, and variance threatens the well-established organizational arrangements and, more importantly, those in control of those arrangements. As the system suppresses emergent properties, it can become more and more out of sync with its environment. Negative feedback allows the system to perform necessary corrections to its linear processes in an effort to produce useable outputs for its environment. When systems ignore environmental negative feedback long enough, they become so out of sync with their environment that they must be transformed to survive. Transformation is much more difficult to lead than course corrections over time (Schneider & Somers, 2006).

Feedback, when coded and interpreted properly, allows the system to communicate with its environment to produce goodness of fit. If the feedback is not coded and interpreted properly, the system runs the risk of producing outputs that the environment does not need. If this process is not corrected, the system becomes more and more misaligned with its environment and, over time, entropy sets in. Entropy indicates a high level of internal disorganization (Schneider & Somers, 2006).

THE CONGRUENCE MODEL

Understanding performance within healthcare organizations requires an assessment and analysis of its systems components and the interaction and fit (congruence) among those elements (Nadler, Tushman, & Hatvany, 1982). Organizational outcomes result from alignment of each of the components of performance: structure, people, culture, and tasks (Mercer Delta, 2012; Nadler, Tushman, & Hatvany, 1982). The greater the congruence among these elements, the greater the performance of the organization. The model (**Figure 13-1**), originally developed by Nadler and colleagues (1982), views the organization as a sociotechnical system with four components or subsystems that contribute to the transformational process within organizations: (1) the work; (2) the formal organization (structural or technical); (3) the people; and (4) the informal organization (social).

Input from both internal and external sources informs corporate and business strategy to translate the organization's vision and objectives and its decisions for operations, provision of resources, operational structures, and policies and procedures into the system's outputs (products and services).

Figure 13-1 The congruence model

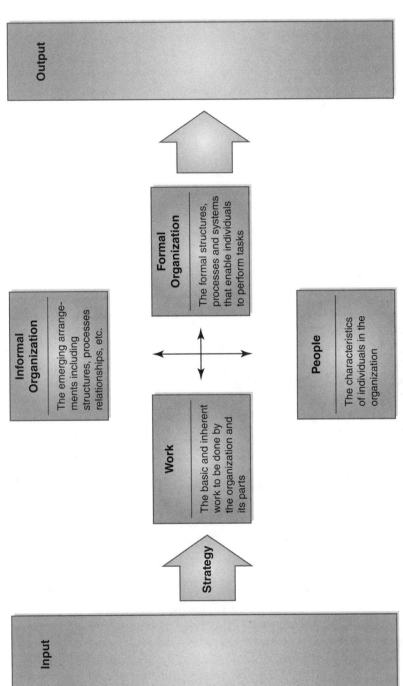

Model source: Nadler, Tushman, & Hatvany, N. G. (1982) from Nadler, D. A., Tushman, M. L. & Hatvany, N. G. (1982). *Managing organizations*. Boston: Little, Brown. *Image source:* Mercer Delta Consulting (2012). Reprinted from *Organizational Dynamics* 9(2), Autumn 1980, David A. Nadler and Michael L. Tushman, A model for diagnosing organizational behavior, pp. 35–51, Copyright 1980, with permission from Elsevier.

The external environment shapes operations and outputs of the organization by imposing economic, social, and legal constraints. Demands from an organization's consumer base shape the organization's scope and business model, create its market opportunities, and influence cost and profit decisions. Legislative and legal constraints shape internal operations, requiring compliance to public and business policies and practices as well as consumer protection and safety standards. The organization's social and community responsibilities and commitments also influence the system's goals and priorities.

Resources available to the organization include the assets of financial capital, employees, equipment and technology, information, the organization's reputation, and its history. The history component of the model represents both legacy and recent-past influence. "There is considerable evidence that the way an organization functions today is greatly influenced by landmark events that occurred in its past" (Mercer Delta Consulting, 2012, p. 12). Well-established reputations, declared commitments to the mission, and social and community obligations of the organization direct the organization's philosophies and operations. Recent-history effects are shaped by current and near-past administrations and their views, vision, leadership expertise (or lack of it), and strategic priorities imposed on the organization by virtue of their titles, positions, and granted authority.

At the center of the congruence model is the transformation process (**Figure 13-1**), which draws input from both internal and external sources and transforms those inputs into outputs (organizational, group, and individual performance). In healthcare organizations, the work component represents the delivery of patient care services. The people component represents the employees—their knowledge, skills, abilities, performance and productivity, and relationships with the organization itself and with others in the work environment, all of which potentially contribute to outcomes (system output). The informal component of the system represents the processes and relationships that emerge from doing the work as interactive, interdependent, task-oriented teams. The formal organization includes the sanctioned design of hierarchy and reporting structures, policies, procedures, and operational systems that enable task performance. Output is the organization's delivery of products, services, revenues, profits, community contributions and impact, and fulfilling the mission and objectives of the enterprise.

The congruence model is essentially about the concept of fit. The performance of the organization as a whole is dependent on the fit or alignment of each component of the system to achieve its mission, vision, and goals. The systems framework of the congruence model suggests that the interaction and synergy of all components is more important than any one component in realizing the organization's *raison d'être*. When all components of the system are in harmony and congruent with the organization's mission, performance and productivity are high and the system is effective. When elements are not congruent, it is incumbent on leaders to facilitate processes that identify and respond to misalignment of system components; individual and group non-performance; needs for knowledge and skill development; adjustments of methods, policies, procedures, and structures to enable improved performance; and the need to foster widespread innovation in thinking and doing.

Use of the congruence model by healthcare leaders provides a systematic way to consider the elements that drive organizational performance and provide insights not only to understand, but also to predict operations, and patterns. . . of organizational behavior and performance (Mercer Delta Consulting, 2012). In complex organizations, the tendency among managers is to target interventions and change based on the symptoms of problems instead of seeking to understand the root causes. Specifically, the model affords leaders a framework to identify potential and actual problems that impact performance and effectiveness (and those who may solve the problems); gather data on performance gaps and the dynamic interaction of context, process, behaviors, and relationships; discover opportunities to initiate and determine the impact of innovation and change; and monitor and manage the system's response to innovation process and systems outcomes. The astute leader not only looks for what is *not* working well (i.e., what is *not* goodness of fit among the system components), but also what is currently well coordinated or congruent and supports continuation of those practices. Maintaining the goodness of fit among components of the system contributes to the sustainability of innovation, performance, and productivity of the organization.

Case Example: Implementing a new practice procedure

Ann Jones, RN, PhD, had been in her first chief nursing officer (CNO) role for 5 months and was eager to have a quick win early in her tenure. Her PhD dissertation was focused on the benefits of hourly rounding, and she wanted the knowledge she gained in her research put into action in an effort to decrease falls and increase patient and family satisfaction, both of which are issues of concern for the chief executive of the medical center. In Dr. Jones' weekly meeting with the head nurses and divisional directors of this 350-bed inner-city medical center, she presented a form she developed based on her research, along with a policy to enforce the new procedure. She also announced that the form and procedure should be implemented in the next 7 days. The first data from each unit, confirming the new procedure was implemented and used, would be due in 30 days. The nurse managers raised concerns that although the idea was a good one and was supported by the best available evidence, the manner in which the new procedure was being introduced would result in pushback, especially from the intensive care unit nurses who spend about 90% of their time at the patient's bedside. Dr. Jones, noting the concerns, announced that the change in procedure and documentation would proceed as planned by her, regardless of the context and location of care.

The first data on the procedure demonstrated a 38% compliance rate in the intensive care unit, the neonatal intensive care unit, and the pediatric intensive care unit.

Questions

1. What inputs did Dr. Jones appear to ignore when she first introduced the change in practice to the directors and head nurses?
2. Considering the elements of the transformation process, how would you assess congruence between the goal for the desired change and the process Dr. Jones used to design and implement this change in practice?
3. The first data set revealed a 38% compliance rate in the intensive care units. What advice would you offer Dr. Jones for how she could have used the congruence model to guide her original plan for change?

WHOLE-SYSTEMS SHARED GOVERNANCE

Shared governance has been closely associated with nursing systems. Shared governance systems have allowed registered nurses to fulfill their role as part of the primary professional group that links all aspects of patient care to the healthcare organization's mission, vision, and values. Whole-systems shared governance is a decentralized and accountability-based system that allows the entire healthcare organization to be linked, interconnected, and, more importantly, focused on meeting the healthcare needs of all it serves while simultaneously ensuring internal and external goodness of fit with its environment. A whole-systems shared governance organization operates from its core where its mission, vision, and values should be most visible.

At the core of whole-systems shared governance is an infrastructure to support patient care delivery that is intended to enhance outcomes and productivity. Outcomes and productivity realized at the point of service define the purpose of the healthcare organization. All workers have both the obligation for accountability and the right to contribute to decisions that impact their work (Porter-O'Grady, 2009). Horizontal structures must be the dominant model to support effective working relationships and integration of all components and processes involved in delivery of the product, in this case patient care.

Governance is about sharing power, influence, control, and authority. In shared governance, practitioners and staff are the organization's primary resource for providing care. Therefore they must have influence and control over their professional practice. Structure is vital to shared governance (Hess, 2004). Shared governance provides both a structure and an environment to empower staff, legitimizes control over professional practice, and permanently extends influence to staff and practitioners in areas previously controlled exclusively by managers (Hess, 1994; Westrope, Vaughn, Bott, & Taunton, 1995).

Whole-systems shared governance is a professional practice and governance model of empowerment that is based on the principles of equity, partnership, ownership, and accountability (**Box 13-1**). The whole-systems framework on which shared governance is based affords many benefits.

Box 13-1 Principles of Leadership in Whole-Systems Shared Governance

Partnership:

- Expectations are negotiated, clearly defined, and communicated.
- There is equality among individuals.
- Interdisciplinary relationships are based on shared risk.
- Measures for contributions are established.
- Horizontal links, practices, and processes are well defined.

Equity:

- Each contribution is understood by all.
- Payment for contribution reflects value to outcomes.
- Role is based on relationships, not status or given title or position.
- The team defines service roles, relationships, and outcomes.
- Methodology is defined and established to manage conflict and service issues.
- Assessment and evaluation of team outcomes and contributions are conducted.

Accountability:

- Accountability is internally defined by the person in the role.
- The role defines accountability, not the job or task.
- Accountability focuses on evidence-based care outcomes, not processes.
- Accountability is linked and leads to defined and desired results.
- Processes are overt, observable, and evident.

Ownership:

- All team members are invested in the enterprise.
- Every role is a stakeholder in the outcomes.
- All members are associated with a team.
- Processes support relationships and are not limited to supporting tasks.
- Opportunities are based on demonstrated competence.

Data from Porter-O'Grady, T. (Ed.). (2009). *Interdisciplinary shared governance: Integrating practice, transforming health care* (2nd ed.). Sudbury, MA: Jones and Bartlett Publishers.

Box 13-2 summarizes the characteristics and features of a whole-systems orientation.

Whole-systems shared governance council members, and specifically chairs and cochairs of the councils, are composed of staff, practitioners, and managers from across the healthcare organization. Their primary focus is to ensure that the healthcare organization provides barrier-free, gold-standard care to patients and families.

Porter-O'Grady says that "90% of decisions made in the organization should be made within the context of service pathways" (2009, p. 55). Within healthcare organizations, a service pathway is where patients and care providers meet (i.e., the point at which the work is done). Decisions made at the point of service involve the stakeholders with vested interest and accountability for outcomes. Locating accountability and the authority for making decisions at the point of service requires a value for, and commitment to, shared decision making by staff, practitioners, and managers. Shared decision making supports the empowerment of those who do the work.

Decentralized authority for decision making empowers and engages each member of the healthcare team to partner in interactive and iterative processes that support planning, implementation, and evaluation of care processes that are designed around the needs of the patient (Porter-O'Grady, 2009). If stakeholders are located everywhere in the healthcare organization and are supported in making decisions at the point of service, a mechanism must be in place that enables them to interact to ensure that their decisions are mutually supportive and to facilitate the achievement of desired

---

Box 13-2 Characteristics and Features of Whole Systems

- The whole always defines the parts.
- Each element or component supports the whole system.
- Problems and failures in performance and outcomes impact the whole system.
- The heart of system (where it lives) is at the level where service is provided.
- All roles and functions serve the customer or support somone who does.
- Design and strucutre must be centered on the point of service.
- Form must always follow function.
- All members in the system are stakeholders and are invested in outcomes.
- Managers are facilitators, integrators, coordinators of processes, or support the work or providers. They do not control and decide.
- Outcomes always define the value of the processes and performance (function is subordinate to purpose).

Modified from Porter-O'Grady, T. (Ed.). (2009). *Interdisciplinary shared governance: Integrating practice, transforming health care* (2nd ed.). Sudbury, MA: Jones and Bartlett.

outcomes. This is a critical function served by the infrastructure of whole-systems shared governance.

Traditionally, true partnerships in healthcare organizations are often limited to the practices of physicians and consultants (Hendel, Fish, & Berger, 2007; Kramer & Schmalenberg, 2003; Patterson & McMurray, 2003). Patient care staff and those who provide support services are often excluded from these partnerships. When point-of-service staff members are limited in establishing partnerships and are not empowered to make decisions related to the care they provide, they are limited in directing their own discipline-specific work, and patient outcomes are potentially compromised. Engagement and empowerment in one's work and the outcome of that work are critical to taking responsibility and accountability for that performance (Kramer & Schmalenberg, 2003; Patterson & McMurray, 2003).

Because the infrastructure in whole-systems shared governance is nonhierarchical and is built on shared decision making, there are increased opportunities for input and decisions to modify operations, standards, and services, which also benefit diffusion of innovation. Because decision making is decentralized and distributed among the various councils in whole-systems shared governance, the governance structure itself provides a series of checks and balances to manage potential conflict and to limit the power and influence of any one person or group. Whole-systems shared governance as an organizing infrastructure facilitates the active participation and investment by all council members as stakeholders in processes, decision making, and outcomes. The stakeholder concept increases the likelihood that decisions will be implemented and outcomes realized without confusion about the locus of control and decision-making authority. When accountability is clearly delineated, determination of expectations for and measurement of performance are facilitated within each context where decisions are made (Porter-O'Grady, 2009).

When those who provide care are partners in problem identification, solution creation, decisions, and evaluation of outcomes and processes, higher levels of care quality are realized, and both patient and staff satisfaction are enhanced (Laschinger & Wong, 1999). "Quality is about achieving sustainable outcomes. Outcomes are what we use to measure the value of processes. Our actions have no meaning separated from the ends to which they are directed" (Porter-O'Grady, 2009, p. 19). Individual expertise and performance alone cannot get the job done; effective partnerships are required for success in contemporary, complex, evolving healthcare organizations.

In vertical, hierarchical systems, the ultimate responsibility is located at the top. In horizontal, complex adaptive systems that are supported by the whole-systems shared governance paradigm, accountability is located where care occurs and decisions are made. Accountability results not from a structural or functional model, but from the interdependent decisions made within various councils and teams who are doing the work. Accountability is generated from within a role and is defined by the associated scope of practice. Accountability cannot be delegated (Porter-O'Grady, 2009). Lack of accountability in any part of the system negatively impacts all parts of the system and, therefore, the enterprise.

Two types of accountability are represented within the whole-systems shared governance paradigm: system accountability and service accountability. System accountability involves activities and operations that are concerned with process and outcome effectiveness, and it ensures the integrity of the system and all its parts (Porter-O'Grady, 2009). Service accountability is concerned with the shared obligations of everyone in the healthcare organization to perform those duties and activities that enable the organization to meet its purposes (Porter-O'Grady, 2009). In healthcare organizations this purpose is clearly the provision of patient care, requiring multiple teams of individuals to carry out this mission and to demonstrate safe, effective, efficient, cost-effective, and population-sensitive patient care outcomes.

Engagement and synergism (both hallmarks of whole-systems shared governance) among all members of the healthcare team facilitate sustainable quality outcomes because they integrate the concepts and behaviors of continuous quality improvement into the expected performance behaviors of everyone in the organization. According to Senge (1990), a system's structure influences behavior patterns. Changing structure can motivate change in behaviors. A structure that empowers staff enhances individual and group influence within the system. Facilitating individual and team accountability for the concepts of continuous quality improvement through the structures of whole-systems shared governance promotes an outcomes and value-added focus among healthcare team members. All stakeholders are involved in a continuous effort to improve the quality of care, manage costs, and enhance the level of services provided by the healthcare organization (Gardner & Cummings, 1994).

Organizational effectiveness is improved in organizations wherein employees self-manage and self-improve their performance in highly flexible teams (Kim, 1992). The whole-systems shared governance structure provides a focus on the organization's mission, purpose, and operations that creates a shared mental model that aligns team priorities and outcomes with those of the organization. Organizations that embrace structures and procedures that are flexible and responsive to both external and internal change realize the greatest organizational success (Gardner & Cummings, 1994). Integrating continuous quality improvement provides the tools for problem solving; it also supports systems thinking and continuous learning.

Councils: Structure, Membership, and Function

In whole-systems shared governance, a council is the location for consultation, deliberation, advice, authority, and decision making. It is the venue for gathering practitioners, staff, and managers together to make decisions. Mitchell, Brooks, and Pugh

(1999) state that the council structure enables staff, practitioners, and managers to jointly question policies, procedures, and practices regarding patient care. Mitchell and colleagues also report that members of the council can "ask questions they previously dared not ask," feel they are equals, and through the council structure of shared governance, "have greater access to information from senior staff" (1999, p. 198). The council chair must ensure that the four elements of the congruence model transformation process (people, informal organization arrangements, formal organization arrangements, and the work) are in harmony to enhance council functioning and outcomes.

Although each healthcare organization must design a whole-systems shared governance framework specific to its needs, there are some general councils that appear with great regularity:

- Coordinating council: The purpose of the coordinating council is to oversee coordination and integration of the work of the other councils and provide a forum for communication, collaboration, and conflict resolution among all the councils.
- Quality and safety council: The quality and safety council has the overall accountability to ensure that national, state, local, and organizational quality and safety standards are integrated throughout the healthcare organization. This includes using evidence-based research and other sources of best evidence to guide the quality and safety processes of the healthcare organization.
- Education council: The education council ensures that the existence of ongoing education and development of all employees is consistent with the mission, vision, values, and strategic plan of the healthcare organization. It is also responsible for providing educational activities that have a particular focus (i.e., leadership and management development programs that support the whole-systems shared governance process). This council establishes and maintains a system-wide educational framework that inculcates the need for continuous learning to every corner of the healthcare organization.
- Resource council: The resource council ensures the optimal deployment and use of human, physical, fiscal, and material resources that directly support the staff, practitioners, and managers in operationalizing the mission, vision, values, and strategic plan of the healthcare organization. The resource council leads proactive fiscal planning and performance accountability, and it makes adjustments based on changes in market factors or subscriber base to achieve goals and provide essential services (Porter-O'Grady, 2009).
- Patient care council: The patient care council defines and integrates a comprehensive approach to patient care services that spans the service delivery continuum and is designed to meet the needs of everyone the healthcare organization serves. "Anything related to the integrated patient care delivery process in the

system as a whole falls within the ambit of authority of the patient care council" (Porter-O'Grady, 2009, p. 63). It ensures that the standards on which care is developed are contemporary and evidence based.

- Innovation council: A new council we are beginning to see is the innovation council. The innovation council is accountable for identifying, investigating, evaluating, and recommending new ideas, technologies, and processes for improving patient care and organizational effectiveness. The innovation council serves as the organization's think tank, where organizational boundary spanners seek out new ways to provide patient care that help the organization remain ahead of the curve. This council resides at the border between now and the future, and it is the catalyst for keeping the healthcare organization nimble and flexible in how it designs, implements, and evaluates innovations in patient care delivery. Whole-systems shared governance provides an excellent vehicle for diffusing any innovation because it is vertically and horizontally integrated. An additional advantage of whole-systems shared governance in the diffusion of innovation process is that councils are populated with staff, managers, and practitioners, thereby ensuring that important stakeholders are at the table.

Empowerment in whole-systems shared governance requires all leaders to develop and practice facilitative leadership. Moore and Hutchison identify seven practices consistent with facilitative leadership: "(a) sharing an inspiring vision, (b) focusing on results, processes, and relationships, (c) seeking maximum appropriate involvement, (d) designing pathways to action, (e) facilitating agreement, (f) coaching for performance, and (g) celebrating achievement" (2007, p. 565). All these leadership behaviors are essential to implement and sustain whole-systems shared governance. Managers are challenged to transform their own leadership behaviors from a focus on controlling and monitoring to a transformational model that is facilitative, participative, and directed at developing successful leadership skills among individuals and groups at all levels of the service line. This change in focus serves to inspire and empower team members to commit to the achievement of mutually developed and mutually achieved goals and outcomes. Most importantly, these leadership behaviors support the healthcare organization to remain adaptable to dynamic variables and to facilitate diffusion of innovation. The participative design of whole-systems shared governance provides the structure for such changes in leadership behaviors among managers, staff, and practitioners with the healthcare organization.

Organizations learn through individuals who learn (Senge, 1990). In contemporary healthcare organizations, problems are complex and the solutions are not always readily apparent to an individual or discipline. The design and structure of whole-systems shared governance promote an integrated, interactive environment to conduct the business of healthcare delivery. It is here where individuals and teams learn to deepen and broaden their understanding to include multidisciplinary perspectives to effectively and efficiently create meaningful change and to respond to clinical challenges.

People are an organization's most valuable and critical resource (Gardner & Cummings, 1994). When an organization is designed as a learning organization (Senge, 1990), where continuing education, exploration, and the quest for new knowledge and understanding are not only encouraged, but supported and funded, employees in that organization become valuable resources. The value added to the system is not generated merely by the enhanced performance of an individual or group (team), but it results from the synergism of interactive, collective experience and action. In a learning organization, contributions emerge from the processes of learning to think in new ways, by reframing past approaches and behaviors, by abandoning path-dependent thinking, and by collaboratively creating solutions and direction for the way forward.

Discussion

During the journey to create, implement, and sustain whole-systems shared governance within a complex healthcare system, what do you anticipate to be the most challenging aspects related to your role as a healthcare leader?

THINK TANKS

Caliva and Scheier define a think tank "as a process for in-depth consideration of issues and challenges whose relevance reaches beyond the individual person or program and the immediate timeframe" (1992, p. 2). McGann (2005) notes that one function of a think tank is to help organizations better understand and make informed choices about issues the organization will likely face in the future.

The concepts of *in-depth* and *beyond* assist the members of a think tank to not only identify possible future challenges, but to deeply analyze those potential environmental factors (internal and external) that may have a profound influence on how the healthcare organization goes about meeting the demands of its environments. The think tank process goes beyond *how* something is to *why is it that way* and from *what* to *what if* (Caliva & Scheier, 1992; McGann, 2005). The bottom line is that a think tank will help a healthcare organization not sacrifice long-term benefits that help it more successfully realize its preferred future in favor of quick, concrete answers.

In essence, a think tank is what Burton and Moran (1995) describe as a future-focused organization. Future-focused organizations are constantly changing and sharpening their focus on purpose and how that purpose will be realized into the future. These organizations understand and act on the idea that an organization's future is where its very existence lies and realize that their future must be discovered. This is why an organization must have many boundary spanners, so that more than one or two sets of eyes are focused on how to better organize the healthcare organization to flourish in the future, no matter what the future brings. Moreover, Caliva and Scheier (1992) and McGann (2005) note that the discovery of future issues and how they are likely to impact the healthcare organization is only part of the discovery process. The healthcare organization must blend the discovery of the future into its plan for operations so it can take full advantage of what the future offers. A healthcare organization's capacity to transform information into knowledge to produce the future service bundles the public wants and values is the hallmark of a future-focused organization. Future-focused organizations "do not sacrifice tomorrow on the altar of yesteryear" (Burton & Moran, 1995, p.1).

Caliva and Scheier (1992) and McGann (1995) note that a think tank endeavors to step beyond the day-to-day practical needs to do the following: (1) create a place for those restlessly creative employees to freely experiment; (2) provide tools for identifying and dealing with deeper and longer-range issues; (3) develop whole-systems thinking skills; (4) balance the need to stimulate creativity and innovation in a domain that also seeks to standardize routines to drive out variations in practice, which often lead to errors; (5) transform ideas and emerging problems into policies that align the healthcare organization with its future environment; (6) provide a place and a forum for the healthy and in-depth exchange of ideas and information among key stakeholders in the policy generation process; and, perhaps most importantly, (7) provide a safe place for collaboration among separate groups to challenge conventional wisdom and business practices in the delivery of safe and effective patient care.

We recommend that for a period of 6 months each member of a whole-systems shared governance council be allotted 20% of his or her council work time to devote to think tank activities. They will use the time to identify a future-focused need and to develop a plan of action with a clearly written outcome goal and timeline. The council members can work alone or in small interest groups, and these groups can be comprised of members from any council. We recommend a limit of five individuals per small interest group. The low number of participants allows the group to be nimble and flexible in their operations focused on solving problems and facilitating innovation. The time frame for identifying an issue and presenting an evidence-based proposal should be 6 months. They give monthly progress reports to the appropriate council, and the role of members of the other council is to positively challenge the individual or small interest group on their assumptions, progress, and outcomes to date. This is meant to be a challenging yet open and friendly process. At the end of the 6-month period, the individual or small interest group makes their final proposal to the appropriate council, and that council then decides to accept, reject, or refine the proposal. Additionally, all activities of the individual or small interest group must be directly linked to, and in direct support of, the healthcare organization's mission, vision, values, and strategic plan.

Devoting 20% of a council member's time to think tank activities is an expensive process. The healthcare organization has every right to expect outcomes that enhance the organization's ability to function with greater flexibility and focus and to provide a return on the investment of time and money allocated to think tank activities. Simply said, innovation should result in actions that better align the healthcare organization with its internal and external environment.

A word of caution: a leader does not one day decide that the healthcare organization will have a think tank and it happens. The leader must prepare the healthcare organization to take full advantage of a think tank. Culture trumps everything; healthcare organization leaders must address this aspect in preparing the environment to accept the purpose and functions of a think tank, or creating the think tank will waste valuable resources. As Malloch noted, the healthcare organization that will reap the biggest benefits for innovations derived via a think tank must have the following cultural attributes: "(a) a high regard for and valuing of creativity, (b) an openness to new ideas, (c) a strong change management process, (c) positive conflict utilization, (d) an expectation to challenge assumptions, (e) understanding of the business case for innovation, and (f) the availability of financial resources for innovation work" (2010, p 39).

As with any endeavor, one must select the right people to participate in the innovation processes and think tank activities. Caliva and Scheier (1992) note characteristics the healthcare organization leader should take into consideration when appointing an innovation team or think tank. Those characteristics are as follows: (1) mature as people (not age); (2) self-disciplined (the ability to work independently and deliver work on time); (3) possesses a willingness to share ideas (even when those ideas are challenged in front of others); (4) have a willingness to take informed risks (risks that are informed by the literature as much as possible); (5) a mix of experienced and inexperienced staff; (6) has demonstrated vision and creativity in their present work; (7) comfortable with unconventional approaches to problem solving; (8) a willingness to question their own assumptions (prior to questioning anyone else's); and (9) seekers of a broader perspective through the use of empathy (the ability to put one's self in another's place is vital to creativity and innovation).

Discussion

What opportunities are available to healthcare staff and management to become boundary spanners within healthcare systems? What challenges are associated with becoming a boundary spanner?

INNOVATION

There is no more delicate matter to take in hand, nor more dangerous to conduct, nor more doubtful in its success, than to be a leader in the introduction of changes. For he who innovates will have for enemies all those who are well off under the old order of things, and only lukewarm supporters in those who might be better off under the new.

—NICCOLÒ MACHIAVELLI

The contemporary healthcare organization is emblematic of a dynamic organizational culture that must be nimble and responsive to rapid change, and it must develop capabilities to adapt its systems and procedures to maintain quality output—in this case, patient care services. With ever-increasing business competition and growing complexity, an organization's survival, and indeed its success, are now determined by using its "competitive intelligence and knowledge as a key asset" and its "rate of learning" (do Carmo Caccia-Bava, Guimaraes, & Guimaraes, 2009, p. 456). Long-term success in contemporary complex organizations now requires responsive, proactive change that is fueled by creativity and innovation. In addition, the organization's rate of change must be faster than the external environment and its competitors (do Carmo Caccia-Bava et al., 2009).

The unrelenting operational and financial pressures, and regulatory mandates for all healthcare organizations to ensure that the golden thread of safety is maintained throughout all operations within their systems, create a formidable challenge to those healthcare organizations wishing to embrace creativity and innovation. "In health care, there is a dearth of innovative cultures because the nature of health care inherently requires behaviors that seek stability and safety" (Jaramillo et al., 2008, p. 31). Innovation challenges conventional thinking because healthcare providers are professionally educated and socialized as convergent thinkers, focused on compliance with evidence-based protocols and policies of healthcare systems that are intended to maintain quality standards and reduce risk to patients and staff, all of which create barriers to full participation in creative, innovative thinking. "Highly evolved systems with deeply entrenched organization layers of decision making create complexity for the innovative process" (Blakeney, Carleton, McCarthy, & Coakley, 2009, para. 19). Some assert that to ensure the viability of healthcare organizations, embracing creativity and innovation is simply no longer an option, and "creating the culture and infrastructure that make innovation a way of doing business is the critical role of healthcare leadership in all places in the system" (Porter-O'Grady, 2010, p. 29).

Discussion

Acknowledging that healthcare systems must be nimble in response to both internal and external factors that stimulate the need for change, what are examples of your workplace culture that impede flexibility and innovation?

In response to this assessment, what actions by leaders will have the greatest impact on the transformation process within the system?

The terms *creativity* and *innovation* are often used interchangeably. Although they are closely related, they have very different meanings in organizations that are responding to continuous change. Creativity is the generation of ideas, solutions, insights, and/or novel approaches to a given situation. It involves perceiving the world in new ways, making connections among seemingly unrelated phenomena, and creating meaningful new ideas or interpretations that are useful to others (Creativity, n.d.; Creativity at Work, n.d.; Franken, 2007). Creativity is about thinking of things, whereas innovation is about doing things (implementation). Being creative facilitates being innovative. Ideas that are creative and imaginative, but are not implemented, are not innovative (innovation is about implementation); however, one can be innovative without being creative (e.g., integrating and implementing an idea that was not your own is innovative action). People are motivated to be creative by the need for novel, varied, and complex mental stimulation, the need to communicate ideas and values, and by their need to solve problems (Franken, 2007). Creativity happens primarily at the early stages of the innovation process. Creativity is the development of ideas, and innovation is the application of ideas (West, 2002b). "Generating creative ideas in a group is relatively easy; implanting new products, processes, or procedures in work organizations is difficult and takes time because of resistance to change, and structural and cultural barriers" (West, 2002a, p. 412).

Innovation within an organization is "the intentional introduction and application within a job, work team or organization of ideas, processes, products or procedures which are new to that job, work team or organization and which are designed to benefit the job, the work team or the organization" (West & Farr, as cited in West, 2002b, p. 357). Blakeney and colleagues (2009) assert that the innovation process has three highly interdependent components: individual or team creativity, the innovation itself, and the environment in which the innovation is developed, introduced, and sustained. The generation of ideas alone is insufficient to initiate meaningful change, and even when implementation follows, innovative change cannot be sustained in environments that lack receptivity for change and support of the innovation process itself (Blakeney et al., 2009).

Disruptive Innovation

The innovation process is one that moves creativity to measurable outcomes, observable actions, products, or process changes within an organization (Blakeney et al., 2009). "Innovation implementation involves changing the status quo, which implies resistance, conflict, and a requirement for sustained effort" (West, 2002b, p. 366). Innovation as a process is not linear, but rather cyclical and iterative, encompassing periods of creativity, implementation of the innovation, adaptation to the change, and stabilization periods (West, 2002b). In fact, innovation itself is disruptive to the organization because those who are initiating the innovation process think differently, ask new and different questions, challenge the status quo and entrenched ideology, and have the potential to significantly impact the entire organization (Blakeney et al., 2009). Disruptive innovation (Christensen & Raynor, 2003), by its very nature, not only challenges conventional thinking and behaviors, but it is also expected to provoke conflict, controversy, and resistance (Blakeney et al., 2009; West, 2002b). It is suggested that this disruption is valuable to the organization as it stimulates dialogue, engages staff in deeper conversations about the impact of change and the actual process of creativity and innovation, and may reveal new solutions that potentially transform the workplace (Blakeney et al., 2009). Benefits of the conflict provoked by engaging in innovation include the following: (1) constructive task-related controversy that improves the quality of decision making and stimulates creativity because it initiates exploration of opposing opinions; (2) frank analyses of task-related issues; and (3) challenges to the status quo (Jackson, as cited in West, 2002b). Moreover, divergent viewpoints, multiple perspectives, and diversity of knowledge, skills, and abilities within work groups not only predict innovation (West, 2002b), but also contribute to the overall impact of the innovation and enhances creativity (Dunbar, as cited in West, 2002b).

Positive Deviance

Those who initiate innovation within systems are sometimes labeled as positive deviants (Jaramillo et al., 2008). Those who employ positive deviance to effect change use behaviors and strategies that are uncommon but honorable and are successful in finding better solutions to a problem than their peers when faced with similar challenges and without extra resources or knowledge (Jaramillo et al., 2008; Tuhus-Dubrow, 2009). "Positive deviance is a method for transforming the culture to incubate creativity and grow innovators from within the organization" (Jaramillo et al., 2008, p. 34). Because solutions to problems are found within the work group, the innovation and behavior changes that result are often sustainable; as one of the principles of change adoption posits, "people do not resist their own ideas" (Jaramillo et al., 2008, p. 31).

Discussion

In what ways can change agents best use the talents of positive deviants to overcome resistance to innovation and change?

CHANGE MANAGEMENT AND DIFFUSION OF INNOVATION

Shift Happens

It is clear that many healthcare organizations are struggling to meet the demands placed on them by patients, families, communities, state and federal governments, insurers, and its practitioners and staff. We believe that the main impediment to meeting these demands is largely due to how healthcare organizations are designed, operated, and led. Much blame has been placed on the dated hierarchical structures still in place in many healthcare organizations that limit their ability to change with the times. Recommendations have been made to flatten these organizational structures to improve effectiveness. Although we believe that organizational structures that are flat (with minimal vertical layers) are most appropriate in contemporary healthcare systems, being flat in no way guarantees that an organization will be flexible enough to meet demands imposed by current and future healthcare needs. Although structure is important, behavior is paramount. A flat organizational structure can produce as many impediments to organizational change as a tall one. Although it is rather easy to flatten an organization's structure, it is much more difficult to change an organization's behavior. The astute leader who does not understand that structural changes must be coupled with behavioral changes, will fall short of creating an organization that is equipped to successfully evolve and change.

What is clear is that long ago the American healthcare system shifted from being a complicated system to a complex system. Numerous factors have created this shift: an aging population, the growing size of our healthcare system, increased numbers of uninsured and underinsured, complex federal and state reimbursement schemes, technology, pharmaceuticals, and increased specialization. Most healthcare organizations continue to be organized, operated, and led as rigid mechanistic hierarchies that are overly bureaucratic and are very slow to change and adapt to changing environmental demands. Today's healthcare leaders are discovering that the mid-20th century models of rigid, hierarchical, industrial, nonadaptive systems that were effective in the past no longer generate the outcomes required today.

Are You Rigid and Frozen in Place?

According to Leonard (1998), rigid organizations exhibit very distinctive characteristics that are the result of extreme insularity.

Limited Problem Solving

Rigid organizations, regardless of their structures, exhibit an overdependence on the strategies of the past to solve the problems of today. This type of rigidity is referred to as *path dependence*. Organizations select the old path to solve problems, even when better alternatives are available (Leonard, 1998). Hammer and Champy warn us that although the familiar path may be more enticing, "the easy way out leads back in" (1993, p. 62).

Inability to Innovate

Rigid organizations become so paralyzed that no amount of energy can bring about meaningful innovation (Leonard, 1998). They suffer from what Barker calls "paradigm paralysis, which is a terminal disease of certainty" (1992, p. 155). These types of organizations are convinced they can continue to do what they have done in the past. In doing so, they believe, or hope, that success is just around the corner. The leaders of these organizations deeply believe that what they need to do is to get their practitioners and staff to do more of what they used to do well, and if they can manage to expand and grow, their troubles will go away. This strategy produces more trouble for the organization because it relies on old strategies to solve new problems (Leonard, 1998). Many of the problems faced by healthcare organizations cannot be overcome by producing more of the same faster. When an organization expands and grows but does not alter its mechanisms of production, it merely produces more of the same thing in the same way. Producing more of something that a healthcare organization's environment no longer requires creates greater misalignment between the organization and its environment.

Limited Experimentation

All, or most, innovation in rigid organizations is believed to be the exclusive domain of its top executives. The problem with this way of leading is that those at the point of service are completely left out of the innovation process. The innovation process is subverted into a top–down, command-and-control maneuver. When experimentation is generated from the apex of the organization and is forced down through the system, failure is almost assured (Leonard, 1998; Rogers, 2003).

Screening Out New Knowledge

Rigid organizations no longer possess the ability to experiment with new methods and processes because the few people who control the flow of external information for internal use literally screen out data and information that does not fit their worldview (Leonard, 1998). Barker calls this malady the "paradigm effect" (1992, p. 153). The organization that suffers from this malady has become so invested in the present paradigm that any talk of moving beyond the present paradigm is immediately rejected. "Stay the course" becomes the organization's mantra.

Discussion

Describe a scenario that represents how your healthcare organization's limited problem solving abilities have negatively impacted patient safety and quality. How has the paradigm effect impacted your healthcare organization's ability to support innovation?

CHANGE AGENT ROLES

Rogers (2003) identified a sequence of roles for the change agent that enhances the likelihood that an innovation will be adopted and sustained. The first role is to develop the need for the innovation. This step in the sequence is much like Lewin's (1935) unfreezing phase of change, where the change agent creates the psychological need for change. If the target audience is not convinced the innovation is essential or required, the innovation is likely to fail. As the agent helps others to see the need for innovation, he or she must simultaneously build confidence that staff and the organization as a whole are quite capable of adopting the innovation; in this way the agent of change begins to create ownership for the innovation's success within the target audience (Rogers, 2003).

The second role of a change agent is to establish trust and an effective information exchange method between the agent and the audience that will need to adopt the innovation. Enough cannot be said about the need for clear, concise, consistent communication in this sequence of the process. There is a very fine line to walk here. Too much communication (even if it is clear, concise, and consistent) can overwhelm the target audience. We suggest that you ask the target audience for their preferences in form and frequency of communication, then honor those choices. Too much communication overwhelms; too little leaves the target audience in the dark. Different segments of the organization often require different levels of content in the communication to keep them enthused about the change or, at the very least, still interested in the proposed innovation. The change agent must be credible, competent, and most of all trustworthy (Rogers, 2003). The messenger must be accepted before the message itself. Acceptance of the change agent is dependent on the trustworthiness of the change agent. Simply stated: no trust, no change.

The third role of the change agent is to diagnose problems the target audience sees as associated with the innovation. The agent must listen carefully to those required to change in order to identify and thoroughly understand all sources of possible resistance to the innovation (e.g., cultural, technical, operational, and what's-in-it-for-me variables). Without completely understanding resistance, the change agent will not be able to accurately diagnose the situation (Rogers, 2003). As Covey notes, the single most important principle in interpersonal relations is to "seek first to understand, then to be understood (1990, p. 237)." An effective agent of change listens carefully and observes closely.

The fourth role of the change agent is to create in the target audience the intent to change, or to accept the innovation. In this role the change agent helps the target audience understand what actions individual audience members can take to achieve the goal; this role is primarily motivational and inspirational (Rogers, 2003). One must remember that there are people who are great at thinking of innovations yet lack the ability to inspire and motivate. The change agent must paint a vivid picture of how the proposed innovation will enhance the ability of the individual and the healthcare organization at large to better meet the needs of all they serve. The goal is to make the innovation something that the target audience cannot live without.

The fifth role of the change agent is to clearly demonstrate how to move from intent to accept the innovation to action (Rogers, 2003). In this role it is imperative that both the change agent and the early-adopter group chosen to help guide the innovation are competent, trustworthy, and credible. These change leaders must demonstrate effective interpersonal skills and the ability to empathize with the target audience without being dragged into any negativity associated with adoption of the innovation.

The sixth role is that of stabilizer. This role is about ensuring the innovation is incorporated and stabilized in daily routines and that the innovation is sustained beyond the initial implementation phase and immediate evaluation period (Rogers, 2003). Rogers notes this role is akin to the refreezing phase of Lewin's (1935) change model. We believe that the last step in Lewin's model should be termed *slush*, not refreeze. The goal of change is acceptance, adoption, and incorporation into daily practice, not to be held as orthodoxy and so deeply frozen that it cannot be unfrozen for the next wave of change. We must convey that nothing is permanent, knowing that humans seek out, and are comforted by, routine, control, and predictability.

The seventh and last role of the change agent is to terminate the relationship. Rogers (2003) notes that the change agent's ultimate goal is to avoid creating dependency. By ensuring the target audience has developed the necessary skills, abilities, and knowledge and will continue their support of the innovation beyond the initial implementation stage, the change or innovation is sustained, and the work of the change agent is completed.

The seven roles of the change agent, as described by Rogers (2003), are presented as a linear process. Change does not unfold in a linear process. Change is an iterative and sometimes messy process. Those leading innovation must realize that the change agent's roles as described by Rogers may need to be used simultaneously and repeated to reach the ultimate outcome of change.

Case Example: Moving from top-down management control to a staff-led patient care unit

Mark Jacobs, MSN, RN, was recently hired to become the third nurse manager in 5 years for a very busy 36-bed cardiac telemetry unit in a major urban teaching medical center. The unit had a current staff turnover rate of 20%. The CNO, who was hired 1 year ago, discussed with Mark during his interview that the organization had a long history of using top–down, command-and-control and punishment "to keep staff in line." The CNO informed Mark that he was interested in moving the nursing division from a management-driven model to a staff-management partnership. Knowing Mark had previous experience with staff empowerment, the CNO requested that his unit become the pilot unit to design and implement a shared decision-making model. Mark agreed with the CNO and accepted the challenge, knowing that the transformation would not be easy. The process Mark decided to use was Rogers's (2003) seven roles of the change agent for introducing the shared decision-making innovation. The roles are operationalized in three phases.

In phase one, the primary goals are to develop the need for change and establish the information exchange relationship between the design team and the staff:

- Introduce the idea of shared decision making, highlighting the evidence and benefits to staff and patients.
- Seek volunteers to participate on the design team, which has credibility with peers. The team members are open to new ideas, are flexible thinkers, enjoy their professional roles, and represent a mix of experienced and inexperienced staff.
- The design team elects its own staff chairperson, develops rapport with staff, and establishes communication mechanisms that reflect the staff's need for information, frequency, and mode or modes of communication.
- The design team diagnoses resistance and identifies facilitators of the transformation.

In phase two, the primary goals are to create an intent to change among staff and to translate that intent into action and commitment:

- The design team presents the plan of action to the staff, seeking feedback for modifications.
- The design team provides staff with information that translates the plan into action.

- The design team identifies roles and accountabilities of all unit staff.

In phase three, the goals are to stabilize the innovation and discontinue the design team's leadership relationship with the staff:

- The design team and the manager stabilize new behaviors by reinforcing the roles and accountabilities that sustain the innovation.
- The design team incorporates new expectations for behaviors into all unit job descriptions and performance appraisals.
- The essential goal in this phase is to put the design team out of business and establish the staff–management partnership.

Mark realizes that successful implementation of an innovation does not sustain it. The role of the nurse manager has now completely evolved from telling people what to do, to encouraging the staff to discover the best mechanisms to provide quality, evidence-based patient care through continuous mentoring and coaching and reinforcing behaviors of self-management and accountability.

Diffusion of Innovation as a Process

Diffusion of innovation is a nonlinear and often complex process in which a few early adopters within a social network identify, refine, and accept an innovation and, over time, influence others to accept the innovation as well (Geibert, 2006; Meyer & Goes, 1988; Plsek, 2003; Rogers, 2003; Valente, 1996; West, Barron, Dowsett, & Newton, 1999). West and colleagues make one of the most important statements found in our literature review when they posit that "adoption is a process rather than an event" (1999, p. 634). They go on to say that without allowing the end user of the innovation sufficient time, autonomy, and support to discuss, challenge, reframe, and refine the innovation, the innovation is likely to fail.

Because most healthcare organizations are operated as hierarchical, linear, mechanistic systems (Crow, 2006), the innovation process is often truncated, or outright omitted, in favor of the event that management uses to introduce the innovation to the staff. Because of this truncation, many innovations fail. Without the engagement of those who are impacted by the innovation, the innovation is likely to be rejected, regardless of its usefulness. When the diffusion of innovation process is subverted into an authoritative forced-decision process, it can further separate management from staff. When management and staff are estranged from each other, organizational effectiveness decreases.

In contrast, a system that is more organic, with a high degree of management and staff interaction that is based on trust, partnership, and equity, allows innovations to arise from anywhere in the system. Diffusion of innovation, when done properly, is an organic process that allows sufficient time for the organization, and its end users, to adapt to the innovation while simultaneously allowing the innovation to adapt to the organization (Valente, 1996; West et al., 1999). These types of organizations are more likely to be successful in adapting to the ever-changing and complex American healthcare system.

Diffusion of Innovation Process Elements

The diffusion of innovation process is a vital element of a healthcare organization's success. When done properly, it can put new tools and competencies in the hands of clinical practitioners and management that have the potential to decrease the costs of care delivery, improve the quality and safety of patient care, enhance patient satisfaction, and engage employees in a participatory leadership model that promotes personal and professional accountability. Whole-systems shared governance provides the structure and process to facilitate these outcomes by supporting the diffusion and successful adoption of innovation and change. Diffusion of innovation is not a top–down, command-and-control process, but rather a horizontal practitioner-to-practitioner influencing process that takes time and astute informal and formal leaders to facilitate. Healthcare organizations, like all organizations, cannot assume staff or managers have all the necessary skills to position the organization for goodness of fit. We believe that whole-systems shared governance is the ideal structure to educate and develop staff, practitioners, and managers who courageously step forward to meet the complex challenges of the American healthcare system. We also believe that the diffusion of innovation process, coupled with whole-systems shared governance, is a powerful and effective way to diffuse one of the most important innovations of the 21st century: managers and staff who have the capacity to successfully lead complex, adaptive healthcare organizations. We believe that in an effort to deal with the increasingly complex American healthcare system, leaders must decentralize power, influence, and control over care processes and resources to point-of-service staff and practitioners and, in turn, have the added obligation to ensure they use this newfound power and influence to benefit the patients and the organization rather than themselves. For this to occur, executives must ensure that staff, practitioners, and managers have the necessary skills, abilities, capabilities, and capacity to lead.

Characteristics of the Diffusion of Innovation Process

Rogers (2003) identifies five main characteristics of the diffusion of innovation process: relative advantage, compatibility, complexity, trialability, and observability of the proposed innovation. These five characteristics, although presented in a linear fashion, are anything but linear. The diffusion of innovation process is an iterative one where each new piece of information informs and reinforces the entire process (Rogers, 2003). The diffusion of innovation process is truly greater than the sum of its parts; however, any single characteristic can derail the entire diffusion of innovation process. Equal attention must be paid to every step and characteristic; failure to do so will certainly place the innovation at risk.

Relative Advantage

The relative advantage of an innovation is its perceived value to the end user. Simply said, perception is reality. The innovation must be perceived as a better fit with the end user's practice than the practice it supersedes. It does not matter if the proposed innovation has a great deal of objective advantage or is based on the best available evidence, the adopter must perceive that the innovation is better. Because an individual's perception about an innovation is that person's reality, time must be allowed to evaluate its usefulness (Rogers, 2003). One must remember that an organization's timeline for diffusion of innovation is not always shared by a department and individual (Geibert, 2006).

Change Agent Role

The change agent's role is to sell the product or process change. At this step the change agent should partner with the healthcare organization's marketing department to identify a strategy to ensure that the organization sees the newest thing or process as better than what it is replacing. The message about the proposed change must be presented in a uniform and consistent manner. At this step in the process, it is useful to have a script. The purpose of the script, and the need for all presenters to stick to the script, is to avoid that all-too-familiar conversation between staff: "When I went to the meeting they never mentioned _____." We all know that two people can attend the same meeting and walk away with different information. To avoid this pitfall, we recommend a printed frequently asked questions handout that conveys the central message exactly as it was presented in the initial briefing. Enough cannot be said about the need to state clearly and consistently the relative advantage of the innovation and the benefits of change.

Origin of Resistance

Staff and management may feel that the innovation could lead to their decreased status in the healthcare organization. Another source of resistance is inadequate information about the basic need for the innovation and how well the innovation fits with the healthcare organization's mission, vision, and values. The change agent must so thoroughly connect the innovation with the enactment of the healthcare organization's mission, vision, and values that everyone can identify the connection. Goodness of fit between the innovation and the healthcare organization is a must. If the change agent cannot accomplish this step, the entire process will be flawed at best.

Response to Resistance
The change agent must first carefully listen to those resisting the change to deeply understand each individual's concerns. Specific feedback should be provided and individual concerns addressed separately (Rogers, 2003). The change agent carefully and thoroughly presents valid and reliable evidence in support of the innovation and how the innovation has a clear relative advantage over what exists currently. The change agent must also be open to alterations to the innovation initially presented to the target audience. Innovations that allow for appropriate alterations in procedures or processes create better goodness of fit among the innovation, individuals, departments, and leadership within the healthcare organization. Strategies that promote goodness of fit must not compromise expected outcomes related to the innovation. Change agents must uphold the underlying principles that guide the intent and implementation of the innovation and identify nonnegotiable modifications that undermine these principles.

Discussion

As the change agent, you are introducing an infrastructure innovation that may threaten the status of individuals whose roles and functions will change. How will you anticipate and respond to this perceived threat?

Compose a five-floor elevator speech that communicates clearly and concisely the value-added benefits of a recent innovation you proposed.

Compatibility

An innovation's compatibility with the needs, professional norms, values, and past experience of those adopting the change must be evident before potential adopters will accept the innovation (Denis, Herbert, Langley, Lozeau, & Trottier, 2002; Ferlie, Gabbay, Fitzgerald, Locock, & Dopson, 2001; Rogers, 2003). Rogers (2003) advises that intended adopters must have the necessary time and autonomy to refine the proposed innovation to increase its goodness of fit with the people who will use it. This process takes time. Determining compatibility cannot occur in one event or one process meeting wherein the innovation is first announced. Not even early adopters are likely to fall for this ruse.

No matter what change is being implemented, those affected (the target audience) must see how the proposed innovation supports (is congruent with) the healthcare organization's mission and values. Additionally, the target audience must have opportunities to provide feedback and suggest modifications that accommodate its local context of care delivery. Once again, the change agent has the responsibility to ensure that modifications to the initial proposal do not violate guiding principles or intended outcomes upon which the innovation is based.

Change Agent Role

The change agent's role in this phase of the diffusion of innovation process is to connect, in a very concrete and overt way, how the innovation will improve the healthcare organization's capacity to operationalize its mission. As mentioned earlier, this does not occur with just one meeting. The change agent needs a plan to introduce and reintroduce the innovation multiple times and in multiple venues with a consistent, scripted message. If individuals within the healthcare organization can see how the proposed innovation supports the organization's mission, vision, and values and also provides them opportunities for participation and contribution to the process and outcome, adoption of the innovation is favored (Rogers, 2003). Just like the incompatibilities encountered following organ transplant surgery, if the host sees the innovation as incompatible, it will be rejected.

Origin of Resistance

The questions and concerns expressed in this step of the diffusion of innovation process are deeply rooted in how the innovation is or is not congruent with the mission, vision, and values of the organization, and with the values of the various professional and technical employee groups within the organization. This is why communications about the proposed innovation must be consistent. If the link between the innovation and the organization's mission, vision, and values is not clearly demonstrated, the target audience has every right to question the efficacy of the innovation. An additional role of the change agent in this step of the process is to be prepared to deal with that age-old response: "We tried that in 1999, it did not work then, and it will not work now!" The best response is not to engage and argue about the past, but rather to clearly articulate that the context and operations of health care have changed and that contemporary conditions require new thinking and new operations. The context in which the innovation was tried in the past is not the context of today, and this insight must be made explicit.

Response to Resistance

Dealing with old ideas and dated mental models among employees within a healthcare organization is one of the greatest challenges for the change agent leading innovation. Mental models are the way we see the world and how we see our place in the world. Undoing a mental model, especially one that is shared within a group, is a monumental undertaking. However, until the old mental model is replaced with a more contemporary one, the target audience for change will simply screen out and resist the innovation as just another flavor of the month and wait for it to pass. Humans rarely discard old ways without a clear understanding of the new way and why a change is necessary. The change agent must present a new view of the contemporary enterprise of healthcare delivery systems. The change agent must be prepared to deliver a consistent message over and over again and not be drawn into arguments about past failures. If the target audience is allowed to continue its focus on the past context and processes, it will not engage as an active member to create the future. The change agent's strategy must be to listen carefully, redirect the conversation and goals, listen and redirect again, and repeat as needed.

Complexity

The complexity of an innovation is concerned with how difficult the proposed innovation is to understand. Innovations that are overly complex or require a great deal of learning are slower to be accepted. If a proposed innovation is labeled as overly complex by early adopters, its chance for acceptance is harmed or outright killed (Rogers, 2003). Maeda informs us that "reaching a balance between how simple you can make an innovation with how complex it has to be to be effective, is not a simple process. The goal of innovation is to develop a process or product that is easy to use, while ensuring that it will do everything that a user might want it to do" (2006, p. 1). We believe that whole-systems shared governance is an excellent platform to negotiate the ideal balance between complexity and simplicity for proposed innovations.

Change Agent Role

When introducing innovation, the change agent must be concerned with complexity in two domains: the complexity of the innovation itself (design, properties, principles, and associated procedures), and the complexity of the innovation's marketing message. The change agent's ability to deconstruct and describe the complexity of an innovation into simple and unambiguous steps is a critical skill whose impact on successful change cannot be underestimated. The marketing message is equally challenging. If the change agent cannot communicate the need for the new thing in a clear and unambiguous manner, the entire process of adoption can be disrupted. If an innovation is both complex to communicate and complex to operationalize, and these two domains of complexity are not well managed, it is likely that adoption of the innovation will fail. This step in the diffusion of innovation process is challenging for all—even the most able change agents.

Origin of Resistance

The origin of resistance in complexity is quite simple. Is the innovation so complex that people feel overwhelmed? The change agent must continually seek to make any change as simple and explicit as possible.

Change Agent Response

The first thing the change agent must do prior to introducing an innovation is to simplify it, reducing the core elements, principles, and intended outcomes (benefits) into a manageable message to communicate both content and process. Complexity is reduced where possible, and clear direction is provided for the steps to success. The change agent designs adequate time for adjustment and training to ensure the target audience can successfully master new skills and procedures required by the innovation. There are times when the process to adopt an innovation is complex, and no matter how effective the plan for change, a target audience may question its ability to master the new process. This is when the change agent must become a coach and mentor whose purpose is to guide, support, and encourage those undergoing the change.

Trialability

Rogers (2003) notes that most staff will not adopt an innovation without first having the opportunity to try it out themselves. Therefore, trialability of a proposed innovation is concerned with whether or not the intended end users have the opportunity to experience what the innovation means to them (Geibert, 2006; Rogers, 2003; Yetton, Sharma, & Southon, 1999). Crow states that "all change is experienced locally, and through this experience the end user gets to identify 'what's in it for me?' (WIIFM)" (2006, p. 239). The WIIFM test for goodness of fit is paramount to acceptance of any innovation. Perhaps Lewin's (1935) change model best explains this characteristic. He identifies three stages of movement during change: unfreezing, moving, and refreezing. In the moving phase, the end user is afforded the opportunity to actually experience what the change means to him or her. A user's ability to experience what the change means to him or her will favorably impact the innovation's relative advantage, compatibility, and trialability. Again, the diffusion of innovation process is iterative, not linear. Trialability is about the experience of the innovation as well as how the usefulness of the innovation is communicated throughout the organization (Rogers, 2003).

An example of not managing the trialability phase is provided by one healthcare organization's experience during the introduction of an electronic health record. As the electronic health record was being introduced, staff members in training classes were put in front of a computer, and one of the first things the instructor said was, "Now, your screen in your clinical area will not look like the one on the screen in front of you." This example identifies a serious failure in managing the trialability phase. To provide staff members an individual experience of the impact of the proposed change, they must experience the actual product in an authentic context and performing a realistic process. Without this personal change-impact experience, the following problems are generated: (1) opportunities are missed to demonstrate the need and benefits of the innovation, (2) new skills will not be learned, (3) additional training will be required to develop essential competencies, (4) missed go-live deadlines are likely due to inadequate user preparation, and (5) the end result is generation of widely held negative attitudes toward the innovation itself and the process of change to adopt it.

Change Agent Role

The change agent's role in this phase of the diffusion of innovation process is to ensure that everyone who is expected to use the new thing or process gets the opportunity to observe that it works better than the thing or process it is replacing (Rogers, 2003). This is akin to the moving phase in Lewin's (1935) change model. This is the phase wherein the target audience gets to experience what the change means to it individually. In this phase, it is critical for the change agent to ensure the design of effective training, opportunities for guided practice with feedback and corrections, and time to develop confidence and positive perceptions of the efficacy of the innovation.

Origin of Resistance

This is where the question arises, whether asked or not asked, WIIFM? This is a fair question, and the change agent must have thought of this before the innovation process begins. WIIFM is a normal human response to change. When confronted with change, we evaluate its relative value by asking WIIFM. Resistance to change in this phase could be a function of the change agent not clearly connecting the WIIFM inquiry, the innovation itself, and the way it supports the mission, vision, and values of the organization. Lacking these connections, the innovation will fail.

Change Agent Response

The change agent must ensure that the education and training associated with the innovation are focused on allowing each member of the target audience to have adequate time to actually use the new thing or process. This is not a one-time education and training session. Reinforcing the education and training and building performance confidence may take numerous sessions. In this phase, the users of the innovation should be allowed to alter the innovation for the context of care without ignoring or altering the underlying principles associated with the innovation. How something is used may be negotiable; however, the underlying principles and expected outcomes are nonnegotiable.

Observability

The observability associated with the innovation is concerned with how visible the advantages of the innovation are to the potential adopter. When potential adopters can actually see the results of the innovation, and those results are clearly associated with increased value and performance, the innovation is more likely to be adopted (Geibert, 2006; Rogers, 2003; Yetton et al., 1999). The need to see how an innovation will aid the practitioner to improve patient care, increase patient satisfaction, and control healthcare costs are powerful ways to increase the likelihood that the innovation will be adopted. The observability characteristic of the diffusion of innovation process provides late adopters the opportunity to observe how the early adopters demonstrate the innovation's advantages (Rogers, 2003).

Change Agent Role

Observability is associated with the visibility of the innovation's advantages as perceived by the individual or group who is expected to adopt it. Observability is an extremely important component of the diffusion of innovation process. In this phase the change agent *must* make visible the various advantages promised by the innovation. The change agent positions those most satisfied with the innovation out front to assist with dissemination of the marketing message and to highlight the positive benefits and advantages of the innovation. Not just anyone will do for this role. The change agent should carefully and thoughtfully select the most articulate, credible, and respected super users who demonstrate consistent competence in both deeply understanding and using the innovation. These super users must possess the ability to absorb the frustrations of a diverse population of learners without being drawn into their negativity, have strong listening and coaching skills, and demonstrate the ability to redirect learner frustration to productive attitudes and actions that will prepare them for successful adoption of the innovation and new practices.

Origin of Resistance

The majority of resistance at this last stage of the diffusion of innovation process will be from the laggards in the healthcare organization. Rogers (2003) describes laggards as living in the past. Their mental model traps them in the past. When staff can only focus on the past, they are not likely to adopt the innovation. The change agent must remember that routines and consistency bring staff comfort and are not easily changed. Resistance could also arise if people in the healthcare organization have been successful at derailing change simply by protesting its existence.

Change Agent Response

The change agent must endeavor to refocus the individual or group on the present. We believe it is helpful to listen to what these individuals have to say; however, at some point the laggards will have to demonstrate that they have internalized the innovation and are prepared to use it in their work or practice, as designed. There will be times when the innovation or change is so dramatic that the individual may no longer have goodness of fit between themselves and the healthcare organization. At this point, the employee is unwilling to change even after coaching and mentoring—it may be time for such an employee to separate from the organization.

SUSTAINABILITY OF INNOVATION

All organizations are faced with the challenge of implementing new practices or processes (innovations) at one time or another; however, many of the innovations that are initially successful fail to become part of the long-term habits and routines of the host organization. Understanding how, why, and under what conditions innovations are sustained are of vital importance to all leaders of healthcare organizations. For the purposes of this chapter, sustainability is defined by Rogers (2003) as "the degree to which an innovation continues to be used over time and after a diffusion program ends" (2003, p. 183).

Organizations no longer sustain a competitive advantage by maintaining practices and processes that are inadequate for the times. Most innovative endeavors will fail without a strong organizational strategy to identify and use innovations. The organization must have a culture that will allow new ideas to be implemented and maintained, and it must have support from the informal and formal organizational arrangements (e.g., the stakeholders in all whole-systems shared governance councils).

Novotna, Dobbins, and Henderson (2012), Scheirer (2005), and Stirman and colleagues (2012) note that there is a near absence of research on how organizations sustain innovations past the implementation phase of change. A quick Google search using the keywords "managing organization change" resulted in 94,900,000 hits, and the keywords "sustaining organizational change" resulted in 3.2 million hits. Many of the citations under sustaining change confuse the implementation phase of innovation with sustaining the innovation; or they confuse institutionalization of the innovation with sustaining the innovation. Stirman and colleagues (2012) note that sustainability of innovations must be studied as a separate phenomenon from implementation and institutionalization.

A review of several current best-seller business books regarding the management of change and innovation found only scant mention of sustaining innovation. Scheirer (2005) posits that one of the difficulties in measuring sustainability is that it requires further data collection to determine whether or not the activities and benefits of the implementation phase continue to be realized over time. Many organizational leaders believe that successful implementation is the cardinal sign that the innovation has been accepted and will continue. Authors do Carmo Caccia-Bava and colleagues (2009), Edwards and Roelofs (2006), Martins and Martins (2002), Novotna and colleagues (2012), Scheirer (2005), Stenmark, Shipman, and Mumford (2011), and Stirman and colleagues (2012) agree that more work needs to be done to operationalize the concept of sustainability because operationalizing a concept leads to measuring the concept.

Factors that increase the likelihood that an innovation will be sustained are associated with the innovation itself, the capacity of the organization to embed the innovation in day-to-day routines past the implementation phase, and a strong history of successful innovation (Edwards & Roelofs, 2006; Shediac-Rizkallah & Bone, as cited in Scheirer, 2005; Stirman et al., 2012). These authors posit that if an organization has these characteristics, sustaining innovation will be more likely.

Scheirer (2005) notes that components of the innovation, such as the project design, organizational factors, and support from the broader community, are factors that determine the innovation's sustainability. The aspects of the project's design include the design process, the involvement of key stakeholders, the ability of the target audience to modify the innovation to meet local needs, and whether or not the implementation data demonstrate that the innovation led to improved performance.

Organizational factors include the innovation's champion and the degree to which the target audience believes the innovation is a good fit with the organization's mission and operating procedures. The champion of any innovation should be highly placed in the organization and well respected and trusted by colleagues. If an innovation cannot be connected to the healthcare organization's mission and to how the innovation assists the healthcare organization in better demonstrating its mission to the community, it will likely fail (Scheirer, 2005).

Sustainability factors associated with a healthcare organization's environment are the socioeconomic environment, market forces, and the legislative actions taken by state and federal governments that mandate healthcare organizations coordinate and seek support from the community it serves for innovations that impact healthcare services delivery. This is why we recommend that community members be a part of all whole-systems shared governance councils and any think tank activities.

Discussion

In the 1870s, Joseph Lister introduced the practical application of germ theory and disease to sanitation practices in medical settings. Knowing that 150 years later we have not effectively sustained the basic practice of hand washing to prevent the spread of disease, how will you sustain complex innovations in your organization?

CONCLUSION

Fostering and sustaining organizational innovation has emerged as an important issue for healthcare leaders. The ability to innovate is a core process that every organization must master to retain its viability as a community resource. Some leaders of healthcare organizations believe that the community needs them more than they need the community. Nothing could be further from the truth. An organization is sustained by its community; if it gets too far out of alignment with the community it serves, there is no need for the healthcare organization to exist. When this occurs, the healthcare organization has drifted from its mission. This misalignment of purpose, operations, and community does not happen overnight. It is a slow and insidious process—one that, without attention, can overtake a healthcare organization before it realizes it is no longer a viable community resource.

Successful innovation in health care requires that healthcare organization leaders have a thorough understanding of the innovation process. Moreover, healthcare leaders must ensure the organization has designed into its operating procedures the capacity to absorb innovations with the least amount of disruption. We believe that whole-systems shared governance with the added function of an internal think tank is a synergistic combination that can ensure organizational success as it continually adapts to its ever-changing environment.

REFERENCES

Barker, J. A. (1992). *Paradigms: The business of discovering the future.* New York, NY: Harper Press.

Blakeney, B., Carleton, P., McCarthy, C., & Coakley, E. (2009). Unlocking the power of innovation. *The Online Journal of Issues in Nursing, 14*(2), Manuscript 1.

Burton, T. T., & Moran, J. W. (1995). *The future focused organization: Complete organizational alignment for breakthrough results.* New York, NY: Prentice-Hall.

Caliva, L., & Scheier, I. H. (1992). *The think tank technique.* Retrieved from http://academic.regis.edu/volunteer/ivan/sect03/sect03b.htm.

Christensen, C., & Raynor, M. (2003). *The innovator's solution: Creating and sustaining successful growth.* Cambridge, MA: Harvard Business School Press.

Covey, S. R. (1990). *The 7 habits of highly effective people: Powerful lessons in personal change.* New York, NY: Fireside.

Creativity. (n.d.). In Dictionary.com. Retrieved from http://dictionary.reference.com/browse/creativity

Creativity at Work. (n.d.). What is creativity? Retrieved from http://www.creativityatwork.com/2014/02/17/what-is-creativity/

Crow, G. L. (2006). Diffusion of innovation: The leader's role in creating the organizational context for evidence-based practice. *Nursing Administration Quarterly, 30*(3), 236–241.

Denis, J. L., Herbert, Y., Langley, A., Lozeau, D., & Trottier, L. H. (2002). Explaining diffusion patterns for complex health care innovations. *Health Care Management Review, 27*(3), 60–73.

do Carmo Caccia-Bava, M., Guimaraes, C. K., & Guimaraes, T. (2009). Testing some major determinants for hospital innovation success. *International Journal of Health Care Quality Assurance, 22*(5), 454–470.

Drucker, P. F. (1995). *Managing in a time of great change.* New York, NY: Turman Talley Books.

Edwards, N. C., & Roelofs, S. M. (2006). Sustainability: The elusive dimension of international health projects. *Canadian Journal of Public Health, 97*(1), 45–49.

Ferlie, E., Gabbay, J., Fitzgerald, L., Locock, L., & Dopson, S. (2001). Evidence-based medicine and organizational change: An overview of some recent qualitative research. In L. Ashburner (Ed.), *Organizational behavior and organizational studies in health care: Reflections on the future.* Basingstoke, England: Palgrave.

Franken, R. E. (2007). *Human motivation* (6th ed.). Belmont, CA: Thomson Wadsworth.

Gardner, D. B., & Cummings, C. (1994). Total quality management and shared governance: Synergistic processes. *Nursing Administration Quarterly, 18*(4), 56–64.

Geibert, R. C. (2006). Using diffusion of innovation concepts to enhance implementation of an electronic health record to support evidence-based practice. *Nursing Administration Quarterly, 30*(3), 203–210.

Hammer, M., & Champy, J. (1993). *Reengineering the corporation: A manifesto for business revolution.* New York, NY: Harper Business Essentials.

Hendel, T., Fish, M., & Berger, O. (2007). Nurse/physician conflict management mode choices: Implications for improved collaborative practice. *Nursing Administration Quarterly, 31*(3), 244–253.

Hess, R. G. (1994). Shared governance: Innovation or imitation? *Nursing Economics, 12*(1), 28–34.

Hess, R. G. (2004). From bedside to boardroom: Nursing shared governance. *Online Journal of Issues in Nursing, 9*(1), 2–2.

Jaramillo, B., Jenkins, C., Kermes, F., Wilson, L., Mazzocco, J., & Longo, T. (2008). Positive deviance: Innovation from the inside out. *Nurse Leader, 6*(2), 30–34.

Kim, D. H. (1992). *Toward learning organizations: Integrating total quality control and systems thinking.* Cambridge, MA: Pegasus Communication.

Kramer, M., & Schmalenberg, C. (2003). Securing good nurse physician relationships. *Nursing Management, 34*(7), 34–38.

Laschinger, H. K. S., & Wong, C. (1999). Staff nurse empowerment and collective accountability: Effect on perceived productivity and self-rated work effectiveness. *Nursing Economics, 17*(6), 308–316, 351.

Leonard, D. (1998). *Wellsprings of knowledge: Building and sustaining the sources of innovation.* Boston, MA: Harvard Business Press.

Lewin, K. (1935). *A dynamic theory of personality.* New York, NY: McGraw-Hill.

Maeda, J. (2006). The laws of simplicity. Cambridge, MA: MIT Press.

Malloch, K. (2010). Creating the organizational context for innovation. In T. Porter-O'Grady & K. Malloch (Eds.), *Innovation leadership* (pp. 33–57). Sudbury, MA: Jones and Bartlett Publishers.

Martins, E., & Martins, N. (2002). An organizational culture model to promote creativity and innovation. *South African Journal of Industrial Psychology, 28*(4), 58–65.

McGann, J. G. (2005). *Think tanks and policy advice in the US.* Public Administration, 87(1), 148–149.

Mercer Delta Consulting. (2012). The congruence model: A roadmap for understanding organization performance. Retrieved from http://ldt.stanford.edu/~gwarman/Files/Congruence_Model.pdf

Meyer, A. D., & Goes, J. B. (1988). Organizational assimilation of innovations: A multilevel contextual analysis. *Academy of Management Journal, 31*(4), 897–923.

Mitchell, M., Brooks, F., & Pugh, J. (1999). Balancing nurse empowerment with improved practice and care: An evaluation of the impact of shared governance. *Journal of Research in Nursing, 4*(3), 192–200.

Moore, S. C., & Hutchison, S. A. (2007). Developing leaders at every level: Accountability and empowerment actualized through shared governance. *Journal of Nursing Administration, 37*(12), 564–568.

Nadler, D. A., Tushman, M. L., & Hatvany, N. G. (1982). *Managing organizations.* Boston, MA: Little Brown.

Novotna, G., Dobbins, M., & Henderson, J. (2012). Institutionalization of evidence-informed practices in healthcare settings. *Implementation Science, 7*, 1–9.

Patterson, E., & McMurray, A. (2003). Collaborative practice between registered nurses and medical practitioners in Australian general practice: Moving from rhetoric to reality. *Australian Journal of Advanced Nursing, 20*(4), 43–48.

Plsek, P. (2003). *Complexity and the adoption of innovation in health care.* Paper presented at Accelerating Quality Improvement in Health Care: Strategies to Accelerate the Diffusion of Evidence-Based Innovations, Washington, DC. Retrieved from: www.nihcm.org/pdf/Plsek.pdf.

Porter-O'Grady, T. (Ed.). (2009). *Interdisciplinary shared governance: Integrating practice, transforming health care* (2nd ed.). Sudbury, MA: Jones and Bartlett Publishers.

Porter-O'Grady, T. (2010). Leadership for innovation: From knowledge creation to transforming health care. In T. Porter-O'Grady & K. Malloch (Eds.), *Innovation leadership* (pp. 1–31). Sudbury, MA: Jones and Bartlett Publishers.

Rogers, E. M. (2003). *Diffusion of innovations* (5th ed.). New York, NY: Free Press.

Scheirer, M. A. (2005). Is sustainability possible? A review and commentary on empirical studies of program sustainability. *American Journal of Evaluation, 26*(3), 320–347.

Schneider, M., & Somers, M. (2006). Organizations as complex adaptive systems: Implications of complexity theory for leadership research. *The Leadership Quarterly, 17*, 351–365.

Senge, P. M. (1990). *The fifth discipline: The art and practice of the learning organization.* New York, NY: Doubleday.

Stenmark, C. K., Shipman, A. S., & Mumford, M. D. (2011). Managing the innovation process: The dynamic role of leaders. *Psychology of Aesthetics, Creativity and the Arts, 5*(1), 67–80.

Stirman, S. W., Kimberly, J., Cook, N., Calloway, A., Castro, F., & Charns, M. (2012). The sustainability of new programs and innovations: A review of the empirical literature and recommendations for future research. *Implementation Science, 7*(17), 1–19.

Tuhus-Dubrow, R. (2009, November 29). The power of positive deviants: A promising new tactic for changing communities from the inside. *The Boston Globe.* Retrieved from http://www.boston.com/bostonglobe/ideas/articles/2009/11/29/the_power_of_positive_deviants/?page=1

Valente, T. W. (1996). Social networks thresholds in the diffusion of innovation. *Social Networks, 18*(1), 69–89.

West, M. A. (2002a). Ideas are ten a plenty: It's team implementation not idea generation that counts. *Applied Psychology: An International Review, 51*(3), 411–424.

West, M. A. (2002b). Sparkling fountains or stagnant ponds: An integrative model of creativity and innovation implementation in work groups. *Applied Psychology: An International Review, 51*(3), 355–387.

West, E., Barron, D. N., Dowsett, J., & Newton, J. N. (1999). Hierarchies and cliques in the social networks of health care professional: Implications for the design of dissemination strategies. *Social Science and Medicine, 48*(3), 633–646.

Westrope, R. A., Vaughn, L., Bott, M., & Taunton, R. L. (1995). Shared governance: From vision to reality. *Journal of Nursing Administration, 25*(12), 45–54.

Yetton, P., Sharma, R., & Southon, G. (1999). Successful IS innovation: The contingent contributions of innovation characteristics and implementation. *Journal of Information Technology, 14*, 53–68.

CHAPTER 14

Evidence-Based Education for Healthcare Innovation

Sandra Davidson

CHAPTER OBJECTIVES

Upon completion of this chapter, the reader will be able to:

1. Understand the current context and challenges in health professions education.
2. Describe the historical progression and developments in health professions education.
3. Explore the current evidence base in adult education and emerging educational theories that can inform the educational experiences of future healthcare practitioners.
4. Discuss the emerging trends, innovations, and possibilities for transforming healthcare education.

INTRODUCTION

This chapter is a compilation of questions, issues, evidence, innovations, and a vision for the future and how care providers could be educated to create the preferred future of health care. It builds on many of the themes that are interpreted within an educational context. There is a Buddhist saying that is helpful in framing the discussion in this chapter: If you want to know your past, look into your present conditions. If you want to know your future, look into your present actions.

The chapter will start with an overview of the current contextual challenges and opportunities in health sciences education. I will use the discipline of nursing as an exemplar to parse the historical backdrop and influences that have shaped the educational experiences of healthcare practitioners. We will then turn our attention to the emerging edge of the future. What do emerging trends, evidence, innovation and andragogy tell us about how we might act to transform the education of health disciplines?

REFLECTIONS ON WHAT IS

As I reflect on what is, I am reminded of the words of Czech president Václav Havel from a speech he gave in 1994: "It is as if something were crumbling, decaying, and exhausting itself—while something else, still indistinct, were rising from the rubble" (Havel, as cited in Scharmer, 2007, p. 1). Scharmer elaborates further: "The crisis of our time reveals the dying of an old social structure and way of thinking, an old way of institutionalizing and enacting collective social forms. Frontline practitioners—managers, teachers, nurses, [and] physicians . . . share a sense of the current reality. They can feel the heat of an ever-increasing workload and pressure to do even more" (2007, p. 2).

I believe this characterizes the vibe in healthcare education today. Health professions faculty (as both practitioners and teachers) are doubly aware of the pressures to do more with less and the ultimate futility of continuing to educate and practice as we have in the past. In this section I will highlight some of the contextual challenges, debates, and pain points that permeate the current reality of healthcare education. The pressure to do even more, I believe, comes from the friction created when old ways of being and doing rub up against the new. The faculty themselves may feel conflicted and bewildered as they try to make sense out of the ambiguity of what has been versus what is becoming. In an effort to cover all the bases (often out of fear and uncertainty), faculty end up doing double work—maintaining the practices of the past while attempting to engage with new educational innovations, ideas, and practices. As a result of spreading our time, attention, and energies too broadly, we often feel that nothing gets done particularly well. How do we make decisions about what educational practices to let go of, what to keep, and what is worth developing? We will return to this question later.

And what of students? What is the experience of our students who have arrived in our classrooms (both physical and virtual) full of purpose and excitement? Health professions students often arrive with an idealized view of the profession they seek to join. As students progress through their programs of study, they become increasingly aware of the frenetic nature of both healthcare education and practice. They see faculty trying to cover all the content and find themselves cramming for tests. In their learning experiences in clinical settings, they see care providers who are trying to do more with less. Rarely do they see their clinical mentors step off the treadmill long enough to catch their breath. Students' idealized visions of their profession are quickly replaced with cynicism and trepidation as they are immersed in the brine of toxic healthcare workplaces and as they absorb their mentors' professional malaise.

Of course, education does not occur in a vacuum. Health professions faculty and students teach and learn within complex contextual structures, namely the educational system and the practice environment. Each of these structures is constituted of unique processes, policies, and personalities that make up the overall environment. Our current organizational realities are dominated by hierarchy and mechanistic structures in both practice and education. A common metaphor used to describe the structures and hardened divisions in these organizations today is that of the silo. In these columnar and encapsulated structures, there is little communication or diffusion between practice and educational contexts. Is it any wonder that the literature and research in healthcare education is replete with references to the education–practice gap?

Even within each silo, there are layers and levels of division. At each level, we find ourselves separated by the siloed distinctions: surgery unit or medical unit, inpatient or outpatient services, clinical course or theory course. We are habituated to organizing and constructing our world around what makes us different. It is not surprising, then, that we struggle to find common ground, to collaborate, or to seek synergies. **Figure 14-1** depicts the contextual silos and the intersilo distinctions that perpetuate this divisive mindset. Although there is some communication and movement among the grand silos (for example, students who graduate from the educational system move to the practice context), there is a disconnect (gap) between the silos because they function as closed systems. This model is representative of current mainstream health care and healthcare education, and it is emblematic of our mechanistic and Newtonian legacy. To use an industrial analogy, our machines are obsolete. They still function quite well, but their purpose and form are suited to a bygone era. Before exploring the social, organizational, and learning technologies that are state of the art, let us delve a little deeper into our current predicament.

Figure 14-1 Education and practice silos

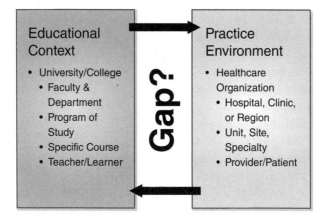

In 2008, the Association of Academic Health Centers (AAHC) published a report on the state of the health workforce (2008). The report is aptly titled *Out of Order, Out of Time*. It provides an excellent overview of the contextual challenges in health professions education. I will use some of the key findings of the AAHC report to frame the discussion that follows here.

THE CANARY IN THE MINE SHAFT: DISSATISFACTION IN HEALTH CARE

To start with, the healthcare industry has experienced waning workforce satisfaction for several decades. Healthy workplace environments and overall work life satisfaction are crucial for both the recruitment of future health professionals and for the retention of existing providers (Association of Academic Health Centers [AAHC], 2008). However, numerous surveys across all disciplines point to growing dissatisfaction. In an international study conducted among hospital-based nurses, almost one in three nurses younger than the age of 30 reported that they were planning to leave their jobs within the year (Aiken Clarke, Sloane, Sochalski, Busse, 2001). In a 2014 survey, 66% of pharmacists rated their workload level as high or excessively high. Further to this, forty-five percent of pharmacists reported that their current workload had negative or very negative effects on mental/emotional health. (Midwest Pharmacy Workforce Research Consortium, 2015).

Overall, six workplace characteristics have been identified as the most prevalent barriers to the recruitment and retention of healthcare providers (AAHC, 2008):

- The healthcare system is too hierarchical, with too much rigidity or little room for growth or innovation.
- The work is too traditional; new graduates, particularly, find practice environments to be antiquated and stifling.
- The work is too physically demanding.
- The 24/7 nature of many healthcare settings results in undesirable schedules for some health professions. There is still a negative stigma about shift work.
- Financial remuneration may be low or has plateaued.
- The pace of work is demanding and stressful.

The healthcare system, as it is currently experienced by many providers, feels untenable, yet there is no distinct resolution or relief in sight. From a health professions, education perspective, the challenges are many. How do educators recruit prospective students into health professions yet still present an appealing (and realistic) vision of what their future professional practice will be like? How do educators manage the tensions among textbook idealism, preparing the practitioners of the future, and the often-grim reality of current practice environments? What is the quality and effectiveness of clinical experiences for students, given the widespread dissatisfaction and role strain of practicing healthcare providers? These are just a few of the countless questions that keep many educators up at night.

Learning Activity

In small groups, spend 15 to 20 minutes addressing the following three questions:

1. How do educators recruit prospective students into health professions yet still present an appealing (and realistic) vision of what their future professional practice will be like?
2. How do educators manage the tensions among textbook idealism, preparing the practitioners of the future, and the often-grim reality of current practice environments?
3. What is the quality and effectiveness of clinical experiences for students, given the widespread dissatisfaction and role strain of practicing healthcare providers?

Please share your own experiences (as students, providers, leaders) in relation to these issues. Are there best practices you could suggest?

CREDENTIAL CREEP: RAISING THE BAR AND ADVANCED PRACTICE

The elevation of minimum credentials across many health professions has created tensions both within and among disciplines. A potpourri of issues—such as rising healthcare costs; patient safety; disciplinary turf, scope, and prestige; and changing career options and career ladders for students—have been discussed and debated. What many have termed *credential creep* is at the heart of many debates. There are two primary aspects of credential creep: increasing entry-level educational requirements for health disciples, and the proliferation of terminal degrees that prepare providers for advanced clinical practice.

The evolution of physical therapy programs is one example of creeping entry-level education. In the early 20th century, physical therapy programs were comprised of on-the-job training and a 3-month program of study resulting in a certificate. At the dawn of the 21st century, all physical therapy degree programs are expected to be at the doctoral level by 2020 (AAHC, 2008). Advocates of raising entry-level requirements suggest that more education will result in better patient care outcomes and that given the increasing complexity and explosion of knowledge in health care, more education is warranted. On the other hand, many prospective students see increased years of education (and the added costs) to enter a health profession as a barrier. There is the potential that elevating entry requirements will result in further shortages of care providers in many disciplines.

At the other end of the spectrum, there has been a proliferation of terminal clinical (doctorate) degrees that prepare practitioners for advanced practice. Nursing is an excellent example of this phenomena. Over the past decade, clinical doctor of nursing practice (DNP) programs have proliferated rapidly in the United States. Advocates of the DNP suggest that this represents another rung on the career ladder for nurses and that DNP-prepared providers will be better positioned to contribute to the development and use of clinical research to improve evidence-based care (AAHC, 2008). However, there are also concerns within nursing that the DNP will provide an added burden to the already dire faculty shortage. That is, faculty with doctorates will be increasingly needed to teach in DNP programs, thus reducing the overall number of doctorally prepared faculty to teach in other programs and possibly decreasing the capacity to educate sufficient nurses for entry to practice positions. Still other critics suggest that the market demand for clinical doctorates is less than the number of providers being educated at that level (supply is greater than demand). These critics characterize the trend as self-serving and motivated by the quest for prestige and higher salaries, which, in turn, raises healthcare costs (AAHC, 2008).

Obviously, there are no easy answers, and the debate rages on. For the purposes of this chapter, the phenomena of credential creep represents a set of complex, multilayered, and multisectoral issues and interests that no one discipline (or sector) can address independently. In fact, unilateral decision making and action (of the past), based on our siloed ways of thinking and oversimplification of complex problems, have contributed to the current situation.

QUALITY AND CONSISTENCY OF EDUCATION AMID FACULTY SHORTAGES

Faculty shortages are present and intensifying across all heath disciplines. The shortages are driven by a number of factors. Prominent among them are the aging of the existing faculty workforce, coupled with the declining pipeline of future faculty to replace them upon retirement.

In nursing, the age of faculty members has been increasing steadily. The average age of doctorally prepared and masters-prepared faculty is 53.5 and 54.5 years, respectively (American Association of Colleges of Nursing, 2006). As a result, large numbers of nursing faculty are retiring. In a 2006 publication, the National League for Nursing (NLN) projected that two thirds of nursing faculty would retire or resign over the next 20 years. Similar trends are present in dentistry, pharmacy, and allied health professions such as nutrition, respiratory therapy, dental hygiene, and radiography (AAHC, 2008).

These mass retirements across all health disciplines necessitate a focus on the recruitment and development of new faculty. However, retiring faculty are not being replaced at a rate sufficient to even maintain current enrollment numbers, not to speak of future growth of educational programs (AAHC, 2008). The reasons for the paucity of qualified new faculty are many. Salary inequities are prime among them. Across all disciplines, clinical salaries are higher than academic salaries. Given that most health disciplines require faculty to have at least a master's degree and ideally a doctorate, the added time and expense of earning this advanced education (e.g., lost wages due to prolonged study, along with tuition and student loans) tends to diminish the financial appeal of academic work even further.

There also seems to be a general lack of enthusiasm for academic healthcare positions. Just as in the clinical realm, low job satisfaction has been reported among health professions faculty. "Stress, unrealistic job expectations, and difficulties managing academic life and personal life contribute to this problem. There is evidence that many junior faculty members have difficulty securing the research grants that are necessary for promotion and tenure" (AAHC, 2008, p. 46). Unfortunately, and mostly unconsciously, healthcare faculty tend to role model the less desirable aspects of academic life for students. If students perceive the work of academics to be characterized by burdensome teaching schedules, nonexistent work–life balance, the constant scrambling for scarce research funds, and impossible publication expectations, there is little mystery as to why so few students are interested in academic healthcare positions.

With respect to the quality and continuity of health professions education, the combination of aging and retiring seasoned faculty and the lack of qualified new faculty to replace them constitutes a crisis not only of numbers, but also quality. In an article in *The Chronicle of Higher Education*, Dr. Pascarella, a professor at the University of Iowa, was quoted as saying, "It took me a while to become a decent teacher. I just hate to think of the students I've screwed up" (Berrett, 2013). Many faculty in the health disciplines today would echo Dr. Pascarella's sentiments.

Becoming a good teacher requires a substantial investment of time and effort to develop one's abilities. Particularly in health sciences, there exists another challenge toward achieving good teaching. The majority of health professions faculty are not formally educated to be educators. That is, our primary discipline is not education; we are physical therapists, physicians, nurses, social workers, and pharmacists who have figured out how to teach, largely through informal learning, such as trial and error, self-study, and student feedback. New faculty who are fortunate enough to have good mentors may have had a somewhat less tumultuous introduction to teaching. However, with the impending retirements of many seasoned faculty, health professions are also losing those who can most wisely mentor and support new educators. Dr. Valiga, in her address to the NLN's National Advisory Council on Nurse Education and Practice in April 2002, summed up the situation:

> *Without preparation in the faculty role . . . without role models and mentors to help them manage the unique issues one faces in that role . . . without strong commitment to a role where teaching is primary and one's own clinical practice is secondary . . . and without a science to undermine their practice, individuals whose preparation was as a nurse practitioner or clinical nurse specialist struggle to implement the faculty role. They often teach only as they were taught (which, by the way, typically uses strategies that are being shown to be quite ineffective with today's learners). They fail to innovate. And they are likely to prefer to engage in a clinical role that fits much more closely to what they went to graduate school for in the first place . . . and where they are likely to earn more money! The crisis, therefore, is real, and the potential for it to grow in severity very soon is high. (Valiga, 2002, p. 4)*[1]

INTERPROFESSIONAL EDUCATION AND PRACTICE: THE KEY TO MEETING FUTURE NEEDS?

A wide variety of national and international groups have highlighted the need for and promise of interprofessional education and practice over the past 25 years (AAHC, 2008, 2013; Institute of Medicine, 2001, 2011; Interprofessional Education Collaborative Expert Panel, 2011; Tresolini and Pew-Fetzer Task Force, 1994; World Health Organization, 2010). As evidenced by this broad array of reports, it is evident that dialogues have been occurring for several decades around interprofessional education and practice. In light of these long-running interests in interprofessional activities, one might wonder why we are not further ahead.

---

[1] Dr. Thersa Valiga, in an address to NLN's National Advisory Council on Nurse Education and Practice (NACNEP), April 2002. Reprinted by permission.

Interprofessional or multiple disciplinary education, more generally, tends to occur in isolated pockets, and initiatives seem to be short term. It is often the case that an interprofessional education initiative flourishes for several years under the auspices of a grant or research project, but institutional interest and resources wane after the project period ends (AAHC, 2008; Interprofessional Education Collaborative Expert Panel, 2011). Again, many of the identified barriers to true collaborative practice and interprofessional education programs can be traced back to our siloed and hierarchy-heavy organizations and professions. The following is a summary of the major barriers to interprofessional education (Interprofessional Education Collaborative Expert Panel, 2011; World Health Organization, 2010):

- Institutional-level challenges: Leadership support, buy-in, and resource allocation
- Practical concerns: Scheduling, space, synchronizing multiple curricula
- Faculty development: Teaching interprofessional process is different than traditional discipline-specific didactic methods
- Lack of collaborators: One discipline may want to participate, others may not; single-discipline schools may not be able to provide interprofessional education opportunities
- Regulatory challenges: Discipline-specific regulators may not view interprofessional competencies as essential for practice
- Assessment: What exactly is being assessed (knowledge, skills, and behaviors), and how do we assess interprofessional learning?

Our organizational structures, mind-sets, policies, and long-held assumptions about the nature of health care and education are the biggest impediments to change. In other words, we are getting in the way of our own success.

However, there is reason for optimism. Slowly but surely, there is progress. There are individuals, teams, and even organizations that are leading the way in overcoming these traditional barriers to interprofessional education and collaborative practice. In relation to the themes and focus of this text, healthcare innovation is just one type of collaborative practice. There is great synergy between interprofessional education and educating the future leaders of healthcare innovation. Innovation is a team sport, so to speak. It follows, then, that the basic knowledge, skills, and attitudes that enable teams to be innovative are also the foundation of high-functioning collaborative care teams. Innovation theory and practice may well be the vehicle that propels us from teaching through the past the past toward preparing the next generation of healthcare providers who are fully capable of transforming health care. Before we get back to the future, let us take some time to better understand the historical legacies that have contributed to our current circumstances.

There is value in examining how we have arrived at the present. There may be important learnings in terms of not repeating mistakes of the past. Additionally, exploring our history provides perspective and can help us appreciate how far we have come in health care and education. Because it would take the entire chapter to fully trace the educational developments across all health disciplines, I will use nursing as an exemplar and draw attention to particular eras and developments that influenced education across multiple disciplines and higher education in general.

WHERE HAVE WE COME FROM? A BRIEF HISTORY OF NURSING EDUCATION

The vast majority of educational programs for healthcare providers today still retain the mechanistic blueprint handed down from the time of the industrial revolution. Education in the industrial era was focused on the preparation of students to take their place as cogs in the grand industrial machine (e.g., factory workers). Hospitals, much like other organizations of the late 19th century, were being designed for efficiency and mass production. To educate the volume of workers needed to move the industrial age along, education took on a mass production model. It was important that each cog (or student) be educated in exactly the same way so they could all perform to certain specifications and essentially be interchangeable.

Because textbooks and paper were expensive, it was necessary for teachers to disseminate the information from books to students by means of lecturing or speaking the contents of the texts aloud. Thus, the teacher was placed in a powerful position of knowing, and students were in a position that was subservient and reliant upon the teacher to provide knowledge.

Florence Nightingale undertook her work in the midst of England's Industrial Revolution. The birth of modern nursing occurred in the late 1800s in England at the hand of Florence Nightingale and her School of Nursing at St. Thomas Hospital. Nightingale's program consisted of 1 full year of training and a 3-year service obligation (Bevis & Watson, 1989). Nightingale's curriculum was highly structured and well organized. As Bevis and Watson suggested, "It was an idea whose time was right" (1989, p. 21). Indeed, the Nightingale curriculum, and even the ward structure of St. Thomas Hospital, was influenced by modernity and industriousness that were transforming the world at that time.

In the late 19th century, the Nightingale curriculum was imported to North America. Soon after, nursing schools proliferated without regulation or external oversight, and this often resulted in the exploitation of student nurses within hospital environments (Bevis & Watson, 1989). At this time, nursing education was entirely hospital based. All the instruction and training took place within the hospital, and funding was supplied by hospitals (Pringle, Green, & Johnson, 2004). In the likeness of Taylor's scientific management which was widely influential in the early 20th century in 1911, hospitals had a vested interest in controlling the training of nurses and other healthcare workers. Just as factories set forth specific training for their workers, so did hospitals.

At the beginning of the 20th century, there began a slow migration of hospital nurse training programs toward university- and college-based programs of nursing education. So that nursing might develop into a recognized profession, there was a need for autonomous control of nursing practice, education, and research (Bevis & Watson, 1989). The move to university-based education provided this opportunity. The first true university-based nursing education program was founded in 1909 at the University of Minnesota (Bevis & Watson, 1989). In Canada, the University of British Columbia (UBC) established the first nursing degree program in 1919. It may not be a coincidence that the president of UBC at that time had come from the University of Minnesota (Pringle et al., 2004).

In this same era, the League for Nursing Education addressed the lack of consistent control and regulation of nursing programs in the United States by publishing the Standard Curriculum in 1917. The book listed objectives, content, materials, equipment, and methods for instruction needed to run a standardized, effective school of nursing. This document was revised in 1927 and 1937 (Bevis & Watson, 1989). In Canada, an education professor from UBC, George Weir, was commissioned by the Canadian Nurses Association to complete a report on the state of nursing education. The report was published in 1932. In the report, he was scathing in his review of the practices in many schools at the time. Among these practices were admitting students who had little, if any, high school education, schools that had no teachers, and the heavy focus on hospital service provision over actual education (Pringle et al., 2004). The report led to improved standards and practices in nursing education and resulted in the closure of many of the smaller schools that had proliferated in the absence of external regulation and quality control (Pringle et al., 2004).

The next great developments in nursing education were not until the 1950s. In that decade, there were great advancements and a proliferation of research in many areas, including medicine, education, and the social sciences. **Figure 14-2** summarizes a sample of the prominent researchers and theorists whose work has had a lasting influence on education. Many of these names are well known because the concepts and theories developed in the 1950s and 1960s are still used today.

Of particular importance to nursing education was the Tyler Rationale. Tyler's work was rapidly taken up by the accrediting bodies that regulated nursing schools in the United States as the way to educate nurses. Indeed, the Tyler Rationale was broadly adopted and institutionalized among both higher education and K-12 educational systems throughout North America. Bevis and Watson suggested that what Tyler intended to be a mere guide for education morphed into "laws so immutable as to make the Ten

Figure 14-2 Overview of research from the 1950s that influenced education

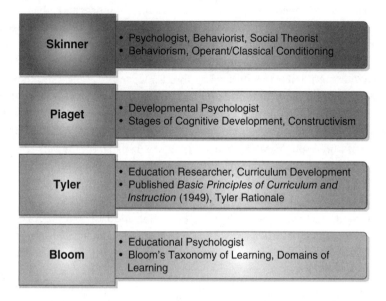

Commandments easier to break without bringing down organized condemnation and punitive consequences" (1989, p. 31). I further suggest that behaviorism, together with the Tyler Rationale, have been forged into a kind of hegemony that functions to perpetuate a bygone era of health professions education.

The 1980s saw the first substantial challenges to the dominance of behaviorism and the Tyler Rationale in nursing and the broader realm of higher education. In their seminal work, *Toward a Caring Curriculum: A New Pedagogy for Nursing* (1989), Bevis and Watson made a compelling case for revising the behaviorist-laden curricula. Their Caring Curricular model drew upon feminist and critical pedagogy, constructivism, and andragogy and applied these multiple pedagogical approaches to nursing education. Bevis and Watson highlighted nursing as a human science and were critical of the behaviorist approach, stating that it did not address the seemingly immeasurable aspects of nursing practice, such as caring, compassion, clinical judgment, creativity, self-reflection, and ethical comportment in practice. What now seems like foreshadowing, Bevis and Watson admonished that what behaviorism "cannot do is to support the changes necessary to keep pace with society's changing demands and the natural evolution of nursing as a profession" (1989, p. 32).

In the early part of the 20th century, knowledge doubled every 30 years; by the 1970s, the world's knowledge (historical information, books, and electronic files) was doubling every 7 years. It is now estimated that knowledge doubles every 13 months. The involved observer soon sees the inadequacy of behaviorism alone to prepare health professionals for current and future practice environments. Clinical reasoning, creativity, multiple disciplinary collaboration, evidence-based practice, and leadership amid complex systems are but a few of the competencies deemed essential in 21st century healthcare practice. These new competencies and realities for practitioners require that we transform the ways in which individuals are educated for and enter into health professions in the knowledge era and beyond.

Although behavioral aspects are still pervasive in both the design of programs and teaching practices today, nursing and other health professions education has entered a phase in which multiple educational philosophies and andragogic approaches are used. Constructivism and learner-centered approaches currently shape many of the curricular revision efforts. Education needs to continue to move beyond its habits of teaching to the past. For this to happen, faculty need to embrace current and emerging educational philosophies, evidence, and practices. The default position of teaching as we were taught will keep health professions education perpetually in the past.

WHERE DO WE GO FROM HERE?

Benner, Sutphen, Leonard, and Day (2010) published the most significant work on the transformation of nursing education since Bevis and Watson's work in 1989. Through their research, Benner and colleagues crafted a compelling, and at times scathing, exposé of the current realities and inadequacies of nursing education in light of the state of the U.S. healthcare system and the clinical settings in which nurses practice. The following are the four transformational "shifts for integration" (2010, p. 82) that arose in their study:

- "Shift from a focus on covering decontextualized knowledge to an emphasis on teaching for a sense of salience, situated cognition, and action in particular situations" (2010, p. 82).
- "Shift from sharp separation of clinical and classroom teaching to integration of classroom and clinical teaching" (2010, p. 83).
- "Shift from an emphasis on critical thinking to an emphasis on clinical reasoning and multiple ways of thinking that include critical thinking" (2010, p. 84).
- "Shift from an emphasis on socialization and role taking to an emphasis on formation" (2010, p. 86).

This list is yet another reminder of the pathologies of either/or, mechanistic, and siloed thinking that has led to the current situation in healthcare education. In the view of Benner and colleagues, "to become a good nurse, one must develop not only technical expertise but also the ability to form relationships and engage in practical ethical and clinical reasoning" (2010, p. 86). These findings point to the need for more relational ways of being and learning. More and more, the work of nurses and all healthcare providers is relational in nature, so the value of creating a learning environment that allows students to learn and practice in relational ways seems self-evident. However, to accomplish this means that we must (in many instances) reinvent our relationships in health professions education and health care. That encompasses relationships with students, academic peers, clinical colleagues, leaders, patients, communities, and regulators.

REVISITING THE ORGANIZATION AS CONVERSATION

Organization as conversation is a useful way to reframe our thinking about what happens in our day-to-day interactions in the places where we work and learn. This perspective is theoretically grounded in complexity science (complex responsive processes, to be specific) and social constructionism. From this relational complexity perspective, reimagining our constellation of relationships starts with new language. New language is a powerful tool for creating the potential for novelty and change. If we want to transform healthcare education into something beyond the mechanistic, siloed, either/or, and boundaried reality, a change of language may be useful in generating new ways of being.

Language is conduit for shared meaning making. That is, the ways that people talk together and the language they use can dramatically shape how they perceive their circumstances. Perception then comes to bear on the actions we choose and the attitudes we adopt in response to our perceived circumstances. Language is the foundation of the stories (narratives) we tell and the metaphors we use to make sense of the world around us; reciprocally, our experience in the world is shaped by the stories and metaphors we choose. Take, for example, the language used earlier to describe the existing dynamic between education and health care: the education–practice *gap*. As we perpetuate this narrative of disconnection and division, the gap becomes more real as we continue to behave accordingly. What would happen if we spoke about the education–practice *connection*? Imagine if we began to act into that connection rather than widening the gap? Another example of how language serves to reinforce our experiences of the world is the analogy of the discipline, unit, or specialty as a silo.

Palmer suggested that we must endeavor to "debunk the myth that institutions are external to and constrain us, as if they possessed powers that render us helpless—an assumption that is largely unconscious and wholly untrue" (2007, p. 3). This raises another facet of the power of language. Narratives and myths can serve to either enable

Learning Activity

1. Individually reflect on the idea of analogies and metaphors as a way to describe our experiences. What metaphors or analogies have you heard, or used yourself, to describe the following?
   - Clinical practice (unit culture, interprofessional practice, hospital administrators, etc.)
   - Educational experiences (e.g., teaching, learning, assessment, labs)

   Take a few minutes to write down the analogies and metaphors that came to mind.
2. Share your analogies and metaphors with a peer or in a small group. Were your metaphors similar? Can you discern an overall theme across them?
3. Take some time to discuss what you think this collection of analogies and metaphors tells us about health care and education.
4. With a peer or in a small group, share your personal visions of what you want the future of health care and healthcare education to be like.
5. Try to generate metaphors or analogies that would capture what that preferred future would look and feel like. You may want to share and compare your future focused analogies and metaphors in a large group discussion.

or constrain our actions. Have you ever heard a peer or colleague say, "I should have done X, but the system would not let me," or perhaps, "I was only following policy." In other words, we may use policies, processes, or other organizational constraints to abdicate our personal responsibility for unprofessional behavior. Rather than continuing to tell victim stories about how we have been done wrong by the system, we can choose to view ourselves as the organization (education or practice or both) that we are a part of. Said differently, the system is not some faceless overlord or mythical force that keeps us under a spell. Instead, from a complex relational perspective, the organization is made up of people (you and me) working together toward a common purpose or goal. In this sense, we are the system, the system is us. This vantage point places the power to change the system in our hands. The language we use, the relationships we foster, and the day-to-day choices we make can act as vectors that help us move toward the preferred future of health professions education.

In the sections that follow, we will explore various facets of healthcare education in hopes of discerning a way forward. The relational complexity perspective described in the previous section brings a new layer of meaning to the Buddhist saying shared at the beginning of this chapter: if you want to know your future, look into your present actions. We have a choice in each and every moment. We can choose to perpetuate the past, in which case the future will yield more of the same; or we can choose different ideas, relationships, theories, and narratives that will bring about something new. The concepts, theories, practices, and research highlighted in the rest of this chapter are meant to provide incitement for readers to engage further with new or different ideas and perspectives. I urge you to talk about, try, question, tinker with, and add to them from whatever your particular vantage point in health care happens to be (student, teacher, practitioner, leader, or patient).

THE NATURE AND AIMS OF HEALTHCARE EDUCATION REVISITED

Given the contextual aspects of the current state of health professions education outlined earlier, it seems reasonable to start by reexamining the goals of healthcare education. Slattery suggested that "the demoralization of educators, disenfranchisement of students, and the dissatisfaction of stakeholders [in healthcare education and practice] are all indications that something is terribly wrong" (2013, p. 285). It is clear that we cannot keep doing what we have always done. Returning to the idea that we seem to be always trying to do more and more, and the question of how we decide what to let go of, let us first explore the function of content in health professions education.

The premise of teaching in the past has been driven by covering content. Like many other practices of the previous century, the assumption that teachers cover content is ingrained and indeed part of the professional identity of many educators (Weimer, 2013). Covering the content is another metaphor that shapes our perceptions. "Thinking that content is there to be 'covered' does not cause us to use the content in ways that promote learning or develop important learning skills" (Weimer, 2013, p. 117). Tied in with covering content are long-held assumptions about content, such as that more is better, or that course quality is determined by how content rich it is. In fact, we have ample educational research from the past 30 years which states that what is transmitted to students through covering (lecturing) is not retained beyond a few days or weeks (Finkel, 2000). Faculty are often reticent to give up favorite topics or content. The irony is that in merely covering the content, we have already been giving them up (Weimer, 2013).

As an alternate metaphor, Weimer asked, "what if our introductions to our fields were characterized by the features of a good introduction of one person to another? A good introduction offers a few details about the new person that makes her sound interesting—someone you'd like to meet and possibly get to know" (2013, pp. 117–118). Of course, this analogy is doubly appealing because it frames content relationally. We want our students to develop relationships with the content of our beloved disciplines. Although we as educators may be responsible for the initial introduction to the discipline, we hope that students develop their own friendships and connections with the content of health care.

What is the function of content, then, if not to be covered? First, content is (and always has been) essential to develop a knowledge base around a specific topic or discipline. Surgeons could not practice surgery without the requisite knowledge base. However, we must assist our students to engage in the content in a deeper way to develop an enduring knowledge base. Concept-based, problem-based, and context-based learning strategies are a few examples of deeper ways to engage students in the content. Second, content acts as a medium for learning how to learn and also for helping students understand the work of a discipline. Content is necessary for students to engage in cognitive apprenticeship (learning to think like a pharmacist, doctor, or social worker). Learning to learn is especially noteworthy and tied to another important aspect of the nature of content in healthcare education. That is the exponential growth and short life span of content (knowledge) in the 21st century.

TEACHING IN THE KNOWLEDGE ERA: LEARNING IN A WIRED WORLD

Since the 1990s we have been living in the knowledge era. All health disciplines have experienced an unprecedented explosion in the generation and availability of research and information in general. More and more practitioners see themselves as knowledge workers rather than task-driven care providers. The exponential growth of knowledge and the ubiquitous access to it has been enabled by amazing advancements in technology. Access to an ocean of information is literally at our fingertips. Clinical apps for our phones (such as drug guides, clinical practice guidelines, and yes, even Google), vast research databases, and access to experts and networks of peers are as close as our pocket. The knowledge era has presented us with a new dynamic between information and learning, and we must overcome long-held assumptions about how we think about information, knowledge, and learning.

The life span of relevant knowledge has greatly diminished. For instance, the amount of new technical information produced doubles roughly every 2 years. This means that for students who are in a 4-year degree program, half of what they learn in their first year of study may be outdated by their third year (Tucker, 2008). The shortening half-life of information further suggests that focusing on covering content is less useful than using content to learn how to learn. This also means that healthcare education programs must prepare students to engage in life-long learning and ongoing professional development to remain competent.

Knowledge is no longer a commodity, but it has become an application to be accessed and used as needed and purged when no longer useful (Brown, 2005). Brown used the term *navigationism* as a way to frame how we might educate students to thrive in the knowledge economy. He described information navigation as a new type of literacy for the 21st century: "I believe that the real literacy of tomorrow will have more to do with being able to be your own private, personal reference librarian, one that knows how to navigate through the incredible, confusing complex information spaces and feel comfortable and located in doing that" (Brown, 2006, p. 112).

Brown suggested that the learning paradigm is shifting beyond constructivism (knowledge production) to knowledge navigation. **Table 14-1** Compares the landscape of learning as seen from different paradigms.

Siemens (2005) suggested an additional learning theory that aligns with and builds upon navigationism. Siemens integrated principles from chaos, network, complexity, and self-organizing theories and applied these into learning in the knowledge era.

From this integrated complexity perspective, Siemens described learning as actionable knowledge that is focused on connecting specialized information sets, "and the connections that enable us to learn more are more important than our current state

Table 14-1 Characteristics of Knowledge and Learning from Three Perspectives

Paradigms	Past (knowledge adoption)	Present (knowledge production)	Future (knowledge navigation)
Learning	Memorizing, studying. Aim is a change in behavior of the learner.	Inquiry and research, active learning. Aim is the construction of new personal knowledge and meaning.	Exploring, connecting, evaluating, manipulating, integrating, and navigating knowledge.
Nature of knowledge	Knowledge creation was for elite experts. Knowledge was already there and ready to be learned.	Previous (existing) knowledge is built upon. Active learning enables the creation of new meaning or knowledge.	Sources of knowledge are everywhere. The focus is on navigating the vast amounts of information and making sense of it.
Learner	Focused on gaining knowledge.	Constructs new meaning by actively engaging with knowledge.	Solves contextual real-life problems via active engagement, networking, communication, and collaboration.
Teacher	Sage on stage. Subject expert, primary source of knowledge.	Guide on side. Not the only source of knowledge, guide both what and how to learn.	Coach in touch. Coaches and mentors in skills of sense making, information facilitation, knowledge configuration.

Modified from Brown, T. H. (2006). Beyond constructivism: Navigationism in the knowledge era. *On the Horizon, 14*(3), 108–120.

of knowing" (Siemens, 2005, p. 5). The principles of connectivism (Siemens, 2005; Brown, 2006) are described as follows:

- Learning is a process of connecting specialized nodes or sources of information.
- The capacity to know more is more critical than what is currently known.
- Nurturing and maintaining connections is needed to facilitate continual learning.
- The ability to see connections among fields, ideas, and concepts is a core skill.
- Currency (accurate, up-to-date knowledge) is the intent of all connectivist learning activities.
- Decision making is itself a learning process. Choosing what to learn and the meaning of incoming information is seen through the lens of a shifting reality. Although there is a right answer today, it may be wrong tomorrow because of changes in the information climate that affects decision making.

It is also important to highlight our shifting understanding of valid sources of knowledge (evidence) in light of emerging learning paradigms, technology, and the knowledge era. In the past, it was easier to discern reputable sources of knowledge, mostly because there were fewer of them. Knowledge production was much slower, and the means for knowledge production and dissemination were available only to experts (e.g., elite academics and researchers). There was a time in the not-so-distant past that information presented in a textbook could be assumed to be expert and up to date. Recall that in the first half of the 20th century, knowledge doubled every 30 years. The concern of textbooks being obsolete almost as soon as they are printed would have seemed ludicrous to publishers in the 1920s.

However, today that is a reality. In response to the exponential growth of knowledge, many of our more traditional sources of knowledge and evidence have adapted by moving to online publishing processes that are faster and more nimble. Many peer-reviewed professional journals have leveraged technology to accelerate the peer review process and shorten the time between submission of a paper and its publication. Most journals today have electronic version and use online and early release features to expedite the dissemination of new research.

The traditional sources of evidence and knowledge (books and journals) are now one of many sources. The rise of Web 2.0 technologies has democratized the access to knowledge production. Almost everyone with an Internet connection has the ability to self-publish a book, create a website or blog, participate in social media conversations, and generally contribute to the ongoing production of knowledge. This means that the critical appraisal of the electronic sources of evidence (and knowledge sources in general) becomes an important skill, not just for healthcare professionals, but for everyone.

The term *digital literacy* has been used to describe and enumerate the skills, attitudes, and knowledge needed to be an active and informed participant in the digital world. Digital literacy is "the ability to use information and communication technologies to find, evaluate, create, and communicate information, requiring both cognitive and technical skills" (Visser, 2012, para. 2). Specific to healthcare education and practice the ability to "use diverse technologies appropriately and effectively to retrieve information, interpret results, and judge the quality of that information" (Visser, 2012, para. 4) is critically important in the current learning paradigm and also the future paradigm (navigationism and connectivism). Coaching and mentoring students to develop their digital literacy is a role that health professions faculty must be ready to take on. This means that faculty themselves must develop and practice digital literacy.

Discussion

Digital literacy is described as a set of skills that are both *technical* and *cognitive*. This includes the actual mechanics of using technology to access information and thinking about it in sophisticated ways (e.g., clinical reasoning and critical, creative, and ethical thinking).

- What barriers have you experienced to developing and using digital literacy skills?
- Were they mostly technical or cognitive?
- How did you overcome them?
- How might you partner with others in your organization to create an environment that supports the ongoing development of digital literacy?

Another aspect of digital literacy that is of particular importance in health care is e-health literacy; that is, the ability to find, understand and appraise health information from electronic sources and apply the knowledge gained to address health problems (Norman & Skinner, 2006). Not only do future healthcare providers need to be e-health literate, but they must also have the skills to coach and mentor others (patients, peers, communities) in this endeavor. Active learning opportunities that help students to develop their e-health literacy and digital literacy skills are critical and should be integrated into health professions education.

Learning Activity

In this chapter we have discussed the need to rethink the function of content in healthcare education programs. Keeping in mind the aspects of navigationism and e-health literacy, consider the following:

1. How might you develop a learning activity that would use content as a vehicle to help students solve a real-world problem? For example, have a student

collaborate with a newly diagnosed type I diabetic patient who is experiencing low blood glucose levels in the morning (content). The patient and her family do not understand why this is happening, and they have asked about a suggestion they read in an online patient chat room for new diabetics (real-world problem).
2. Have the student and patient work together to find, understand, and appraise health information from electronic sources (digital literacy) and apply the knowledge gained to address health problems (e-health literacy).

TEACHING INTO THE FUTURE: RELATIONSHIP-CENTERED CARE AND INTERPROFESSIONAL PRACTICE

It has been suggested that interprofessional practice and relationship-centered care may hold the potential to be transformational forces in health care. For this potential to be tested and hopefully realized, future healthcare providers need to be educated in ways that are resonant with these practices. This section presents emerging learning theories, and teaching and learning practices that create the context for students and educators to develop relational competence.

Relational Education

Relationship-centered healthcare has been described by Tresolini and the Pew-Fetzer Task Force (1994) in terms of three pivotal relationships in health care: the patient–provider relationship, the provider–provider relationship, and the provider–community relationship. Each type of relationship requires the provider to apply specific knowledge, skills, and attitudes for positive relationships to be formed and maintained. Gergen (2009) likewise asserted that there are relationships (or circles) that enable relational education:

Circle 1: Teacher and student
Circle 2: Relationships among students
Circle 3: Classrooms and community
Circle 4: Classrooms and the world

Indeed, as Gergen (2009) added, there are actually unceasing circles or relationships that may be envisioned in relational education (e.g., teacher to teacher, administrator to teacher, regulators to administrators, administrators to students, etc.). The point of describing and highlighting certain relationships is simply to illustrate the idea that when we focus on relationships (as opposed to individuals) as the organizing feature of health care or healthcare education, we can envision new possibilities and potential.

Social construction theory posits that knowledge and reason can be viewed as relational achievements rather than entities held in the minds of individuals. From this standpoint, the "primary aim of education is to enhance the potentials for participating in relational processes—from the local to the global" (Gergen, 2009, p. 243). Most of our educational systems are built upon the individualist, siloed mentality and traditional hierarchies that place knowledge in the minds of individuals. From this view, learning is something that can be managed, measured, and precisely orchestrated using tools such as a curriculum, course syllabus, and meticulous lesson plans. In this traditional (behaviorist) view of learning we draw a clear distinction between the "knowing teacher and the ignorant pupil . . . and we presume that a knowing mind is good preparation for a successful future" (Gergen, 2009, p. 241). From a complex relational point of view, learning is a relational process of communicative interaction. It is participative action rather than mere reproduction of memorized steps (mimicry). Knowledge arises in the participative communicative interactions that take place among people in moment-to-moment interactions (Stacey, 2001).

A helpful analogy for this socially constructed and complex relational view of learning is education as a rhizome (Cormier, 2008). Cormier suggested that in collaborative learning, "knowledge becomes negotiation" (2008, p. 1) in that the learning process itself is ongoing negotiation. A rhizome is plant that has no center no boundaries; rather, it is constrained only by the limits of its environment (habitat). Rhizomes are comprised of a number of semi-independent nodes that are each capable of growing and spreading on their own (Cormier, 2008). When this analogy is applied to education, knowledge can only be negotiated. The contextual and collaborative learning experience is a social and personal process of knowledge creation "with mutable goals and constantly negotiated premises" (2008, p. 1).

In the rhizomatic model of learning, the curriculum is not driven by predefined inputs from experts; it is constructed and negotiated in real time by the contributions of those engaged in the learning process. This community acts as the curriculum, spontaneously shaping, constructing, and reconstructing itself and the subject of its learning in the same way that the rhizome responds to changing environmental conditions (Cormier, 2008).

For all health professions to engage in the healthcare transformation that is called for, educators will need to take up new ways of teaching and participating in educational processes. Tresolini and the Pew-Fetzer Task Force (1994) highlighted that the educational environments we construct serve to reinforce the underlying assumptions about both learning and care. As such, relationship-centered care is reflected in learner-centered education. "The caring relationship between practitioner and patient is modeled by the nurturing environment that students, faculty, and practitioners themselves create through the quality of their relationships" (1994, p. 42). Similarly, learning goals that are mutually established by a community of teachers and learners can be used to teach the parallel process of collaborative goal setting in provider–patient relationships (Tresolini & Pew-Fetzer Task Force, 1994).

From a collaborative practice and interprofessional perspective, the same logic applies. Collaborative practice is reflected in collaborative learning experiences. A wide array of collaborative learning processes exist (communities of practice, learning collectives, self-organized learning environments, etc.). Any type of collaborative learning configuration leverages the power of coconstructed knowledge and social meaning making. Collective learning also provides opportunity to develop relational competence (for example, emotional intelligence, self-regulation, deep listening, improvisation, and authentic presence).

Figure 14-3 visually represents how the various ideas and perspectives on teaching and learning discussed in this chapter might come together. A brief description of the elements in the figure is as follows:

- Learning is not solely content driven, but content provides a context for learning both technical skills and relational skills. It is about learning to learn while learning how to be (in the profession).
- There are multiple sources of evidence and information (some are technology enabled, others are relational); for example, electronic databases, clinical applications, and texts that could be technology enabled. Peers, practitioners, patients, and teachers are also sources of knowledge (relational).

Figure 14-3 Learning in the knowledge era

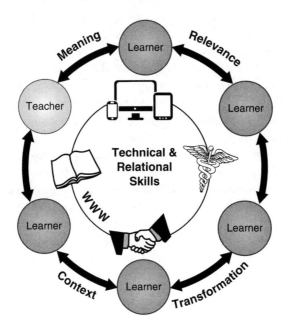

- Digital learning resources and technology are integrated into learning in a way that helps students understand how practitioners can (and do) use technology to solve real-world problems. Digital literacy and e-health literacy are integral to learning in the knowledge era.
- Student and peer knowledge contributes to learning. Peers learn from each other and cocreate new meaning together. The teacher's knowledge is not privileged as the only source. The teacher is a colearner and participates in the meaning-making process.
- Student-centered learning environments are context rich. Learning is situated in ways that make it relevant to the learner and to his or her future practice.
- Learning is collaborative and inherently relational. Meaning and knowledge are socially constructed. Participation in learning creates new patterns of meaning and patterns of relating that have the potential to transform both the individual and the system (we are the system).

Safe Learning Environments Celebrate Failure

Failure is an essential element of learning. However, students, educators, and practitioners typically view failure as negative and something to be avoided. We know that deep (enduring) learning occurs when we are active and engaged in doing learning. In passive education, there is no skin in the game, so to speak. There is less risk of failure, and there is also less learning. When we are engaged in trying, tinkering, and testing new ideas, of course there will be mistakes. Those mistakes are the source of learning! Through ongoing engaged involvement in the learning process, we begin to develop mastery. Chapter 11 focuses on failure as an essential component for innovation.

Mastery develops more quickly in an environment where active engagement is high, mistakes are recognized as part of the process of learning, and students receive just-in-time formative feedback about their learning. This feedback can come from multiple sources (especially in the knowledge era). For instance, a student's own self-reflection and self-awareness are powerful sources of feedback. Peer feedback is also critical and is readily available, especially in collaborative learning environments. Patients, preceptors, mentors, and teachers are also sources of feedback. One of the largest barriers to students tapping into the many sources of feedback and thus improving their learning is a mental construct that is often perpetuated from outdated learning paradigms. That is, the teacher (expert) is the only valid source of feedback. As previously noted, in the knowledge era this is simply not the case. However, many of us have been habituated into paying attention to the teacher (expert) and the hierarchical mindset that students are subservient to the all-knowing expert. This mindset causes us to tune out other useful and important sources of feedback that are literally everywhere.

Grades and assessment practices have also contributed to the prevalent fear of mistakes. In most grading structures, mistakes are punished with lower grades. In traditional educational models, the proxy measure for learning has been grades (based most often on summative, formal evaluations, such as exams). Summative measures alone do not provide feedback about performance until after the fact. Exams, high-stakes testing, and other forms of summative evaluation provide no opportunity to learn from mistakes or develop mastery. Summative evaluation provides only a snapshot of the current state of performance, knowledge, and mastery. These assessments are useful and necessary in certain instances (such as determining if a medical or nursing student has accumulated the requisite knowledge and skills to enter the profession). However, an overreliance and use of summative evaluation has contributed to a prevailing sense of fear and trepidation about both assessment processes and mistakes. This is manifested in a variety of different ways that all function to shut down learning and diminish performance. A classic example is test anxiety.

Emerging theories of cognition are revealing that the process of learning is not a logical and progressive sequence. Rather, learning consists of processes that are nonlinear, intuitive, and emotional. The brain does not separate emotion from cognition structurally or perceptually (Caine & Caine, 1991). In essence, the emotion of fear that is often related to evaluation processes and mistakes impedes our ability to access our higher-order thinking (reasoning, critical thinking, problem solving). The prevailing belief in education for many years has been that we were capable of getting over our emotions and bracketing them out of the learning equation. Brain and learning research is now showing that emotions are integrally important in learning. Just as negative emotions can have a detrimental impact on our learning, positive emotions associated with learning experiences can have a powerful positive influence.

Educators can integrate this new evidence about emotion and learning to create more conducive learning environments. Creating a sense of emotional safety in a learning environment can enhance a student's ability to access higher-order thinking and more fully engage in the act of learning. From a relational point of view, safe and welcoming environments also support the development of relationships and improve collaboration. Safe learning environments can replace the fear of making mistakes with curiosity and excitement about failures. As such, students remain engaged in the learning process and open to feedback that will move them toward mastery.

I have not failed. I've just found 10,000 ways that won't work.

—Thomas Edison

WHAT DOES EVIDENCE-BASED INNOVATION IN EDUCATION LOOK LIKE?

The potential for synergy between evidence-based practice and innovation in healthcare education is extremely promising. We have discussed at length (in the early part of the chapter) the dissatisfaction and dysfunctions and disconnects that make up the current healthcare education context. There is growing acknowledgement that we can no longer simply rearrange the deck chairs on the Titanic. We need to create new patterns of interaction and meaning, new ways of being, and new language that resonates with the current and emerging realities of 21st century health care.

It is very apropos to use the Titanic analogy here. When the Titanic sank in April 1912, it was state of the art and represented the highest achievement in engineering and design at the time. In many ways, our education system is like the Titanic: it was state of the art at the beginning of the 20th century! However, the education system did not meet with an icy adversary as the Titanic did. Instead, it has been lovingly cared for, maintained, and kept in working order for more than 100 years. Perhaps every decade or so, it has received a new coat of paint or its fixtures have been updated based on latest fashion. Educators have reconfigured an assessment here, or a learning strategy there. But, under all the embellishments, it is still a large boat with a steam-powered engine (linear, content-laden, behaviorist education). It is time to adopt a new mode of travel that is more representative of where we want to go.

The Futurist magazine publishes its annual outlook list in December each year. The list is a compilation of forecasts collected by the World Future Society. Of course, it is not intended to predict the future, but rather to provoke thought and inspire action for building a better future starting today. The 2015 outlook list included this statement: "teleportation is getting closer, photon by photon" (Scott, 2014, Innovation and Exploration section). Scott elaborated further:

Moving physical matter from one place to another has long been the impossible dream of science fiction, but physicist Juan Yin of the University of Science and Technology of China claims to have teleported entangled photons over a distance of about 60 miles. While vacationers should make more-traditional travel arrangements for the foreseeable future, teleportation technologies will advance over the next several decades. (2014, Innovation and Exploration section)

Figure 14-4   The mess of healthcare innovation

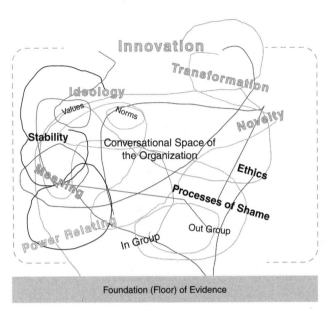

Imagine what we might accomplish in healthcare education if we were to adopt this metaphor to guide our way forward.

In this section I will present some ideas, issues, and opportunities for how the evidence-innovation dynamic can beam healthcare education into the future. To start with, let us revisit the relationship between evidence and innovation from a complex relational perspective. **Figure 14-4** is presented here as a reminder of the socially constructed meaning-making space that exists within our systems: the hurly-burly of organizational life. In the knowledge era, we have access to a wide range of sources of evidence (both formal and informal). In the knowledge era, evidence acts as the foundation upon which educational practices, policies, processes, and programs should be based. Just as in practice environments, there is always the danger of slipping back into habitual and unexamined practices on the grounds that we have always done it this way. It is in the conversational spaces of the organization (in this case, universities, colleges, programs, and classrooms) that meaning about and from evidence is made. The relational dynamics may result in adoption, adaptation, or even avoidance of evidence-based practices, depending on the ebb and flow of enabling and constraining patterns of meaning. Adaptation of evidence often occurs in several ways that can lead to innovation.

First, the foundational evidence may be partial or incomplete, or gaps may exist. For example, there may be compelling and high-quality evidence that suggests gamification is an effective learning strategy, but the population used in the research may not be second-year pharmacy students. Educators would then need to interpret and extrapolate what the utility of these research findings might have in their population of learners. Through conversations, educators might consider and deliberate about learner preferences and characteristics and local best practices, or they may engage experts to provide consultation. Suppose that the educators in this example decided to adapt the gamification learning strategy in ways they believe could best meet the needs of their students. In so doing, an educational innovation occurs. As the educators monitor the impact on student learning, satisfaction, and feasibility (cost, ease of use, etc.), local evidence is generated. From here, further cycles of innovation may occur to further tailor and fine-tune the educational intervention, or if the initial innovation was deemed successful, the educators may decide to publish an article sharing the intervention and associated outcomes. Thus, what was an innovation becomes evidence.

A second scenario for innovation may arise out of a void in the evidence. Perhaps the conversational space of the organization is filled with dissatisfaction with a current practice. For example, perhaps a traditional learning activity (such as lecture) is being used by educators who are charged with teaching pharmacotherapeutics to a class of 100 students. The educators have noted that students' achievement of learning outcomes (and probably satisfaction) is wanting. Perhaps the educators explore the literature and find that there is not strong evidence to suggest that lecture is an effective learning strategy. But what could they do with a large class that would be more effective? For this example, let us say that they are unable to find evidence that provides guidance for how to effectively teach pharmacotherapeutics to large classes of undergraduate nursing students. In other words, there is a void in the available evidence.

Instead of continuing to teach using a practice that is not evidence based (lecture), the group of faculty who team-teach this course might explore literature about adult learning and student-centered learning principles (theory). From this basis, they may use their innovation skills (such as design thinking, experience mapping, and prototyping) to develop an innovative teaching strategy that is founded on sound theory and student preferences and values. This might be a combination of using technology (social media) and student learning collectives, for example. Perhaps it takes several iterations of this teaching approach before improved outcomes are noticed. This is the ongoing process of tinkering (another innovation strategy). Eventually this teaching strategy may become a local best practice for teaching large classes in the nursing program and shared among faculty in the community of practice.

These two examples are just two of the infinite possibilities of how the evidence-innovation dynamic might be actualized from a complex relational perspective. **Figure 14-5** is an adaption of Melnyk and Fineout-Overholt's well known evidence-based practice framework (2005). I have adapted it to illustrate how these same considerations and contextual awareness can be applied in healthcare education. This is useful graphic organizer for educators seeking to engage in evidence-based education.

Figure 14-5   The merging of science and art: Evidence-based practice within an educational context

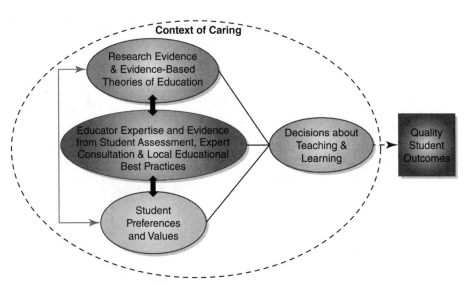

Modified from Melnyk, B. and Fineout-Overholt, E. (2005). *Evidence-based practice in nursing and healthcare*, p. 15. Philadelphia, PA: Lippincott, Williams & Wilkins.

STRENGTHENING THE PRACTICE–EDUCATION CONNECTION

Leaders who work with complex systems in today's world must develop a set of competencies to effect the changes they aspire to make. These competencies are: understanding the evidence–innovation–leadership dynamic, self-leadership, innovation capacity, communication and connection, and building momentum for change.

The development of such competencies is essential for leaders to strengthen the practice–education connection. Existing leaders in health care may undertake additional formal education (e.g., a master's or doctoral program) to develop these competencies. In doing so, they become enmeshed again in the education setting and can cross-pollinate their clinical perspectives and realities that will inform the development and refinement of formalized education programs that are more attuned to practice needs and realities. Of course, leaders in education systems need to develop these competencies as well. Education leaders who develop these competencies will be more attuned to the changing needs of the healthcare system and also build their capacity to begin to change the stagnant ivory tower thinking that is still prevalent in many institutions of higher education. Ideally, with a concerted focus on these competencies, we will create a relationship that no longer resembles two individual silos, but a

Figure 14-6 The education–practice dynamic in health care

© Chuhail/iStockphoto

relational structure that represents the practice education dynamic (**Figure 14-6**). In essence, there is integration, not separation. From a complex relational perspective, the individual and the social (larger organization) are one and the same. Similarly, education and practice are aspects of the same phenomena: health care.

It is not just leaders who need to support and live in the education–practice dynamic. Each of us, from whatever our vantage point in health care, needs to take up more integrative and connected ways of talking and relating. A critical opportunity to strengthen the practice–education dynamic can be found in changing how we relate to the next generation of healthcare educators. Currently, there is reason for much concern; there is a faculty shortage across many health disciplines, and academic careers seem less appealing in the eyes of potential new educators. How can we change this? Focusing on strengthening the practice–education dynamic may be the place to start. In short, if we view our organizations from this dynamic, rather than a siloed, perspective, it is a whole new game. Continuing to socialize incoming faculty into an outdated and overmatched academic culture serves only to put healthcare programs further behind. Even the most thorough, well-crafted new faculty orientation program and mentorship by the most seasoned faculty become counterproductive if they are based on our traditional, mechanistic ways of being. In this new era healthcare education, we are all novices in some way. In fact, our greatest hope for transformation within health care may lie with those we now call novices. New faculty who have

Table 14-2 Summary of the Current Shifts in Healthcare Education

From	Toward
Teacher centered	Learner centered
Knowledge as a commodity	Knowledge as an application
Lone learning	Collaborative learning
Decontextualized facts	Context-based application, solving real-life problems
Technical skills	Technical and relational skills
Silos	Rhizomes
Practice–education gap	Practice–education dynamic
Covering content	Learning to learn, navigationism, connectivism

current knowledge of clinical realities and existing relationships with practitioners could offer a wealth of insight and potential for the integration of healthcare practice and education (**Table 14-2**). We have much to learn from each to other (students, peers, leaders, patients, and colleagues). We need only to take the time to connect, listen, and talk with each other. Transformation may only be a conversation away.

New language can open up the experiential space and create opportunities for re-framing our day-to-day interactions in healthcare education. Bolman and Deal provided a poignant reminder of the value of reframing: "For those with better theories and the capacity to use them with skill and grace, it is a world of excitement and pos-sibility. A mess can be defined as both a troublesome situation and a group of people who eat together" (2003, p. 40). It is my greatest hope that through ongoing collabora-tive dialogue and cultivation of relational practices, healthcare education will look and feel more like the latter.

REFERENCES

Aiken, L. H., Clarke, S. P., Sloane, D. M., Sochalski J. A., Busse, R., Clarke, H., . . . Shamian, J. (2001). Nurses' reports on hospital care in five countries. *Health Affairs, 20*(3), 43–53. doi:10.1377/hlthaff.20.3.43

American Association of Colleges of Nursing. (2006, June). *Nursing faculty shortage fact sheet.* Washington, DC: Author. Retrieved from www.aacn.nche.edu/Publications/issues/IB499WB.htm

Association of Academic Health Centers. (2008). *Out of order, out of time: The state of the nation's health workforce.* Washington, DC: Author.

Association of Academic Health Centers. (2013). *A call to action. Out of order, out of time: The state of the nation's health workforce 2013.* Washington, DC: Author.

Benner, P., Sutphen, M., Leonard, V., & Day, L. (2010). *Educating nurses: A call for radical transformation.* Stanford, CA: Jossey-Bass.

Berrett, D. (2013). Teaching clearly can be a deceptively simple way to improve learning. *The Chronicle of Higher Education,* 1–4, November 22, 2013 (online version). Retrieved from http://chronicle.com/article/Teaching-Clearly-a/143209

Bevis, E. O., & Watson, J. (1989). *Toward a caring curriculum: A new pedagogy for nursing.* New York, NY: National League for Nursing.

Bolman, L. G., & Deal, T. E. (2003). *Reframing organizations: Artistry, choice and leadership.* San Francisco, CA: Jossey-Bass.

Brown, T. H. (2005). Beyond constructivism: Exploring future learning paradigms. *Education Today, 2,* 1–11.

Brown, T. H. (2006). Beyond constructivism: Navigationism in the knowledge era. *On the Horizon, 14*(3), 108–120.

Caine, R. N., & Caine, G. (1991). *Making connections: Teaching and the human brain.* Alexandria, VA: ASCD Press.

Cormier, D. (2008). Rhizomatic education: Community as curriculum. *Innovate, 4*(5). Retrieved from http://nsuworks.nova.edu/cgi/viewcontent.cgi?article=1045&context=innovate

Finkel, D. L. (2000). *Teach with your mouth shut.* Portsmouth, NH: Boyton/Cook.

Gergen, K. J. (2009). *Relational being: Beyond self and community.* New York, NY: Oxford Press.

Institute of Medicine. (2001). *Crossing the quality chasm: A new health system for the 21st century.* Washington, DC: National Academies Press.

Institute of Medicine. (2011). *The future of nursing: Leading change, advancing health.* Washington, DC: National Academies Press.

Interprofessional Education Collaborative Expert Panel. (2011). *Core competencies for interprofessional collaborative practice: Report of an expert panel.* Washington, DC: Author.

Melnyk, B., & Fineout-Overholt, E. (2005). *Evidence-based practice in nursing and healthcare.* Philadelphia, PA: Lippincott, Williams & Wilkins.

Midwest Pharmacy Workforce Research Consortium. (2015, April 8). *Final report of the 2014 national sample survey of the pharmacist workforce to determine contemporary demographic and practice characteristics and quality of work-life.* Minneapolis, MN: Author. Retrieved from http://www.aacp.org/resources/research/pharmacyworkforcecenter/Documents/FinalReportOfTheNationalPharmacistWorkforceStudy2014.pdf

Norman, C. D., & Skinner, H. A. (2006). E-health literacy: Essential skills for consumer health in a networked world. *Journal of Medical Internet Research, 8*(2), e9.

Palmer, P. J. (1998). *The courage to teach.* San Francisco, CA: Jossey-Bass.

Palmer, P. J. (2007). A new professional: The aims of education revisited. *Change: The Magazine of Higher Learning,* (November/December). Retrieved from http://www.changemag.org/archives/back%20issues/november-december%202007/full-new-professional.html

Pringle, D., Green, L., & Johnson, S. (2004). *Nursing education in Canada: Historical review and current capacity.* Ottawa, Canada: Nursing Sector Study Corporation.

Scharmer, C. O. (2007). *Theory U: Leading from the future as it emerges.* Cambridge, MA: Society for Organizational Learning.

Scott, G. (2014). Outlook 2015. *The Futurist, 48*(6). Retrieved from http://www.wfs.org/futurist/2014-issues-futurist/november-december-2014-vol-48-no-6/outlook-2015

Siemens, G. (2005). Connectivism: A learning theory of the digital age. *International Journal of Instructional Technology and Distance Learning, 2*(1). Retrieved from http://www.itdl.org/Journal/Jan_05/article01.htm

Slattery, P. (2013). *Curriculum development in the postmodern era: Teaching and learning in the age of accountability.* New York, NY: Routledge.

Stacey, R. D. (2001). *Complex responsive processes in organizations: Learning and knowledge creation.* London, UK: Routledge.

Tresolini, C.P., & Pew-Fetzer Task Force. (1994). *Health professions education and relationship-centered care*. San Francisco, CA: Pew Health Professions Commission. Retrieved from http://www.rccswmi.org/uploads/PewFetzerRCCreport.pdf

Tucker, P. (2008, December). Forecast #6: Professional knowledge will become obsolete almost as quickly as it's acquired. *The Futurist*. Retrieved from http://blogs.britannica.com/2008/12/forecast-6-professional-knowledge-increasingly-obsolete

Valiga, T. M. (2002, April 11). *The nursing faculty shortage: National League for Nursing perspective*. Retrieved from http://www.nln.org/research/facultyshortage.html

Visser, M. (2012). Digital literacy definition. Retrieved from http://connect.ala.org/node/181197

Weimer, M. (2013). *Learner-centered teaching: Five key changes to practice* (2nd ed.). San Francisco, CA: Jossey Bass.

World Health Organization. (2010). *Framework for action on interprofessional education & collaborative practice*. Geneva, Switzerland: Author. Retrieved from http://www.who.int/hrh/resources/framework_action/en/

Building Diverse Partnerships in Health Care and Industry: How Organizations Must Partner to Build Disruptive Futures

Denise Duncan, Joshua Rutkoff, and Jerry E. Spicer

CHAPTER OBJECTIVES

Upon completion of this chapter, the reader will be able to:

1. Describe the nature of successful labor and management partnership behaviors in healthcare organizations.
2. Define the three paradoxes of labor–management innovation.
3. Discuss examples of innovative partnerships and how they inform healthcare change.

Health care in the United States is going through a period of great change, much of it driven by the multiyear rollout of the Patient Protection and Affordable Care Act (PPACA) and its mandates for who and under what structure individuals will be covered by health insurance. The authors of this chapter are perhaps uniquely situated to forecast the challenges this period of change will present to the U.S. healthcare industry and to recommend strategies for meeting those challenges; they are veterans of the trailblazing labor–management partnership between Kaiser Permanente and the Coalition of Kaiser Permanente Unions, itself a partnership composed of 27 union locals representing 105,000 employees—80% of Kaiser Permanente's unionized workforce. The partnership was born as a response to financial difficulties faced by Kaiser Permanente during the 1990s, which drove innovation in improving the quality of care while simultaneously cutting costs. As Kaiser Permanente has grown in physical facilities and lives covered, and its quality ratings have risen, it has arguably been seen as a model for the more integrated systems of healthcare delivery anticipated to be the likely adaptations that the U.S. healthcare industry will need to make to meet the PPACA's mandates on cost and quality. The partnership was at the heart of the changes in Kaiser Permanente, and it has been well studied within academia. The authors come from each side of the partnership—Kaiser Permanente management and union leadership—and have been intimately involved in its origin, growing pains, and successes.

Additionally, this chapter will review the challenges facing the healthcare industry and labor movement, respectively, the paradoxes that must be engaged to innovate, and several of the notable innovations accomplished by the Labor/Management Partnership (LMP).

CURRENT STATE OF THE HEALTHCARE INDUSTRY AND LABOR UNIONS

Healthcare Industry: Current Challenges and Misconceptions

On March 23, 2010, President Barack Obama signed the PPACA into law. The intended outcome of the legislation is to provide mechanisms through which uninsured individuals in the United States can secure access to healthcare insurance. It is the most significant expansion of U.S. healthcare since the advent of Medicare in the 1960s. In April 2014, the Congressional Budget Office (CBO) and the Joint Committee on Taxation (JCT) estimated that the PPACA will reduce the number of individuals without insurance by 26 million by 2024 (Congressional Budget Office, 2014). This is a dramatic change. Before the advent of the PPACA, it was estimated that more than 46 million Americans did not have basic health coverage. Because of these numbers, the law represents a significant capacity challenge to healthcare organizations across the country, potentially stressing an infrastructure that already faces issues with overcrowded emergency departments and lack of a truly integrated healthcare delivery model. Hospitals and health systems must do their best to provide high-quality and safe patient care in an environment of declining reimbursement and rising costs. Kaufman (2011) estimated that as a result of the PPACA, most healthcare systems will be required to reduce their current cost structures by 10–15%. Specifically, Medicare payments to hospitals will be reduced under PPACA if they are unable to reduce their readmission rates for selected high-cost ailments; experience avoidable hospital conditions, such as patient falls with injury or nosocomial infections; or find themselves in the top quartile of facilities with defined avoidable hospital-acquired conditions. Such PPACA mandates regarding quality will compel hospitals to focus their attention on the most costly areas of traditional inpatient stays and identify ways to provide high-quality care at lower costs.

Although the benefits of the PPACA landmark legislation could impact millions of uninsured Americans, the responsibility for ensuring the continued viability of today's healthcare institutions rests with its leadership and diverse partnerships with nontraditional organizations such as labor unions. Even before the advent of the PPACA, Morrison (2000) suggested that the lack of effective leadership is the largest issue facing healthcare organizations in the new millennium. Effective and competent leadership and diverse partnerships are essential to overcoming the challenges presented by healthcare reform and the PPACA.

It is perhaps worth noting that although the PPACA does contain mandates on healthcare quality, its mechanism for driving quality improvements is largely through reforms in the structure of payment for care—what gets paid for and how. For instance, if a hospital's patients suffer from pressure ulcers—a symptom of poor-quality care, because patients with pressure ulcers have in general not been well-enough attended by the staff who are charged with checking on them and moving them frequently—that hospital will not receive reimbursement from the Centers for Medicare and Medicare Services (CMS) for the care of that condition. If a patient acquires pneumonia while in the hospital, the hospital—not the patient's insurer or own finances—must pay for the resulting treatment of pneumonia. These reimbursement changes shift the financial and quality model of health care from volume and fee-for-service to a more value- and outcomes-based reimbursement model. The shift from volume to value is a significant one because it requires new ways of partnering among providers, insurers, hospitals, and communities to achieve significantly better and more affordable care outcomes. The PPACA has been structured to push more payment toward proactive and integrated care models to encourage the U.S. healthcare industry to evolve toward a focus on wellness and prevention rather than on sickness and cure. Reforms in care quality, including scientific advances, are anticipated to be a by-product of payment reform and the pressures on the system from the expected influx of newly insured people, as well as to be self-reinforcing as the law and its effects continue to roll out. Regardless of any new legislation that might overturn the specific mandates of the PPACA, the healthcare industry has begun the shift to value-based care. To meet the new pressures of affordability, quality, and population health, organizations must work together, in partnership, to innovate solutions for the industry. This affords management and labor new opportunities to develop collaborative relationships; some would argue that it requires interdependency. Without this, it will be impossible for either entity to be successful in navigating the new reality of healthcare reform.

Labor: Current Challenges and Innovation

Today's context for considerations of partnership and innovation as trade union strategies is highly dynamic and complex. The challenges are stark: unions represent just 6.7% of workers in the private sector (Henwood, 2015), down from a peak of about 35% in the mid-1950s. Throughout the 20th century, unions engaged in collective

bargaining with employers to negotiate and improve wages, hours, and working conditions for their members. For decades this model proved successful, allowing unions
to create good jobs and standards of living for their members. Today, with union
membership at its lowest level since the Great Depression, "traditional collective bargaining has all but vanished from the economic landscape—taking raises, benefits,
job security and much of the American middle class with it as it goes" (Meyerson,
2013). Although unions represent 35.7% of public sector workers, recent attacks from
political opponents have rolled back public sector union rights in traditional union
strongholds such as Wisconsin and Michigan. In its 2014 ruling on *Harris v. Quinn*,
the Supreme Court decided that home care workers do not have to pay any fees to
the unions representing them, stripping them of rights enjoyed by other public sector
workers (Greenhouse, 2014). Not just within the healthcare industry, employers (both
unionized and nonunion) do not typically look to unions as drivers of innovation; in
fact, they too often characterize them as obstacles to change. The economic backdrop
for this set of challenges is profound income inequality and wage stagnation, characterized by a growing economy in which working people are not reaping financial rewards for the productivity gains they are helping to achieve for the organizations they
work for. Couple these macro-economic trends with the attendant loss of collective
voice, security and respect that unions help create at work, and the results resemble
the broader conditions in which the kind of workplace speak-up culture required for
creating innovation is suppressed. Detert and Edmondson (2007) describe how in
environments in which workers are forced to focus on their own self-preservation,
"we found the innate protective instinct so powerful that it also inhibited speech that
clearly would have been intended to help the organization." This is one dynamic that
places a divide in how organizations and workers partner to create novel solutions and
can specifically impact how well healthcare organizations can adapt to the changing
environment of quality and cost.

At the same time, in the context of the environment previously described, the labor movement has responded with a willingness to experiment with a broad and vibrant array of revitalization strategies. Labor is embracing innovation and adapting
to current challenges through novel operating structures. Worker centers, such as the
Restaurant Opportunities Center, the National Domestic Workers Alliance, and the
National Guest Worker Alliance, do not yet engage in collective bargaining, but they
nevertheless advocate for and give voice to workers in various industries, including
winning economic judgments for workers from employers. Unions are also leading
broad-based, long-term campaigns to raise standards of living for low-wage workers.
The Fight for 15, which calls for a wage of $15 per hour and the right to form a union, is
mobilizing workers, often through strikes, in industries including fast food, warehous-
ing and logistics, and home care. Strikes (legally protected actions in which workers

withhold their labor) were an integral part of how the labor movement grew strong in the middle of the 20th century in the face of massive, and sometimes violent, resistance from U.S. industry. Geoghegan (2014) describes a major distinction between the often open-ended, lengthy strikes that helped shape industries such as auto, steel, and mining and today's quick and broadly distributed actions targeted at the low-wage service sector. The latter "did nothing to move McDonalds. But these losses put the issue at the top of Obama's 2014 State of the Union address" (2014, p. 37). And unions have helped lead coalitions that won new $15 per hour minimum wage laws in cities including Seattle, San Francisco, and Los Angeles, which will apply not just to union workers, but also to the community at large.

David Rolf, president of Service Employees International Union (SEIU) Local 775, is explicit about the imperative for organized labor to embrace innovation:

Progressives should take a cue from business and enter an era of innovation, leveraging labor's significant institutional resources to create organizations dedicated to studying the future of organizing and work . . . By striking out into complexity instead of retreating back to what is familiar, progressives can seize this moment of crisis and win enormous victories for workers. However, labor and its allies must be willing to experiment with new models outside traditional collective bargaining, even outside the traditional idea of a union. (2014, para. 7, 13)

The labor and management relationship in health care has had some history of adversarial encounters. Nursing and other healthcare worker strikes or work stoppages have created some polarizing opinions from healthcare professionals, organizations, and patients questioning the intent and operations of organizations and the represented workforce. Traditionally, both labor and management have relied on primarily linear leadership practices that focused on singular interests, like pay, benefits, and work hours, and tried to achieve them by inaction (stalled negotiations, refusal to discuss issues, and inflexibility) or overaction (reductions in negotiated benefits, command-and-control management, work stoppages, and negative ad campaigns). Many situations do not yet possess the conditions for exceeding this traditional zero-sum, adversarial approach. Such an approach, although it may produce short-term gains for either party, may have inherent limitations in the context of the cost and efficiency pressures described by Berwick (2011) in his speech to the Institute for Healthcare Improvement:

Our nation is at a crossroad. The care we have simply cannot be sustained. It will not work for health care to chew ever more deeply into our common purse. If it does, our schools will fail, our roads will fail, our competitiveness will fail. Wages will continue to lag, and, paradoxically, so will our health.

The choice is stark: chop or improve. If we permit chopping, I assure you that the chopping block will get very full—first with cuts to the most voiceless and poorest us, but soon after to more and more of us. Fewer health insurance benefits, declining access, more out-of-pocket burdens, and growing delays. If we don't improve, the cynics win. That's what passes the buck to us. If improvement is the plan, then we own the plan. Government can't do it. Payers can't do it. Regulators can't do it. Only the people who give the care can improve the care.[1]

Therefore, we argue that when and where the right conditions exist, innovative partnerships and more evidence-based, interest-based, and innovative leadership practices will result in a better healthcare system where workers, organizations, and patients benefit from better quality, cost, and care.

In this context of a spectrum of experimental strategies for organized labor, the labor–management partnership at Kaiser Permanente provides an intriguing model of what is achievable through collaboration focused on shared improvement and innovation goals, as well as an example of how unions and employers can, under the right conditions, exceed rather than discard traditional collective bargaining in the pursuit of common interests.

HEALTHCARE INDUSTRY: INNOVATION

U.S. health care and labor intersect in an unpredictable and dynamic environment, including patients, payers, providers, suppliers, and each other. These intersections provide a focused lens to examine how evidence-based innovation can occur when tension, environmental factors, and complex connections are acknowledged and leveraged for success. Given the scarcity of resources and a global economy that is far from

---

[1] Berwick, D. (2011, December 7). The Moral Test. Speech to IHI National Forum. Retrieved from http://www.ahier.net/2011/12/remember-patient.html?m=1

stable, health care and labor separately and together face significant challenges driving a need to innovate. For management and labor, traditionally engaged in an adversarial relationship, coming together in partnership to tackle shared challenges could be seen as a kind of top-level, disruptive innovation from which a cascading series of innovations can follow to most effectively respond to such challenges.

To discuss diverse partnerships that drive innovation we must have a common definition of healthcare innovation. Thakur, Hsu, and Fontenot defined healthcare innovation as the

> *adoption of those best-demonstrated practices that have been proven successful and implementation of those practices while ensuring the safety and best outcomes for patients and whose adoption might also affect the performance of the organization. In other words, innovation in health care is defined as those changes that help healthcare practitioners focus on the patient while helping healthcare practitioners work smarter, faster, better, and more cost effectively. (2012, p. 564)*

Healthcare innovation can take many forms, and although it is widely perceived and accepted to be a positive outcome, it carries a number of trade-offs and paradoxes. These trade-offs and paradoxes are best addressed by partnerships between groups that can coadapt to the unpredictable environment.

Innovation does not necessarily follow a logical and sequenced series of well-rationalized steps. It is important for leaders to recognize this and work to identify new approaches in the identification, adoption, and spread of innovation in health care. Dixon-Woods and colleagues (2011) identified three paradoxes that innovators in health care specifically are likely to encounter (**Box 15-1**).

Box 15-1 Paradoxes of Innovation in Health Care

Paradox 1: Uptake of the dubious, rejection of the good; adoption without evidence
Paradox 2: The wisdom and failings of democracy; stopping innovation through collaboration
Paradox 3: Health systems are never able to keep up; change as a barrier to change

Data from Dixon-Woods, M., et al. (2011). Problems and promises of innovation: Why healthcare needs to rethink its love/hate relationship with the new. *BMJ Quality & Safety, 20*(Suppl 1), i47–i51.

Paradox 1: Adoption without Evidence

Paradox 1 addresses the phenomenon of why some new practices are quickly adopted and spread, even though there is little or no empirical evidence that the practice is effective, or even safe, while other practices from which patients could benefit are never adopted, let alone spread. There are a number of reasons why this may occur. The innovation may simply be the latest fad—that must-have practice or product that is so new that no evidence yet exists to support or refute it. This can often be the case with technology; new technologies experience increased hype as they enter the market, but they may not perform as expected while adoption increases. Adopters and resisters demonstrate several behaviors as new practices are introduced into the environment. Sometimes adopters defend their decision to adopt by pointing out that the innovation is better than doing nothing. Or perhaps the innovation does offer some modicum of face validity or intuitive appeal as a possible solution to the problem, so adoption provides a degree of defense against the accusation of doing nothing. The risk of action without evidence can sometimes work in opposition to the values of healthcare workers, such as do no harm.

Each of these reasons for succumbing to paradox 1 poses the risk that an organization will adopt processes or products that have yet to be fully vetted for efficiency or effectiveness. Conversely, innovation under paradox 1 could result in a failure to spread practices that have been proven effective. As a result, there is potential risk to the organization, its staff, physicians, and, most importantly, the patient. At the very minimum, an innovation under this paradox could result in the disruption or displacement of other beneficial efforts. With paradox 1, innovation crowds out others fighting for a place in a landscape of limited resources, both human and capital. An unproven and hastily implemented solution can crowd out a proven, or even yet-to-be proven, but better solution.

Paradox 2: Stopping Innovation through Collaboration

Paradox 2 speaks to innovation through collaboration. Dixon-Woods and colleagues (2011) assert that although collaborating with other professionals may be an effective way of ensuring implementation and spread of an innovation, it may also be one of the most effective ways of stopping it.

The benefits of actively involving those individuals most likely to be affected by the proposed innovation and who are the most knowledgeable about the situation that the planned innovation is designed to address are apparent, including better-informed decisions and greater collective buy-in to the implementation. Actively involving subject matter experts also increases the identification of further opportunities for innovation. This social movement approach and the role of self-organizing and self-governing networks is gaining popularity in numerous settings and is gaining momentum particularly within the healthcare setting. It promotes the self-management of change, and it works well when the problems being addressed are well-known to the organization and individuals involved. In the healthcare industry, where one is attempting to change the practice of professionals, this social movement approach works well. Professionals are educated and prepared to manage their own clinical practices, which can create a negative reaction to being required to do new practices that do not originate from the individual professional. To overcome the potential resistance of dictating innovation through a hierarchy, leaders can use the social movement approach because the individuals designing and implementing the innovation are the same as those who will have to use the innovation.

Although there are many advantages to the social movement approach, it also presents its share of threats to successful innovation. Group-based, collaborative efforts like this can be and are often undermined from within the group. One of the most common innovation-stopping issues the social movement approach creates is the failure to engage stakeholders in the change process. Another threat occurs when an individual attempts to substitute his or her own agenda for the greater good of the organization and those it serves. Thus, it is critical that the innovation process be as transparent and inclusive as possible. Transparency and inclusiveness can serve to isolate and marginalize an individual who is obstructing the will of the group. Although a social movement approach to innovation in health care has been shown to be particularly successful when engaging professionals like nurses and technicians, professional boundaries and scope of practice law can be another source of contention and possible derailment.

Paradox 3: Change as a Barrier to Change

Paradox 3 is rooted in the fact that improvement requires change, and change will always create its own set of challenges. Quality improvement systems are notoriously unable to keep up with the pace of innovation. By its nature, innovation is a disruptive activity, and by the time quality improvement catches up with the innovation, things have usually changed—again. Failures in the evaluation process can only intensify this problem. The evaluation process is often too narrowly focused on a specific intervention while failing to capture the systemic effects and unintended consequences of the innovation.

The Paradoxes in Summary

In this section we examined the challenges associated with innovation in today's complex and volatile healthcare environment. Dixon-Woods and colleagues (2011) identified three paradoxes—the problems and promises—of innovation. Paradox 1 is innovation for the sake of innovating. In some cases, the innovation that is promoted and adopted is without empirical evidence that it will achieve what it seeks to accomplish. Perhaps the innovation is accepted out of pure desperation or simply to do something, which is believed to be better than doing nothing. Innovation linked to paradox 1 potentially places the entire organization, its patients, and its staff at risk by either producing direct harm or by crowding out alternative, more beneficial innovation.

Paradox 2 considers innovation though collaboration. While the authors contend that this form of innovation may result in better outcomes as the result of active involvement of subject matter experts promoting a motivation for the spread and adoption of the innovation as the result of social mechanisms, it too has problems. Innovation under paradox 2 may result in the undermining of the innovation if the members of the collaborative fail to engage or they substitute their own agendas for the innovation, thereby effectively derailing constructive and meaningful change.

The final paradox cited by the authors considers innovation as disruptive change. Innovation and improvement *is* change. The issue, however, is that the normal quality improvement processes central to the healthcare industry are always lagging the innovation. By the time the quality improvement processes catch up to the innovation, new change has occurred, and the quality improvement cycle must start all over. **Box 15-2** outlines the considerations that should be considered to proactively address these issues.

Box 15-2 Innovation in Health Care: An Agenda for Action

- Assess innovation risk and reward for all innovation activities.
- Develop processes for assessing innovation and technology value to the organization.
- Evaluate innovation in real-time including how the innovation is impacting outcomes.
- Use social science to evaluate pilots as the innovation test of change is in progress. Focus on what resources might be needed to implement the innovation in a production environment.
- Clearly define the roles involved in innovation work and use formal leadership structures to facilitate and manage frontline workers, patients, and other stakeholders in the process.
- Identify unintended impacts of innovation by using a variety of research methods, including clinical trial methods, before spreading innovation across an organization.
- Develop innovation competencies through education, training, and experience to help overcome the barriers to change.

Adapted from Dixon-Woods, M., et al. (2011). Problems and promises of innovation: Why healthcare needs to rethink its love/hate relationship with the new. *BMJ Quality & Safety, 20*(Suppl 1), i47–i51.

EVIDENCE-BASED PARTNERSHIPS IN INNOVATION: THE KAISER PERMANENTE EXAMPLE

The partnership between Kaiser Permanente and the Coalition of Kaiser Permanente Unions (the Coalition), started in 1997, has established itself as the longest-lasting and most successful labor–management partnership in the United States. This comprehensive partnership, which is defined in the national agreement between the parties as a strategy for operational collaboration at every level, has built a track record of success in performance improvement. It provides a number of different mechanisms and processes for interaction between labor and management at every level of the organization—national and regional down to the local facility levels—and each provides for extensive engagement and decisions made by consensus.

Hal Ruddick, the executive director of the Coalition, positions the partnership in the context of a trade union legacy of advocating expanded access to health care:

Our partnership is about providing the best care and quality. In that way, it's in the tradition of the historic mission of the American labor movement, which includes ensuring quality, affordable health care for working families. We are able to do that without sacrificing good jobs with good pay and benefits. Many other affordability strategies sacrifice either quality or good jobs, or both. Our strategy is based on high-quality care, good jobs and affordability. (H. Ruddick, personal communication, June 2, 2015)

In his remarks to the Coalition's annual Union Delegates Conference in 2015, Chokri Bensaid, the Kaiser division director from the Coalition's largest local union, SEIU United Healthcare Workers West, characterized the partnership as creating tripartite benefits that go far beyond the immediate self-interest of union members:

When we do things like bargain the best benefits in the country, we don't just do right by our members. We set the bar in our communities. We set the bar in our industry.

> *The Kaiser contract is the contract every healthcare worker*
> *aspires to have. And every time you improve that, you inject*
> *a little bit of hope in the lives of those working people who*
> *aspire to have the same contract . . . We're dealing with*
> *waste, we're dealing with improvement of workflow, we're*
> *dealing with creative ways of delivering care and being more*
> *personal to our patients, and when you cut waste out of the*
> *system, the company wins, we win, and the patients win.*
> *(Bensaid, 2015)*

At the facility level, where the care meets the patient, Unit-Based Teams (UBTs) are groups of frontline workers, managers, and physicians in a given natural work department (such as a medical–surgical unit, pharmacy, or environmental services department) who work together on improvement projects. Using the Rapid Improvement Model (RIM), UBTs identify issues in their departments, review data together, and develop goals for improvement. This process of continuously generating and evaluating data helps avoid the pitfalls of paradox 1, adoption of an innovation without evidence, because the evidence for or against a given innovation arises nearly in real time.

The UBT goals are informed by the core values of the partnership, which are working together with a focus on the patient or member to achieve the best quality and service, and to make Kaiser Permanente both the most affordable care provider and the best place to work. In the decade since UBTs were first negotiated and implemented, Kaiser Permanente has grown into an industry leader in quality and service. At the same time, the industry-best wages, benefits, and working conditions bargained by the Coalition and enabled by this partnership serve as an example to other unions and employers as a potential standard and even a counterexample to the cuts and reductions characterizing much of the rest of the national collective bargaining environment.

The most thorough history of the first decade of this partnership is provided by Kochan, Eaton, McKersie, and Adler in *Healing Together* (2009). The authors describe the traditional collective bargaining relationship between labor and management, according to federal law through the National Labor Relations Act, as by definition adversarial, with "a clear line of demarcation" (2009, p. 22) between management's rights to run an organization and labor's rights to bargain over the impact of changes to hours, wages, and working conditions. "Such efforts are restrained by twentieth-century thinking about how work is organized, organizations are structured, and goods and services are produced and delivered" (2009, p. 23). In contrast, the partnership at Kaiser Permanente reflects more current thinking:

Rather than dividing people into management and labor camps, contemporary models of work organization stress teamwork among people who bring different, specialized knowledge to bear at tasks at hand. That is the potential creativity that labor–management partnerships in general and the KP [Kaiser Permanente] Labor–Management Partnership in particular, seek to mobilize. (2009, p. 23)

With a foundation of approximately 3,500 UBTs covering virtually every department in Kaiser Permanente that employs members of the Coalition, this partnership has built a solid foundation based on improving established work processes. At the same time, it provides intriguing examples and opportunities for how such a collaborative strategy can be leveraged to implement more extensive innovation as well.

A review of the literature reveals both evidence of the efficacy of the labor–management partnership at Kaiser Permanente and examples of the ways that other healthcare unions and their employers have charted their own courses to collaborate to achieve shared interests. These examples show a growing critical mass of experience and proficiency in partnering around performance improvement and glimmers of what might be possible with increased focus on similar efforts to collaborate on innovation.

Adler and Heckscher (2013) situated Kaiser Permanente in the context of the challenges of organizations operating in complex environments to perform both in terms of innovation or flexibility and efficiency or control. This tension describes well the dynamics that healthcare organizations face. The authors characterize high performance in both domains as *ambidexterity*: "the ability simultaneously to exploit existing capabilities and to explore new opportunities" (2013, p. 35). Organizations dealing with complexity that are not able to develop an integrated approach to this dynamic are likely to be mired in mediocrity. According to Adler and Heckscher, ambidextrous organizations synthesize mechanistic and organic approaches through a collaborative model, a form that

is not only a better mix, but also outperforms one-dimensional organizations at their own games. That is, an effective collaborative system is better at efficiency than a bureaucracy, because it engages members in continuous improvement and problem-solving; and it is better at innovation than a market or decentralized bureaucracy, because it coordinates knowledge more effectively across a wider scope. (2013. p. 43)

In their case study of Kaiser Permanente, Adler and Heckscher cite the labor–management partnership as one example of how the company has met its ambidexterity challenges, supporting the implementation of both management-driven initiatives and frontline improvement ideas, along with the spread of lessons and best practices (2013, p. 45). Kaiser Permanente has achieved "dramatic improvements both in exploration and exploitation dimensions" (2013, p. 47), performing at the top of the industry in core outcome measures and having developed "an impressive capacity for radical innovation" (2013, p. 47).

In a separate study, Lazes, Katz, Figueroa, and Karpur (2012b) observed the labor–management partnership between Montefiore Medical Center and 1199 SEIU in the Bronx, New York, finding a similar interplay between disruptive innovation and adaptive change. Disruptive innovation "enables organizations to create new systems of care, products, or services" (2012b, p. 150), whereas adaptive change "is based on incremental changes that optimize current processes or services by improving efficiencies and eliminating waste. The use of the adaptive change approach can be instrumental in standardizing new processes and procedures that were initially created by a disruptive change approach" (2012b, p. 150).

The study focuses on Montefiore as an example of an organization that, in its efforts to become a more fully and deeply integrated care delivery system, is pursuing both disruptive and adaptive change models. The strategy is based partly on increasing prevention and care management efforts to reduce costly hospitalizations—like the labor–management partnership at Kaiser Permanente, perhaps showing a way forward for the entire U.S. healthcare industry as it struggles to adapt to the mandates of the PPACA. Critical to the strategy's success at Montefiore's Contact Centers has been a "comprehensive labor–management partnership to help design and implement new work systems to provide not only a positive customer service experience for patients and providers, but an exceptional work environment for staff as well" (Lazes et al., 2012b, p. 160).

This capacity to absorb and balance both disruptive innovation and adaptive change through the flexibility of its collaborative processes is how the LMP at Kaiser seems to have largely avoided the pitfalls of paradox 3. Labor and management collaborate at every level of the organization, from top leadership down to the unit level and back up through the hierarchy, with information flowing freely not only upward and downward, but laterally. The RIM used by the UBTs allows the most disruptive innovations to be incorporated in the most intimate ways into the basic everyday tasks involved in direct patient care. RIM and UBTs render ideas of change from abstract concepts to concrete procedures and are able to make the necessary adjustments, or adaptive changes, at that level.

Nixon's study of UBTs at Kaiser Permanente (2012) demonstrates the correlation among staff engagement, team performance, and team development. Kaiser Permanente measures staff engagement through an internal survey called People Pulse. With its database of UBTs, called UBT Tracker, which documents teams' activities and accomplishments, Kaiser Permanente can analyze both team performance on operational goals and team development as measured by an internal rubric called the Path to Performance. The study revealed the link between team development (ranked on a five-point scale ranging from foundational to high performing) and a dozen measures of staff engagement, including perceptions of how a department operates effectively as a team and staff understanding of how their jobs contribute to organizational goals. The data demonstrates the connection between staff engagement and performance on key operational metrics. For instance, staff perceptions of more efficient work procedures in their departments correlate to lower hospital mortality rates and greater patient satisfaction with the hospital experience. Similarly, higher levels of comfort among staff in raising ethical concerns to their managers link to significantly lower staff injury rates. The study makes a compelling case that investment in supporting and nurturing UBTs can drive changes in workplace culture that can lead to improved performance.

Lazes, Katz, and Figueroa (2012a) looked at both Kaiser Permanente and other healthcare systems as evidence of how labor–management partnerships can produce improved clinical outcomes, better work environments, and cost savings. They concluded, "the involvement of healthcare unions, including both leaders and members, in restructuring initiatives affecting the entire delivery system yields concrete clinical improvements. Further, such improvements are directly linked to increased involvement of front-line healthcare workers in the process" (2012a, p. 5). Here, too, we see evidence of improved operational performance through partnership and hints of what might be possible with an increased focus on partnering for innovation. The authors examined a number of UBTs at two Kaiser Permanente medical centers: San Rafael and San Diego. For example, in its broader efforts to improve workplace safety and reduce injury rates, the San Rafael Clinical Lab Scientist (CLS) UBT tackled lab design. The CLS UBT "has harnessed the insight of its staff members to transform a department into a safe and efficient workplace designed by its staff, for its staff" (2012a, p. 16). The authors observed that the two unions at Kaiser Permanente San Rafael, through their work with UBTs, "have become more engaged in discussions around remodeling and have taken an active interest in technology issues" (2012a, p. 18).

At Kaiser Permanente San Diego, the Emergency Department UBT developed and implemented a system for team communication to support adoption of a new technology: "Using a communication tree and a training tracking system to support their work, the team increased the percent of staff that had access to and were trained in iNotes from 10 percent to 94 percent from May to July 2010" (Lazes et al., 2012a, p. 28). Finally, the characterization of labor–management partnership at Kaiser Permanente San Diego describes some of the conditions that are necessary for enabling not just joint performance improvement, but collaboration to innovate as well: "UBT work has enabled employees to access and understand key financial and operations data, allowing for a more engaged and effective workforce" (2012a, p. 29).

Looking again at examples outside of Kaiser Permanente, Lazes and colleagues (2012a) find value in the collaboration between Fletcher Allen Health Care and the Vermont Federation of Nurses and Health Professionals, American Federation of Teachers. This partnership is focused on Model Unit Processes (MUPs), a negotiated "innovative process whereby nurses and unit managers would meet to analyze the needs of patients and determine appropriate staffing levels by unit (p. 33)".

MUPs, which are analogous in some ways to Kaiser Permanente's UBTs, are the vehicle for nurses and their managers in given departments to "become involved not only in determining appropriate staffing levels but also in influencing the way in which units function at Fletcher Allen through the redesign of care delivery and work processes" (2012a, p. 33). As an example, the parties worked together to address an overreliance on traveler nurses, a practice which both eroded union jobs and ran up hospital costs.

In 2006, Fletcher Allen employed at least 125 travelers. The MUP teams pursued new ways of giving nurses a voice in the workplace and made specific changes to work environment and clinical practices. As a result, conditions at Fletcher Allen began to improve. At the time of publication, no travelers have been hired, open positions remain limited, and the hospital boasts a low nursing turnover rate. (2012a, p. 40)

The SEIU reports on its National Hospital Quality Initiative, which was launched in 2014 to expand and strengthen its labor–management partnerships with a range of different local unions and their respective employers (Service Employees International Union, 2015). Each appears to ground its partnership in its own particular culture, experience, and strategy. For instance, SEIU Local 721 and Los Angeles County's Department of Health Services have created Care Innovation Teams (CITs), focused on reducing patient wait times and improving patient experience in ambulatory settings. At Los Angeles County's Martin Luther King Jr. Outpatient Center, staff and managers in the hematology–oncology department were able to reduce wait times, from registration to taking vitals, from 23 minutes to 3 minutes (2014). In Miami, SEIU Local 1991 and Jackson Memorial Hospital have partnered to improve safe patient handling; they project $9 million to $13 million in annual savings from their project (2014). SEIU has established a National Learning Collaborative to share lessons and best practices from these various partnership experiences.

Although a partnership between labor and management is far from the industry standard, an increasing body of evidence shows that a diversity of approaches to collaboration among unions and their employers has yielded measurable improvements in targeted areas of focus, including quality, service, affordability, and staff satisfaction. As healthcare systems and unions grapple with increasingly complex competitive, clinical, and financial challenges, this model of partnership may be particularly suited to the imperative to simultaneously exploit existing capabilities and strike out into uncharted areas of innovation.

INNOVATION IN PARTNERSHIP AND SOLIDARITY: THE ELECTRONIC HEALTHCARE RECORD BACKGROUND AND IMPLEMENTATION

Regulations and incentives within the PPACA that are meant to push the entire U.S. healthcare system toward electronic medical records (EMR), both to cut costs and increase efficiency and effectiveness, have already gone into effect. This is another arena in which Kaiser Permanente has led innovation within the industry as the first major health system in the country to roll out a comprehensive EMR. At Kaiser, pressures to create this system came separately from the very top, at the chief executive officer (CEO) level, as well as organically from the grass roots, the bedside nurses on the front lines of patient care. The LMP can be seen as the metaphorical meeting-in-the-middle point, where the vision from above and the knowledge from below intersected in a productive manner. It provided the processes and methodology to translate overarching vision and everyday knowledge into practical design and implementation.

The account from the grass roots is carried by Kathy Sackman, RN, former president of the United Nurses Associations of California/Union of Health Care Professionals (UNAC/UHCP), who recalls a project within Kaiser Permanente in the late 1990s where paper charts were replaced with flow sheets so nurses could document patient care information faster and in fewer places. "At the time," said Sackman, "some individual Kaiser Permanente hospitals in Southern California had internal computer systems that were being used for outpatient care. As soon as we started that patient documentation project, the nurses began asking when we were going to go electronic with our charts. (Kathy Sackman, RN, personal communication May 4, 2015)." Successive CEOs near the latter end of the same period had similar ideas. Dick Pettingale, Kaiser Permanente California Division President from 1999 to 2002, worked on developing such a system. Pettingale's replacement in 2002, George Halvorson, scrapped Pettingale's EMR to bring in a system he had already worked with called EPIC. This became the new basis for Kaiser Permanente's eventual in-house product, HealthConnect, which rolled out in selected California facilities in 2003.

The government mandate for all health records to go digital would not come until 2004, but Halvorson believed that a patient who visited Kaiser Permanente in any area of the country should have the same experience, with the same access to medical records, as any other. In 2002, a patient in such a situation would have had to get paper copies of all files and take them to any other Kaiser Permanente location, even in the same region, for providers to review them. In addition, inpatient care within the hospital was not connected to outpatient care that might take place in the emergency room or outlying clinics. The challenge was not just to share information internally, but also across the continuum of care.

Another challenge was that some of the technology necessary to make it all possible did not yet exist. Plenty of computer and information technology (IT) professionals could write a computer program for a pop-up box to be shown on a screen or code a universal chart to be shared electronically. But there was no health IT specialty, and any technology expert had a steep learning curve when it came to understanding the healthcare side of the work flow. More prohibitive, it was impossible to rewire many old hospitals, constructed decades before local area networks and the Internet, to share information electronically. Wireless technology, though not yet in widespread use, became the only option for sharing information within most hospitals and clinics.

Three groups of workers needed to be involved to get the EMR project off the ground: clinicians, the people who would actually use the system; business representatives, who needed to look at it from a financial perspective and determine how to change Kaiser Permanente policies to support it; and IT professionals, who needed to develop the technological infrastructure. The collaborative model from the partnership was absolutely critical to fitting all the pieces together.

HealthConnect development went through three layers of decision making. The top level was the national development validation and build delegation sessions, made up of a small group from every region, who worked to ensure that the experiences from every Kaiser Permanente region would be homogeneous. Below that was the regional development build group, modeled after the larger group structure. One representative from every emergency department in Southern California attended the regional build validation sessions, for example. Staff educators were involved, as well as local management across all regional facilities. Finally, at the local level, representatives from different units and worker groups across a single Kaiser Permanente health center participated. This allowed local staff to give their input into how the final product would look. The meetings included employees performing a variety of jobs to be certain that all who needed to provide input would be on one of the build teams. One representative from each local facility then represented that facility at the regional build meetings. A three-level review process gave all who were impacted the chance to correct problems before implementation.

Although HealthConnect carried the blessing and mandate of Kaiser Permanente's CEO and top leadership, there was significant initial resistance from those management level staff that comprised the national team working to build the system—an example of paradox 2 in action. Getting the frontline nurses involved at that level was crucial in changing this dynamic. Those nurses already involved pushed for inclusion at the highest levels so that those who would be interacting with the system the most could help build it. UNAC/UHCP president Kathy Sackman, RN, went to bat for the nurses in conversations with top leadership on the management side. Before long, nurses were sitting at the national table discussing the practicalities of how to make HealthConnect function from a worker standpoint.

"The partnership is a commitment by the employer and by the unions that the workforce will be involved," according to Sackman. "It's recognition that the employer understands that the workers know how to do the work and have ideas on how to do it better. They know how to eliminate waste in the system (Kathy Sackman, RN, personal communication, May 4, 2015)." With a project of this scale, designed to impact the work flow of every staff member who interacts with patients, engaging with the workforce from the very beginning was a necessity.

One nurse on the national build team, Troy Seagondollar, RN, ultimately became the lead for the Kaiser Permanente Southern California rollout. Even as a working RN he had an interest in health informatics. His position was a unique hybrid creation and embodiment of the LMP. He came out of the labor side, as a UNAC/UHCP-represented RN. Even during the project, his office was housed at UNAC/UHCP's headquarters, and he served as liaison for the Coalition of Kaiser Permanente Unions. Yet his salary was paid by Kaiser Permanente.

When it came time to do the rollout in the Southern California region, Seagondollar met with the nurse executives at each medical center to plan training. He explained how many people needed to be trained to do peer-to-peer support, by different job type. These workers who were trained would then explain to others with the same job type what HealthConnect was, how it worked, and how it would impact their job flow.

There was training and some measure of selling the new EMR. This allowed innovators to train a wide range of people, engaging all workers in the process.

Finally, when the rollouts of HealthConnect began, there was another process implemented to help achieve success. This work would start 90 days before going live and continue for 6 weeks after the launch. Three teams would go into a medical center to do a readiness survey: IT, Kaiser Permanente HealthConnect Leads, and Deployment Support. The first team of IT workers assured that the necessary equipment and the technical infrastructure was in place to support using the EMR. The Kaiser Permanente HealthConnect Leads worked with management to assess and mitigate the perceived impact. In addition, they would assure congruence between local policies and procedures with expected work flow changes after the deployment of the EMR. The third team, Deployment Support, performed education and training sessions. In this phase, local staff subject matter experts would be selected to assist with the training and support of their respective peer groups; for example, nurse to nurse, lab tech to lab tech, manager to manager, provider to provider. In most instances, a team of nurses was brought together to form a nursing informatics team.

This team's charter was to continue to support their colleagues after the Deployment Teams left. The deployment of HealthConnect in each health center was just the beginning. Those who had done the peer-to-peer support during rollout were now back to their regular jobs and were embedded. When workers had problems with the system, they knew exactly who to ask for help. The clinicians were also free to keep suggesting ways to optimize HealthConnect. Those who did peer-to-peer support became change agents. They still attend regional meetings and continue working to improve HealthConnect. Their position has transitioned from the initial period of disruptive innovation into the current period of adaptive change, creating a helpful continuity from one phase to the other.

ONGOING INNOVATION

Although paradox 3 codifies the risk that while change that moves too rapidly can become a barrier to further change, well-managed innovation, conversely, opens up numerous pathways to subsequent innovation. HealthConnect has not just given different clinicians who are updating or reviewing a patient's records instantaneous access to the same information. As technology has leaped ahead, it has now allowed patients to review their own information on both the Kaiser Permanente website and a mobile app. Patients can access test results and even submit photos to aid in diagnosis, as well as exchange e-mails with their care provider or a nurse who handles patient advice.

Currently, clinicians are limited to using the EMR at desktop computers, though much of their work happens away from the desktop. A newly formed Nurse Innovation

Team is working on how to make the EMR mobile, whether through tablets or other mobile devices yet to be invented. This opens up multiple questions that will need to be worked through in partnership. For example, after critical information is mobile, how can it be shared with all the care providers who need to see it? What information should be sent under given scenarios, and how can it be transmitted to a care provider quickly and with actionable data?

The final major innovation on HealthConnect has the potential to revolutionize the entire healthcare industry by creating a critical mass of data that can be mined for future evidence-based innovation. With years of data now in the system, it is possible to review and analyze it in aggregate to determine which treatments are most effective, separately and in combination, from exercise to medication. Clinicians will be better able to predict the progress of a given patient's condition using vital signs, emergency room visits during the past year, and other data already entered for similar patients in HealthConnect. Kaiser Permanente can create best practices for how to use the data to anticipate a declining condition or redirect efforts toward patients who are likely to worsen. This aggregation and use of data can be used in the future as a means of heading off paradox 1, providing solid evidence of support or refutation when it comes to further innovation within the organization.

LESSONS IN HEALTHCARE INNOVATION

The collaborative model at Kaiser Permanente also encompasses unions and unionized workers. Unions are an essential part of Kaiser Permanente's business, and they have developed a labor–management partnership that is unique in its scale and ambition (Kochan et al., 2008; Kochan et al., 2009). The parties recognized their interdependence in a landmark partnership agreement, included in the collective bargaining contract in 1997. The collaboration enabled by this partnership has become central to the organization's efforts to meet its ever-intensifying ambidexterity challenges, providing a foundation for combining top–down initiatives by specialized technical staff (e.g., for new computerized medical records) and bottom-up input and involvement by a broad range of personnel for local improvement projects, as well as extensive lateral learning so that similar locations can share lessons learned (Adler & Heckscher, 2013).

How can the lessons from Kaiser Permanente LMP and its EMR implementation be universalized and applied in other healthcare settings, whether union or nonunion, system or facility? The first principle for innovation in a healthcare setting is also the foundational concept of the LMP: workers know best how to do the work. Therefore, their full and free participation is not a luxury, but rather an absolute necessity for innovation to weather the paradoxes that threaten all such change, survive the rough seas of disruptive innovation, and make it through to the relative calm of ongoing adaptive change.

It is perhaps ironic that although unions and management are traditionally seen as oppositional, in the LMP setting it is the very presence of the union that serves to give employees the sense of psychological safety and security, without which true partnership and cooperation are not possible. Therefore, in a nonunion setting, it is even more important that the workers feel truly empowered to participate fully and honestly without fear of retaliation from management. Within the context of the team's focus on a given task, it must be clear to all participants that everyone is equal. Lip service to this principle will not work. If an employee contributes to the task-oriented discussion in a way that offends a manager and suffers consequences, this would be fatal to the collaborative nature of the enterprise.

Lesson: Management must make a genuine commitment to the workers involved that their full participation is encouraged without negative consequences to their standing within the organization, and hold to that commitment.

Within the LMP setting, the union always chooses its own representatives for the given committee, task force, or project. Even in a nonunion, non-LMP setting, it is probably a good idea to allow this. If workers feel that their representatives are hand-picked management favorites, this can undermine trust in the process and its results.

Lesson: Let workers choose their own representatives.

In the LMP process, decisions are made by consensus. Neither management nor labor can overrule a group decision. Consensus decision making can sometimes take longer than simply a vote because any one party can halt the process with a simple thumbs down. However, in a consensus decision-making setting, everyone agrees up front that all will support any decision that allows the whole group to move forward. This means that any initiative that does progress has been thoroughly vetted, and it creates greater buy-in and a more personal stake in the outcome from everyone involved. A hybrid system can also be followed, where ground rules are put in place to allow for a democratic vote under certain conditions, agreed upon up front, where consensus becomes unworkable and brings the project to a dead stop.

Lesson: Consider allowing decisions to be made by consensus for thorough vetting and greater buy-in.

For the Kaiser Permanente EMR project, having a workable collaborative structure already in place was a huge advantage. The structure that had previously been set up through the LMP was modeled for the HealthConnect build. Start with a national body that oversees the project from the 37,000-foot level. Add a middle layer with regional bodies that can make the project work within a particular area. Finish with local bodies at the facility level. The key to this structure is that information should flow both ways—down from the national and regional bodies, and up from the local and regional bodies.

Even within one facility, this multilevel structure can be duplicated, with participatory groups functioning, for example, at the facility, department, and work unit levels. As with consensus decision making, this might seem to add time and complexity to the design and implementation of an innovation, but in practice it ensures that the end product receives input from multiple stakeholders at all levels of the organization and with every type of expertise that must be brought to bear so that it has depth and breadth and is robust and comprehensive.

Lesson: A multilevel structure can be useful, adaptable, and sizeable to any enterprise, from a nationwide health system to a single facility.

Seagondollar, the lead on the Kaiser Permanente Southern California EMR rollout, found that one key to successful change management is understanding how individual personalities function within a group dynamic. He found that most workers fall into one of the following categories:

- Innovators: Those that are looking for change and embrace it
- Middle of the pack: These who will buy in as long as they know what they need to do
- Late adopters: Although they really do not want to do it, they will after the initiative is tried and true
- Resisters: Will not make the change, and if it is forced on them, they may quit

One key to a successful rollout of a significant new initiative is to find and encourage the innovators in the process who want to be part of the change. These are the people that keep pushing when the project has problems, and they make it a reality. They can become the trainers, the subject matter experts, the ongoing resources for their colleagues. And they can become a means of heading off paradox 2, where individuals within a group pursuing their own agendas can derail the group initiative.

Lesson: Innovators are always present. They will often step to the fore on their own. Regardless, keep an eye out for them, find them, and encourage them to participate and even take the lead.

The UBTs at Kaiser Permanente have led to dramatic improvements in company operations (Adler & Heckscher, 2013). Based on the UBT model, HealthConnect has regional nurse domain teams that are specific to health care. For instance, case managers have their own regional nurse domain teams. Emergency nurses were their own domain. There is a domain for every specialty. These teams meet monthly to discuss anticipated changes and determine the best way to integrate those changes into Health-Connect, modify work flow, and train colleagues on the modifications. These groups talk about what is not working and suggest ways to improve. If the decision is made to do a pilot, the scope of the pilot is defined at these meetings as well.

Lesson: In addition to the multilevel decision-making bodies, it can be productive to have lateral groups based on profession or unit that meet on an ongoing basis to synthesize input into the wider process and also carry the work forward. These groups can be key to moving an innovation from disruptive to adaptive change.

LEADERSHIP FOR PARTNERSHIP AND INNOVATION

Along the continuum from incremental performance improvement to radical innovation, a number of factors act as preconditions for effective collaboration. These include cultures and practices in which everyone, whatever their formal role, is encouraged to lead and is empowered to do so, including speaking up in an environment of psychological safety, acting and collaborating beyond the constraints of official hierarchy, and thinking with a systems mindset. A review of recent literature highlights some of the key leadership behaviors and practices that support high performance and innovation.

Kotter (2013) speaks to the limits of hierarchy in a competitive environment characterized by an increase in both threats from a variety of directions and windows of opportunity that open and close quickly. In this context, organizations need to be structured to be reliable and efficient, and at the same time nimble and fast moving; a reliance on only the former will not allow organizations to drive the major changes that such challenges demand. People at every level of the organization need to be empowered to act and collaborate beyond the bounds of formal institutional structure. In other words, both hierarchy and network are required. Similarly, Battilana and Cascario (2013) identify the power of informal networks in driving change. In their study of change initiatives at the massive British National Health Service, they conclude that "Change agents who were central in the organization's informal network had a clear advantage, regardless of their position in the informal hierarchy" (Battilana & Cascario, 2013, p. 64).

Within the partnership between the Coalition of Kaiser Permanente Unions and Kaiser Permanente, the parties have identified a set of 37 behaviors, organized around seven core principles, to guide collaboration (Kaiser Permanente, 2003). Each of the principles calls on managers and union stewards to take shared responsibility for various dimensions of the partnership, including ensuring the success of both parties, providing patients with a superior care experience, and engaging employees in decision making. More recently, Eaton, Konistney, Litwin, and Vanderhorst (2011) conducted a study of high-performing UBTs at Kaiser Permanente. Several findings, among other structural and process factors, stand out. They identify psychological safety as key to high performance, describing "a work environment where everyone was able to speak up and had the courage to have difficult conversations. Employees stated they could say what was on their minds without fear of retaliation or retribution" (Eaton et al., 2011, p. 11). Systems thinking is also crucial: "The most successful teams we studied were interested in how their work and performance were affected by that broader system and were working collaboratively with other departments to achieve common goals" (Eaton et al., 2011, p. 10). Among the leadership dimensions identified by the authors is a shift from traditional, command-and-control management to an approach in which "managers would work to coach and motivate employees instead of micromanaging them. They trusted employees to do their jobs. Managers of the teams stated that once they were able to change how they managed employees, their job actually became easier" (Eaton et al., 2011, p. 8). This transformation is accompanied by another noteworthy aspect of leadership: "On most of the high performing teams we studied, the labor leads—who were generally selected by the unionized employees on the unit—took on such an authentic leadership role that they became essentially interchangeable with their management counterparts" (Eaton et al., 2011, p. 8).

Finally, Bevan and Fairman (2014) provide a thorough examination of how leadership needs to shift to reflect the scope and complexity of contemporary healthcare challenges. Like other authors cited here, they identify the need to marry what they term a dominant approach, characterized by top–down leadership, with an emergent model, marked by shared purpose. The mindset is that transformational change is more likely to happen cross-organizationally than within a single organization and that hierarchical levers cannot drive change across the wider system. From this perspective, large-scale change depends on many partners (2014, p. 18). On the emergent side, they note that "the most important skill that leaders of change need to develop for the 21st century is the ability to build partnership" (2014, p. 18).

The labor–management partnership at Kaiser Permanente reflects broader organizational and industry thinking about how collaboration and distributed leadership can help spur the kind of change and innovation that contemporary circumstances demand. At the same time, this partnership has developed its own specific practices and lessons about what is required to achieve high performance. As this partnership continues to grow and evolve, we expect that it will continue to both draw from and contribute to emerging approaches to innovation leadership.

INNOVATION OUTSIDE HEALTH CARE

Looking at the nexus of labor and innovation beyond health care, The Workers Lab is an innovation incubator and accelerator that was established as an answer to its founders who ask themselves, in the context of a shrinking labor movement and a growing low-wage economy, "why can't we take the dynamism and ingenuity fueling new products, services and institutions, and harness them to advance the interests of low-wage workers? Can we channel that creativity and rigorous experimentation to address the vexing problems facing millions of American workers?" (Maxwell, 2015, para. 3).

The Workers Lab focuses on investing in "organizing strategies, business models, and platforms that will lift wages and transform the lives of US workers" (The Workers Lab, 2015, para. 1). Backed by unions and foundations, it funds a small number of projects aimed at developing and testing new approaches to achieving economic justice for workers in low-wage industries.

Among its first round of projects in 2015, The Workers Lab funded an experiment called Top Server with the Restaurant Opportunities Center (ROC) United and the Everett Program at UC Santa Cruz, which marries workforce development to advanced technology and gamification. The mission of ROC United is to address and improve the low wages and poor working conditions suffered by restaurant workers; its Colors Hospitality Opportunities for Workers C.H.O.W. Institute provides free job training and development for restaurant workers to move into living wage jobs. With funding and support from The Workers Lab, ROC United will be developing an online gaming platform for the C.H.O.W. Institute's restaurant worker members to support their efforts to develop career skills to move into higher-paying jobs in that industry.

In an article in *Fast Company*, The Workers Lab executive director, Carmen Rojas, speaks to the benefit that can accrue to employers when they provide workers with living wages and good benefits: "When these conditions are met, corporations and revenue-generating ventures experience less employee turnover and have increased customer loyalty . . . This is great for their corporations as well as for our economy" (Dishman, 2015).

Such intentional experimentation, including the application of innovation methodologies more commonly used in for-profit endeavors, such as technology startups or big business, represents a significant departure from traditional organizing and collective bargaining strategies and holds the potential to provide rich lessons and insights about how to achieve sustainable and scalable victories for the labor movement in a low-wage economy marked by massive income inequality and declining rates of unionization.

REFERENCES

Adler, P., & Heckscher, C. (2013, 4th Quarter). The collaborative, ambidextrous enterprise. *Universia Business Review*, 34–50.

Battilana, J., & Cascario, T. (2013, July/August). The network secrets of great change agents. *Harvard Business Review*, 62–68.

Bensaid, C. (2015, March). *How our strategy works for all workers*. Speech presented at Coalition of Kaiser Permanente Unions Delegates Conference. Anaheim, CA.

Berwick, D. (2011, December 7). The moral test. Retrieved from http://www.ahier.net/2011/12/remember -patient.html?m=1

Bevan, H., & Fairman, S. (2014). The new era of thinking and practice in change and transformation: A call to action for leaders of health and care. Retrieved from http://media.nhsiq.nhs.uk/whitepaper/index.html

Congressional Budget Office. (2014). *Updated estimates of the effects of the insurance coverage provisions of the Affordable Care Act, April 2014* (CBO Publication No. 45231). Washington, DC: Government Printing Office.

Detert, J. & Edmondson, A.C. (2007). Why employees are afraid to speak. *Harvard Business Review*. Retrieved from https://hbr.org/2007/05/why-employees-are-afraid-to-speak

Dishman, L. (2015, May 8). Meet the woman working to change low income workers' prospects. Retrieved from http://www.fastcompany.com/3046041/strong-female-lead/meet-the-woman-working-to-change-low -income-workers-prospects

Dixon-Woods, M., Amalberti, R., Goodman, S., Bergman, B., & Glasziou, P. (2011). Problems and promises of innovation: Why healthcare needs to rethink its love/hate relationship with the new. *BMJ Quality & Safety. 20*, i47–i51.

Eaton, A., Konistney, D., Litwin, A. S., & Vanderhorst, N. (2010, December). *The path to performance: A study of high-performing unit-based teams at Kaiser Permanente* [white paper]. Publication of Kaiser Permanente Labor Management Partnership.

Geoghegan, T. (2014). *Only one thing can save us: Why America needs a new kind of labor movement*. New York, NY: New Press.

Greenhouse, S. (2014, June 30). Supreme Court ruling on union fees is a limited blow to labor. *The New York Times*. Retrieved from http://www.nytimes.com/2014/07/01/business/supreme-court-ruling-on-public-workers-and-union-fees.html.

Henwood, D. (2015, January). Union membership is down again—but it still pays to be a union member. Retrieved from http://www.inthesetimes.com/working/entry/17567/union_membership_is_down_again_but_it_still_pays_to_be_a_member.

Kaiser Permanente. (2003). Labor management partnership behaviors. Retrieved from http://lmpartnership.org/sites/default/files/lmp__behaviors.pdf

Kaufman, N. S. (2011). Changing economics in an era of healthcare reform. *Journal of Healthcare Management, 56*(1), 9–13.

Kochan, T.A., Eaton, A.E., McKersie, R.B., & Adler, P.S. (2009). *Healing together: The labor-management partnership at Kaiser Permanente*. Cornell University Press: Ithaca, NY.

Kotter, J. (2013, October 18). *Accelerate* [Video file]. Retrieved from https://www.youtube.com/watch?v=o9SxvladTCg

Lazes, P., Katz, L., & Figueroa, M. (2012a). *How labor–management partnerships improve patient care, cost control, and labor relations: Case studies for Fletcher Allen Health Care, Kaiser Permanente, and Montefiore Medical Center*. Cornell University, NY: Cornell University.

Lazes, P., Katz, L., Figueroa, M., & Karpur, A. (2012b). Using adaptive and disruptive change strategies to create an integrated delivery system: Montefiore Medical Center's experience. In S. A. Mohrman & A. B. Shani (Eds.), *Organizing for sustainable health care* (pp. 147–168). Bringley, UK: Emerald Group.

Maxwell, M. B. (2015). Investing in the future: The Workers Lab sows the seeds of change. Retrieved from https://blog.dol.gov/2015/04/30/investing-in-the-future-the-workers-lab-sows-seeds-of-change/

Meyerson, H. (2013, September 13). Harold Meyerson: At AFL-CIO convention, labor embraces the new America. *Washington Post*.

Morrison, I. (2000). *Health care in the new millennium: Vision, values, and leadership*. San Francisco, CA: Jossey-Bass.

Nixon, J. P. (2012, January). *Culture matters: An investigation into UBTs, workplace culture and performance.* Presented at the Executive Committee of the Labor Management Partnership Strategy Group, Oakland, CA.

Rolf, D. (2014, June 18). What if we treated labor like a startup? *The Nation*. Retrieved from http://www.thenation.com/article/180316/omcibator-labor#

Service Employees International Union. (2015). *Improving care, lowering costs: How front-line hospital workers are transforming healthcare*. Washington, DC: Author.

Thakur, R., Hsu, S. H., & Fontenot, G. (2012). Innovation in healthcare: Issues and future trends. Journal of Business Research, 65(4), 562–569.

The Workers Lab. (2015). Innovating for worker justice. Retrieved from http://theworkerslab.com/program/

CHAPTER 16

Moving to the Future of Evidence, Innovation, and Leadership in Health Care

Daniel Weberg and Sandra Davidson

You cannot discover new oceans unless you have the courage to lose sight of the shore.

—Anonymous

CHAPTER OBJECTIVES

Upon completion of this chapter, the reader will be able to:

1. Describe key leadership elements for building innovative organizations in health care.
2. Synthesize core aspects of evidence and innovation in relation to the changing healthcare system.
3. Discuss a new framework for innovation in health care.

Now more than ever, the need for innovation in health care is clear. A shift from volume to value has disrupted the status quo and demonstrated that the models of the past are no longer relevant or sustainable ways to improve the quality, cost, affordability, and experience for the greater population. Healthcare organizations are struggling to combine, align, merge, adapt, reinvent, and even innovate new ways to provide superior quality while reducing the cost to the consumer and the overall system.

ARE WE MOVING TOO SLOWLY?

Many healthcare start-up entrepreneurs think so! In 2014, venture funding to healthcare-focused start-up companies was the highest in history (Gandhi & Wang, 2015). Innovators, many with little formal healthcare experience, are developing software, devices, systems, and solutions to fill the gaps left by the shifting healthcare system or to capitalize on emerging opportunities. Universities, venture capital firms, and large organizations are creating incubators for healthcare start-up companies to spin out solutions focused on digital health, pharmaceuticals, medical devices, and diagnostics.

Consumers are also demanding and purchasing services outside the traditional medical model. MeMD, Teladoc, and HealthTap are technology companies that decentralize care and allow patients to see a clinician from their computer or mobile device in seconds for a low one-time charge. Robots are enabling specialists across the world to examine, operate, and follow-up with patients with solutions from InTouch Health and other companies. Sensor devices are allowing healthcare professionals to amass petabytes of data on patients that could not have been collected previously. These petabytes are expanding the sources of data that can be analyzed and translated into evidence automatically and instantly. In fact, there is so much data produced on a continuous basis that practitioners can easily access, that we do not know what to do with it all. Traditional health professions education has not yet caught up with the available technology or mounds of data. Healthcare providers today have not been taught how to assess, diagnose, treat, and monitor patients based on this data captured millions of times per second. The episodic basis of care-related data (vital signs, activity, diet, medication absorption, etc.) is quickly becoming irrelevant. Technology is challenging old models of care, enabling new ones, and providing the evidence of what works and what does not work.

It seems obvious that the needs of clinicians, healthcare consumers, and populations are rapidly changing due to technology, health policy changes, and innovations. Equally as important is the changing focus and scope of leaders in the healthcare industry. The call for outside-the-box thinking, leading, and organizing is loud and clear. However, there are few frameworks of leadership, innovation, and evidence that help new and experienced leaders understand the complexities of the new world of health care. This text has provided the content and evidence needed to inform a new framework, and this chapter will present a synthesis and starting point on which we might build and refine such a framework. We argue that by thinking more intentionally about the interdependence and connectedness of leadership, innovation, and evidence, and by utilizing the skills, attitudes, and ideas presented in this text, leaders in health care can create a greater impact on the outcomes across the system.

THE PARADOX OF THE BOX: MOVING TO AN INTERCONNECTED FRAMEWORK

What is the box? The phrase *think outside the box* has been used to describe anything from innovation, to visionary thinkers, to disruptive ideas. In many organizational

Figure 16-1 Moving out of the box

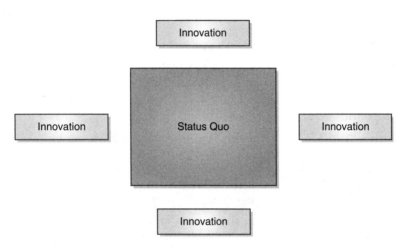

applications, the phrase has been used to describe anything that challenges the normal operating thinking and status quo of the organization. The conceptualization of a status quo box (**Figure 16-1**) that requires people to break their normal routine to disrupt creates a culture of episodic change that may not be responsive enough to adjust to the continuous changes that are impacting health care.

The idea that innovation occurs outside a hypothetical status quo or normal operating procedures box presents conceptual problems that undermine the ability of organizations to implement innovation. By thinking about innovation as something external to the day-to-day workings of an organization, we actually build another silo: the silo of the innovation team. To lead organizations and the health system to new ways of work, it is important to design a system that breaks down silos and reduces fragmentation (Berwick & Hackbarth, 2012). Furthermore, innovation needs to be integrated into the learning experiences and preparation for all healthcare disciplines. It cannot continue to stand alone, or separate and apart, from other dimensions of their learning. In short, innovation needs to take its place among the other core competencies for healthcare practice in the 21st century.

This text has presented content, research, and examples of a three-pronged framework that will help organizations move to a new future of care: evidence-based practice, innovation, and leadership. It is important that we discuss each component, its current status quo, and how the concepts in this text will help disrupt our fragmented system and create more interdependent and relational ways of linking evidence, innovation, and leadership across organizations.

EVIDENCE

Evidence has evolved over time to create rigor, validity, and a rational hierarchy for assessing and appraising research and turning it into insights to improve care outcomes (Melnyk & Fineout-Overholt, 2011). This evolution serves as an excellent and needed foundation on which practitioners can build and incorporate new data into the system and turn it into evidence. Current evidence-based practice hierarchies limit sources of valid evidence to systematic reviews, randomized control trials, and so forth. However, by viewing evidence as generated only from the few sources within the box, we fail to integrate the new emerging sources and insights of evidence, like technology and powerful analytics.

Emerging sources of data that are disrupting existing evidence frameworks include big data technologies, wearable monitors, analytics, continuous patient monitoring, and electronic medical records (EMR) (**Figure 16-2**). These outside-the-box disruptions are signposts for leaders and practitioners to innovate new possibilities for the evidence hierarchy and dynamic. In addition to the technologic possibilities for generating and aggregating evidence, we must also consider the relational and contextual aspects of evidence-based practice. How do we engage patients, communities, and providers in collaborative decision making about the evidence?

Leaders in health care must be able to identify disruptions, challenge current thinking, and begin to facilitate the integration of these new sources of evidence into new ways of clinical decision making.

Figure 16-2 Evidence beyond the box

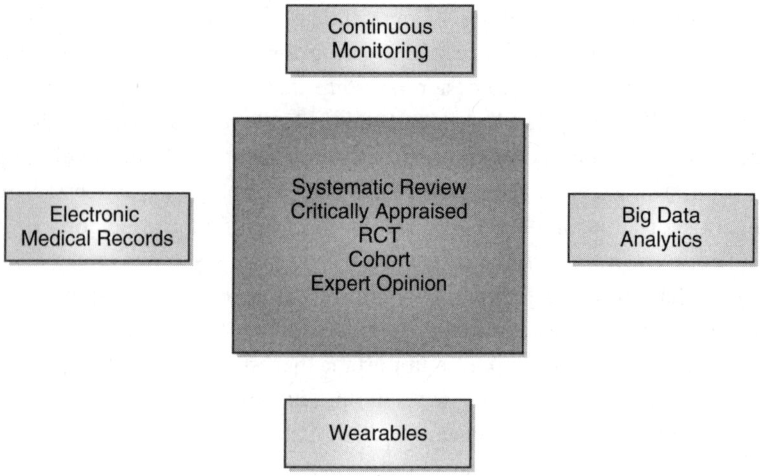

As leaders read the signposts, gather learnings, and test ideas, they will begin to break down the rigid walls of the status quo that organizations build. By connecting evidence to innovation and leadership, a new paradigm of evidence begins to emerge that is fluid, permeable, and able to incorporate out-of-the-box thinking to inform proven methods—in essence, getting rid of the box altogether and creating a more networked and complex approach to linking, trying, and implementing evidence-based practice (**Figure 16-3**). In a networked complex system, the practices informed by evidence begin to connect and incorporate newer sources and insights, thus strengthening the practice and evolving our thinking. This allows us to stay relevant and nimble in how we respond to shifting information and needs. Some practices, such as big data analytics, may have stronger ties to the new sources, such as continuous monitoring. Thus, the fluidity of the new evidence bubble allows practices to shift based on continuous assessment and learnings from innovative testing of linkages among the elements. For example, the ubiquitous adoption of EMRs may signal a need to link the evidence hierarchy to EMR insights and data sources to build new practices, but the use of continuous monitoring may still be in the early stages and have fewer linkages.

It is important to also note that evidence is not a silo. The discussion of evidence presented here is intended to help leaders conceptualize one part of the larger framework discussed throughout this chapter. Accepting new forms of evidence informs expansion and connection building, and it helps us anticipate the future directions of care. It allows us to begin to recognize new patterns. Evidence provides the foundations of innovation and leadership, and innovation and leadership are required to build more evidence. It is an iterative and dynamic system with complex linkages.

Figure 16-3 Emerging sources that further inform evidence-based practice

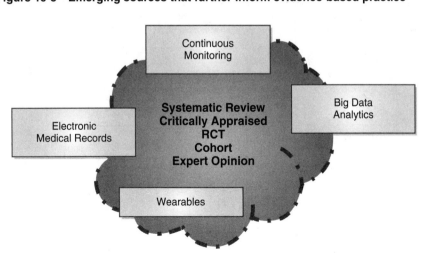

INNOVATION

From a traditional perspective, innovation as a whole is considered outside the box, but from the perspective of an innovator, there are always radical ideas that continue to inform practice and aid in the evolution of new ways of thinking. New and radical technological disruptions are often considered innovation, but other practices, such as process redesign, failure and patient-generated innovations, are not. Even innovation has a cutting edge that continually challenges and moves the practice of innovation forward (**Figure 16-4**).

Disruptive practices that are changing how innovation is practiced include conceptualizing failure as necessary, incorporating and relying on patient-generated innovations, the use of social labs, and building innovation from a foundation of evidence-based practice. These trends in innovation practice rely on the connections among multiple parts of the organization and cannot be accomplished in isolation. Innovation requires a network of people who can collaborate, envision the future, overcome barriers, and generate a new vision and direction for the healthcare system to evolve.

The practice of innovation (in health care particularly) is maturing from the notion of idea generation and radical product creation to a practice that fundamentally derives value and content from the front lines of the organization. Healthcare leaders should be competent in innovation practice, accept failure as part of the journey, and develop their own competencies to support innovators in their organizations by building partnerships across silos and teams. Leaders must continually evolve the innovation practice, looking for new sources of ideas, implementation techniques, and ways to keep change relevant

Figure 16-4 Innovation as its own box?

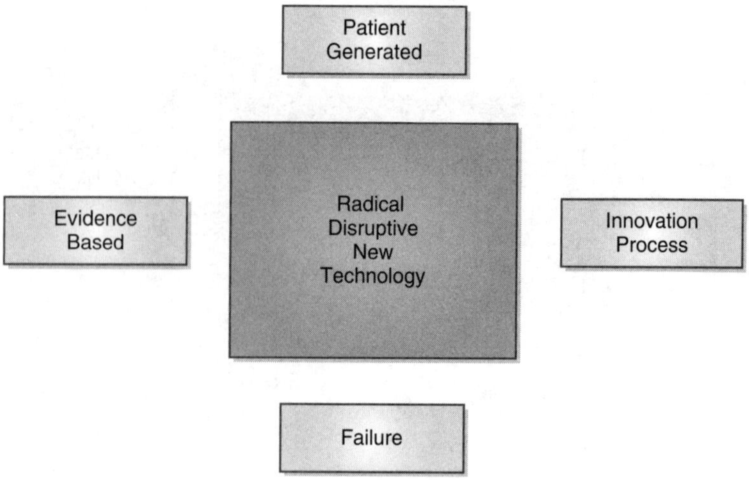

to the organization. Therefore, the innovation practice should continually test and trial new processes of change. Evidence-based innovation will require more leadership energy because many people conceptualize it as separate process. Innovation is often viewed as new, exciting, and future oriented, and evidence-based practice is perceived as steadfast, slow, and present focused. Yet, if you combine the two practices in new ways, such as using evidence as the foundation from which to inform innovation (new practices and process), they actually inform each other and synergize the system change.

The concept of failure can provide a similar example. If failure is viewed through the traditional lens, in which it is punitive, negative, and avoided at all costs, it actually limits the ability of organizations to innovate. By combining the notion of failure and linking it to evidence (knowing what does not work), there emerges another source of innovation rather than a roadblock to it. The failure of practice, process, trials, change, and tests provide a rich source of evidence that can be used as a foundation to improve innovation in the future. Failure should be celebrated for providing insight into all the ways things do not work and providing clues to what is not yet possible. Leaders should strive to fail early and often to rapidly move innovation forward, because failure is the process from which the new replaces the old.

Innovation is the force that propels evidence creation and provides a practice for leaders to use in order to evolve the organization, and it infuses energy into the system to catalyze change. Innovation is not a separate team or event, but rather the life force that keeps individuals, teams, and organizations relevant (**Figure 16-5**). Innovation occurs all the time, at various impact levels, and informs how evidence is created and leadership is practiced. Building a competency in basic innovation concepts and practices is a prerequisite for leaders, regardless of your role in the organization or system.

Figure 16-5 The edge of innovation: New sources and practices

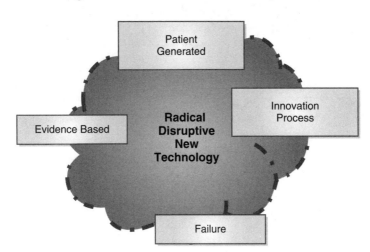

LEADERSHIP

It is possible that the notion of leadership carries with it the most history, misconception, and biggest lack of evidence of all the elements in the innovation, evidence, and leadership framework (**Figure 16-6**). Twentieth century leadership practices built on the ideas of individualistic power dynamics, followership, command and control, and hierarchy still dominate organizations in health care. The disruption of the tradition of leadership thinking and practices is a challenging endeavor that will require evidence, innovation, and significant energy. However, it is an essential element to transform health care. Throughout this text the argument has been made, and supported by evidence, that leadership needs to move toward a distributed, networked, team-based, and relational approach that is supported with the latest evidence and fueled by innovation.

Leadership relies on partnerships, and partnerships are built through networks. To build a network, and thus a partnership, leaders should focus on relationships among colleagues and teams (Porter-O'Grady & Malloch, 2014). The stronger the leader's network, the better the chance that diverse thought and sources of evidence will emerge to inform innovation and change (Weberg, 2013). As the network strengthens, the distribution of decision making can be improved as well. Placing problem-solving and decision-making power at the point closest to the problem allows those with the best connections to relevant evidence to create and sustain solutions (Porter-O'Grady & Malloch, 2014). Distributed leadership requires partnership and team-based models of collaboration to leverage the diverse skill sets of organizations. Partnerships and teams allow groups to leverage their collective expertise and evidence to cocreate innovative changes and move the organization forward.

Figure 16-6 Traditional in-the-box leadership

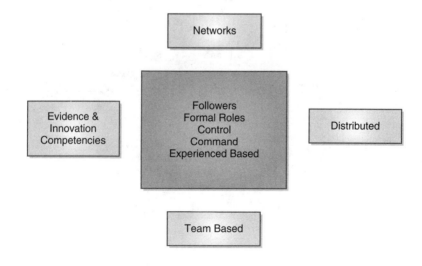

The most important shift in our understanding of leadership is that it is a set of behaviors that helps the organization focus and align time, resources, and energy through relationships and networks. It is not about controlling, but rather facilitating, connecting, and emancipating. Leaders may accomplish this by building relationship-centered cultures and translating information in ways that are meaningful and relevant in local contexts. In essence, leaders can help create the organizational norms that value shared decision making, innovation, and evidence integration. These norms will give rise to a culture that supports evidence-based innovation.

Depending on the current practices of the organization, leaders will need to test and trial new leadership behaviors in different patterns and ways. For example, if the organization has a strong relational and network culture, the leader may be able to more easily try different practices in distributed leadership. If the organization is steeped in hierarchy, the practice of building evidence-based leadership behaviors may be a good use of energy. There is no plug-and-play methodology to change culture and leadership practice other than to innovate, fail, and support decision making with the best data and evidence available. This is the challenge of 21st century leadership. Unlike leadership models of the past that rely on neatly listed steps or recipes for change, transformational and relational leadership embraces the messiness rather than seeking to control and confine it. **Figure 16-7** represents how leadership might look as more collaborative and networked approaches are incorporated. These new approaches will become the new norm, replacing antiquated practices like command and control tactics. The more networked, distributed, and team-based leadership becomes, the more capacity that is created for evidence-based innovation. As the leadership practice matures, the capacity to incorporate more innovative practices will increase.

Figure 16-7 Leadership beyond silos and hierarchy

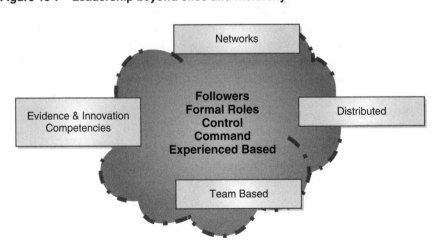

Learning Activity

Reflect on your personal experience with in-the-box leadership and answer the following questions:

1. Have you been in a leadership role in which you were expected to take on the traditional leadership behaviors (e.g., command and control)?
2. Have you been in a staff position in which a hierarchal leadership structure existed? What was your experience of being led by a traditional leader?
3. How do you imagine your experiences would have been different with an innovative or transformational leadership practice?
4. Compare your reflections and thoughts about leadership with a peer.

THE EVIDENCE–INNOVATION–LEADERSHIP FRAMEWORK

The evidence–innovation–leadership framework proposed in this text is an interdependent dynamic that helps leaders frame behaviors, evidence, and change in a way to further organizational evolution in health care (**Figure 16-8**). Often, evidence, innovation, and leadership are seen as disconnected and different, yet this framework describes ways they are synergistic and interdependent. Each concept has been detailed with a description of how organizations have boxed in the notions and created silos around each practice. For example, evidence has been boxed by the rigid use of evidence hierarchy, innovation has been boxed by the expectation for radical change, and leadership has been boxed by the notion that total control is necessary. It is important for leaders to understand the roots and assumptions of these boxes to create new ways of working and integrating concepts that may be more effective.

Building on the boxed assumptions, each concept of the framework has been described in a way that links it to the others and demonstrates their interdependence. This reconceptualization is meant to provide guidance for leaders to build upon and navigate within, to drive evidence-based practice, innovation efforts, and leadership development. Surrounding each of the concepts are the drivers presented throughout this text, including patient-centered care, technology, failure, pattern recognition, and partnerships that keep the framework fluid, informed, and relevant.

Patient-centered care provides relevancy to the framework by grounding it with the viewpoint that patient care is the focus of most healthcare change. Even business model innovations, evidence-based leadership, and technology changes should be done to improve the care experience, health, and safety for the end user of the system: the patient. Relationship-centered care is a framework for thinking about how we engage with patients, providers, and stakeholder communities in the service of patients. Without the

Figure 16-8   The evidence–innovation–leadership framework

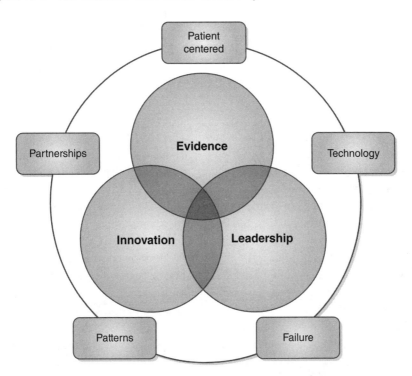

perspective of the patient, there is a risk of focusing energy on evidence, innovation, and leadership efforts that are not aligned with the mission of the organization. Removing the patient-centered care driver from the framework changes the balance of the three core concepts of evidence, innovation, and leadership, and it begins to fragment the system. Patient-centered care and relationship-centered care is discussed in Chapter 4.

The technology driver helps accelerate the framework's rate of change and the ability to gather, interpret, and act on data and evidence. Technology is a cultural norm and expectation that can move a process forward by simplifying complex data for interpretation or providing easy access to information to develop new practices. Technology can also speed up failure in a suboptimal system. Implementing technology on top of a broken process only serves to break the process faster. For example, providing clinicians with mobile devices that can access Google and other data sources without ensuring competency in understanding evidence validity and quality may lead to faster access to inaccurate information. Due to the integration of technology into our everyday lives, technology is quickly becoming the interface that drives care decisions and even patient-centered interactions. We can understand all of the various data points about a patient and at the same time instantly connect them with care team members. Leaders should have an understanding of the impact technology has and the speed at which it changes processes within the evidence–innovation–leadership framework. The technology driver is discussed in Chapters 5 and 8.

The failure driver provides the framework with continuous learning feedback loops and a safe environment to test new ways of work. Continuous learning emerges from tried and failed attempts at change, yet failure is continually avoided in healthcare organizations (Porter-O'Grady & Malloch, 2016). By acknowledging failure and diving deep into the insights that can be gleaned from less-than-successful attempts at change or practice, we can avoid making the same mistakes over and over. Moreover, we get better at failure, and this means we are able to learn more quickly. Celebrating failure can build learning that then cycles back into the organizational knowledge base and continues the iteration and movement forward to novel solutions. Failure is essential in evidence generation (building on research, learning what does not work), innovation work (quickly iterating to create novel solutions), and leadership (understanding the networks and increasing the span of impact). Without the failure driver, leaders condemn organizations to avoid or ignore failure at their own peril, which limits the creation of innovation and the use of novel evidence. Acceptance (even celebration) of failures requires leaders and organization-wide cultures to transcend ego, blame, and punishment to gain insights and grow stronger. The failure driver is discussed in Chapters 3, 7, and 11.

The pattern driver provides a different lens through which to conceptualize evidence, innovation learnings, and leadership signposts. In complex systems, individuals, teams, organizations, and technologies interact in a multitude of ways to accomplish tasks, work, and achieve outcomes (Uhl-Bien & Marion, 2008). The complexity of the system is so high that the impact of individual actions and interactions are nearly impossible to predict by any one leader. Therefore, leaders should look for emergent patterns in the organization to better understand how evidence, innovation, and leadership actions are changing the system. For example, a care practice based on one expert's opinion would be haphazard compared to looking across multiple sources of evidence, such as systematic reviews, patient preferences, and local best practices, for patterns that support a practice change. In innovation, patterns in technological change, consumer needs, and clinician practices provide the context on which to build novel solutions that add value. Patterns in failure also provide evidence that leaders can use to focus innovation efforts, understand what does not work, and search for more evidence to build stronger solutions. Without pattern recognition as a driver in the evidence framework, innovation and leadership become linear endeavors that rely on predictable processes rather than embracing the inherent complexity of relationships and systems. Linear leadership, prescriptive solutions, and a cookbook approach to evidence implementation may result in simpler solutions that lack relevancy and impact in complex environments. Patterns provide the signposts by which leaders can frame evidence and innovation within complex relational systems. The pattern driver is discussed in Chapters 7, 9, and 10.

The partnership driver provides the energy to create and strengthen connections and relationships among the core concepts. A core belief within this framework is the impact that groups of people, teams, and organizations can have in changing a large system. The partnership dynamic provides the tools, energy, and linkages to strengthen these networks and better link evidence to innovation and leadership practices. Without partnership as a driver, leadership can become an individual endeavor, innovation becomes slower and less relevant, and evidence that emerges tends to be less trustworthy or valid and reliable. Partnership improves diversity of thought, evidence sources, and leadership resources so that more diverse solutions are generated and more impactful outcomes can be achieved. One example of this is the use of unit-based teams. Facilitating local teams to source and implement evidence and innovation at the point of care results in greater fidelity and effectiveness of processes and solutions. The practice of engaging unit-based teams to solve problems instead of relying on individual leader solutions has provided sustainable and highly effective changes in some healthcare organizations. The partnership driver is discussed in Chapters 12, 13, and 15.

The evidence–innovation–leadership framework proposed here is focused by the lens of patient-centered care, accelerated by technology, fueled by failure, guided by patterns, and strengthened by partnerships. The framework provides a way for leaders to think about the interdependencies necessary to change the healthcare system and lead evidence-based innovation. The framework is a foundation and a call for a new healthcare system.

USING THE EVIDENCE–INNOVATION–LEADERSHIP FRAMEWORK TO CREATE CHANGE

For an evidence–innovation–leadership framework to exist as a way of doing business and building new systems, certain organizational and role capacities must be established. Leaders in organizations will need to be intentional about the design, development, and focus to create the context that will ultimately support new ways of care, practice, and health care.

The following components must be incorporated in the design of this new system to create an environment in which evidence, innovation, and leadership intertwine and thrive (Malloch & Porter-O'Grady, 2010):

- A commitment to data and information-driven decision making must be made at the very senior levels of the organization in a way that assures the decisions will be generated in alignment with the evidentiary dynamic.

- An investment must be made in the resources needed to build the data and information infrastructure. This includes the appropriation of sufficient hardware and software to assure the utility and effectiveness of information-driven decision making and determination of fixed-process approaches to operational and clinical decision making.
- Meaningful engagement must occur with point-of-service knowledge workers and patients at the outset of the design of management and clinical information infrastructure, software, and processes. This includes using an effectiveness evaluation as a way of assuring a goodness of fit between the proposed data tools and the utility of their application.
- A commitment must be made to ongoing professional development of managers and leaders in the concepts of complex adaptive and responsive systems, role agency, networks, and emergent leadership. Leaders at every level must develop the competencies necessary to ensure that innovation and creativity are embraced as the way of being in the organization.
- Ongoing engagement must occur with health professions education programs to continually strengthen the practice–education connection. Leadership needs to support connection and integration at every level of the organization. This includes supporting individual practitioners and teams to participate in mentoring and teaching students to aligning leadership activities at the highest levels.
- Reconceptualize healthcare organizations and hospitals as complex systems composed of networked relationships. Multifocal interactions, interdependence, and relational processes become the organizing framework, replacing vertical decision models, operating silos, and nonaligned departmental configurations.
- Eliminate discipline-specific locus of control in favor of interdisciplinary processes, teams, and collaborative decision making, resulting in an integrated model of evidence-driven decision making, practice, and impact evaluation. This includes the acknowledgment that sustainable outcome-oriented, evidence-driven practice represents the synthesis and coordination of the effort of all stakeholders, as opposed to focusing only on unilateral measures of incremental impact (isolated, nonaligned, discipline-specific outcomes).
- Embrace and leverage the organization as conversation perspective to strengthen relationships, communication, alignment, and transparency across the organization.
- Invest leaders time and energy into building quality relationships, resilience, and capacity in all three domains: innovation, evidence and leadership.
- Construct and develop a strategic plan and targets for transforming the system environment from a fixed operational model to a fluid, data-driven organizational framework supporting evidentiary systems, structures, processes, applications, and evaluation. This includes consonance among evidence-driven strategic trajectories, resource capitalization, management and operational reconfiguration for leading, and clinical facilities for execution.

These considerations provide starting points or levers that leaders can use to influence their teams, organizations, and broader networks to support movement toward a value-focused healthcare system. The application of these concepts and the evidence–innovation–leadership framework will require risk taking, adaptation, vision, opportunity, facilitation, information, and technology (Weberg, 2013). This means that at an individual level, the leader's own capacity for apprehending these various aspects will determine his or her effectiveness and reach. There are specific competencies leaders can develop that will increase their capacity for changing the system.

COMPETENCY 1: UNDERSTAND THE FOUNDATIONS OF THE INNOVATION, EVIDENCE, LEADERSHIP DYNAMIC

Leaders who wish to change the system must first have an understanding of the complexities and history that are driving current behaviors and the barriers and benefits that allow that behavior to continue (Porter-O'Grady & Malloch, 2016). Specifically, understanding the foundations of evidence, innovation, and leadership in the context of health care is very important.

The foundations of evidence consist of the evidence framework, critical evidence appraisal models, and evidence-based practice models, such as the Disciplined Clinical Inquiry model. Understanding these core concepts and practices allow the leader to quickly and accurately gather evidence to inform decision making, leadership, and innovation. Evidence can inform the change in practices and the beginnings of innovation processes, and provide context for the healthcare system as a whole.

The foundations of innovation consist of innovation methodologies like design thinking, innovation frameworks that include failure as normative, and innovation leadership behaviors that support the practice. Understanding basic innovation methodologies allows the leader to view change as normative and develop behaviors that support teams in problem solving. An innovation mindset also provides a lens for leaders to view new sources of evidence, test new ideas and practices, and develop new models of care to change the entire system. Innovation competence is often overlooked by organizations, but it is an essential skill in remaining relevant and driving improved outcomes in health care.

The foundations of leadership are rooted in leadership theories such as trait, style, transformational, relational, and complexity. By understanding the sources of decision making, power, accountability, and the variety of lenses available through which leaders across the system may make sense of their work, the available solutions and directions become more generative rather than prescriptive. The evidence-based and innovative leader can then develop strategies to overcome resistance, build networks, and create teams that are wired for system change. Understanding that leadership itself is a complex set of interactions and information that is grounded in relationships, evidence, and innovation is key to building the future of health care.

Each of these foundations provides the starting point for research, learning, and the growth of leaders in health care. The beginnings of each of these concepts are presented in this text with specific examples and tools for change. Additionally, leaders should read seminal texts, articles, and search for new evidence to continually build their knowledge and skill. The point is to not silo one's competency in one discipline, but to see the patterns and connections among all the disciplines of change. Additional topics that should be studied, including culture, communication, health policy and law, business operations, and basic technical and informatics knowledge.

COMPETENCY 2: LEADING YOURSELF

Leadership, especially in health care, requires significant energy, reflection, and networking. It can be easy for leaders to focus energy on others, the organization, or the work without regard to their own health and family. Leading yourself includes the concepts of creating your own context for action and balance. Energy management, nutrition, wellness, reflection, and renewal are concepts that professional athletes use for peak performance, and similar concepts can be translated to leadership peak performance. Leaders should make time to build energy through physical fitness and proper nutrition and snacking routines. Wellness and renewal activities, like vacations, deep breathing between meetings, and making time for friends and family, allow leaders to stay grounded in all aspects of their lives and maintain energy throughout the day. Additionally, leaders are visible role models to others in the organization. By modeling self-leadership and encouraging self-care in others, leaders can have a secondary positive effect on the health and resilience of the wider organization. Leaders can also build mental and emotional capacities through emotional intelligence work, mindfulness, and reflection. All these skills help you as an individual engage fully in leadership behaviors. It is necessary to build your own endurance and capacity to weather the stress of challenges that are an inevitable aspect of change and innovation.

Discussion

What self-leadership practices do you currently engage in? What do you think are the biggest barriers to self-leadership? Are there self-leadership behaviors and practices that you want to start? How can you set yourself up for success? Are there peers and/or mentors that you could invite to join the journey toward self-care with you?

COMPETENCY 3: BUILDING AN ADVANCED INNOVATION SKILL SET

After leaders have a good foundation in evidence, innovation, and leadership and have begun to reflect on their leadership journey, more advanced innovation competencies can be introduced. These include advances in design thinking, risk taking, strategic alignment, and culture building skills that can further develop an ecosystem of innovation across departments, organizations, and systems. Concepts such as systems thinking, complexity leadership, and network interaction theory are examples of advanced innovation perspectives that leaders can use to shape change and create lasting innovation structures.

Innovation competency for leaders is not the ability to generate significant numbers of ideas, but rather the ability for leaders to create safe conditions for risk taking and leverage resources to support teams to create novel ideas. Rather than the leader acting as an innovator (which may be the case at a basic competency level), this advanced innovation competency for leaders is about creating the conditions for innovation to happen through the actions of others. Leaders with advanced innovation skills can view complex systems as interconnected wholes and recognize emergent patterns that guide evidentiary and innovation dynamics. Complex adaptive and complex relational perspective taking can result in the creative emergence of new ideas and information. Leaders must be in tune with what is coming into being on the emerging edge of the future and respond accordingly. The advanced innovation leader has multiple streams of information, learning, and insight that help inform decision making. These can be informal sources, such as friends, coworkers, and perspectives outside health care social media and popular culture; or they can be formal, such as journals, research, or organization-specific channels of knowledge dissemination like clinical practice guidelines, intranet resources, and special interest groups. Advanced leaders should have competency in developing and accessing both formal and informal networks.

Viewing the system in novel ways is important, but equally important is measuring the impact of innovation and evidence. Leaders of innovation need to understand and look for ways to assess, measure, and otherwise illuminate how new evidence and innovations are changing and influencing the system. This requires an understanding of metrics. For example, failed innovations may be unsuccessful from an individual project standpoint, but the ripples of failed projects or patterns of innovation activity can open new opportunities, break down previous barriers, or inform others to change efforts in the organization. These impacts are complex and at times difficult to see, but advanced innovation leaders can utilize their networks and pattern recognition to gather diverse sources of information and translate this information into meaningful measures of evidence and innovation.

Building relationships across networks requires leaders to create connections beyond the span of their everyday work and to develop the capability to communicate with diverse groups for information and knowledge sharing. Building your network occurs on two levels: informational and relational. First, the leader should create ways for information to be shared between their teams and other teams. Connections enable sharing information through e-mails, conversation, technology, and interaction. For example, a SharePoint site that is accessible by multiple teams who may be working at a physical distance would be a connection for sharing information. The second level of building a network is to develop relationships. The leader's relationships determine the quality, strength, and longevity of connections that are made. By building strong relationships, the leader increases the likelihood that the information exchanged between the teams will be of better quality, accuracy, and relevance. It also increases the likelihood that team members will develop relationships with counterparts of other teams. Of course, mutual respect, trust, and valuing the expertise of others are foundations of relationship building. Creating connections, building relationships, and knowing how and when to mobilize them is a key advanced innovation skill.

Finally, advanced innovation leaders foster high-performing cultures, and this enables innovation. Cultures are the accumulation of behaviors and interactions that occur among people in an organization. Behaviors turn into norms, and these norms turn into subconscious (unspoken) rules that govern future behavior (Schein, 2004). Leaders have the ability to influence behavior by creating the conditions and structures that foster, for example, open communication and acknowledging and learning from mistakes.

The complex relational perspective is also useful in fostering high-performing cultures. Leaders can begin to transform patterns of meaning and patterns of relating in ways that will support and align with the innovation–evidence–leadership framework. Patterns of meaning within organizations can be influenced by paying attention to what people are talking about, what is rewarded, or what energy and resources are focused on. If leaders discern that patterns of meaning are not in alignment with the framework, they can begin to change the patterns of meaning by shifting the attention, rewards, and language in ways that are more generative and aligned with the importance and value of innovation and evidence. Patterns of relating are equally as powerful. Leaders should be aware of the reasons, issues, and events that people organize their interactions around. For instance, if there is a monthly full-day meeting that brings stakeholders together to discuss a certain topic (e.g., risk management), leaders should evaluate if that topic and the intended purpose of the meeting are time and energy well spent. If the organization wants to foster innovation and empower providers at the point of care to engage in tinkering and process improvement, a full-day meeting spent scrutinizing deviations from the status quo and consistency might be sending the wrong message. Leaders should seek to align patterns of meaning and relating with the

Table 16-1   Advanced Innovation Competency

	Skills
Complex adaptive systems view	• Pattern recognition • View complex interrelationships among teams and systems • Establish strong feedback loops with formal and informal sources
Measure system-level outcomes	• Recognize impacts of innovation and evidence across the system • Determine appropriate metrics to understand impacts
Relationships across the network	• Boundary spanning across organizations • Influencing the network • Model effective network development
Create high-performing cultures	• Align energy and resources to match organizational goals • Model and facilitate open communication • Notice and leverage patterns of meaning and patterns of relating

organization's highest aspirations and priorities (Suchman, 2011). **Table 16-1** summarizes the requisite skills associated with advanced innovation competency.

COMPETENCY 4: COMMUNICATING AND CONNECTING

Leaders who wish to transform systems must be masters at communicating and connecting across networks, teams, and organizations. Communication competencies include the ability to build relationships and networks, as discussed previously, and also the ability to communicate vision and information in a way that influences others to change. The term *influences* is intentional in this context. Leadership is the influencing of others to adapt and change in the face of complex and unpredictable situations (Weberg, 2013). To influence teams of people, leaders must be able to articulate rationale, evidence, data, meaning, and impact clearly; and link those elements to the broader mission of the team or organization. This act is different from motivation. Leaders are influencers more often than they are motivators.

Another important competency related to connecting and communicating is the notion of transparency. In organizations, information is interpreted, analyzed, and acted upon at each level. For example, uninformed rumors of an organizational change can lead people to quit preemptively, look for other opportunities, or launch negative campaigns before official announcements are made. Leaders who value transparency and can communicate effectively are able to anticipate or gain insight about these rumors and work with their teams to communicate and connect concepts in a more focused and meaningful way. For example, the leader may learn of the rumor from his or her professional network and hold a staff meeting to answer questions openly and honestly, providing information proactively. A noninnovative leader would shy away from such conflict and allow team energy to be spent on anxiety-generating activities, thus pushing productivity down and chaos up.

Relationship-centered care comes to bear in our discussion of communicating and connecting, which are of course elemental aspect of effective relationships. Relationship-centered care is supported by what Suchman (2011) described as relationship-centered *administration*. In essence, if we as leaders want care providers to engage patients and families in respectful, honest, and deeply engaged relationships, we must communicate and connect with care providers and patients in ways that resonate with those very same qualities. It is the epitome of walking our talk. Of course, communicating and connecting is not only about talking. Leaders must also be astute listeners. The skills of deep listening (empathically and emergently) are essential for fostering high-quality relationships that ensure connections (Scharmer, 2007). The concept of relationship-centered care is discussed in Chapter 4.

Communicating and connecting is a competency that innovation leaders must hone and continually demonstrate. Deep listening, influencing, transparency, and relationship building are critical to fostering a culture where evidence and innovation are valued and seen as resources for creating high-quality patient care experiences.

COMPETENCY 5: BUILDING MOMENTUM AND INITIATING CHANGE

The final competency for healthcare leaders is the ability build momentum that results in system change. This requires skillful synthesis of the previous four competencies. The important part of this competency is not the magnitude of change or innovativeness of the change, but rather that the leader builds confidence and comfort in trying new things. This also extends to fostering self-efficacy for change and innovation among your team and the larger organization. From a complex relational perspective, even the largest of changes begins with a single step (so to speak). Often, there are also missteps and steps backwards in this process toward change. Perseverance, learning from (celebrating) mistakes, and failing forward are all important elements of building momentum for change. Leaders who are new to this way of being may be frustrated because they expect that change needs to happen on a grand scale to be meaningful, or they might be anxious because change may not be a controlled process. The following are some points to ponder for leaders seeking to build momentum:

- Any movement in the right direction is worthy of celebration. Celebrating small wins creates energy and visibility, which in turn creates momentum for change.
- Think of a flywheel, where accumulated small incremental movements can eventually lead to the release of tremendous momentum that reinforces itself, and the pace of change accelerates when a critical mass is reached.
- Small steps that occur over a longer period of time may be more sustainable than taking larger steps too quickly (go slow to go fast).
- Leverage the organization as conversation perspective to gain momentum. How can you use rhetoric and patterns of relating and meaning to move change along?
- Fail often to succeed sooner. Reframe failures into learning. Do not pass up an opportunity to learn from something that did not work.
- Do the work of translation. Listen to your stakeholders to understand what the change means for them. Align your messages about change with their needs and interests (help them see what is in it for them).
- Leverage high-quality relationships and robust networks to communicate about the true nature of change. Replace rumors with transparent, open communication about change.
- Change requires endurance and optimism. Good self-leadership helps leaders to maintain focus, energy, and remain committed to the change.
- Continued practice at change and successful implementations of smaller change projects can build momentum for further innovation and change on a larger scale.

SUMMARY

The complexity of transforming health care is daunting to even the most seasoned executives and clinicians. The traditions, culture, and knowledge base of the existing system are deeply rooted in the symbols, language, and behaviors of mechanistic, linear, and hierarchy-based organizational ways of being. Leaders of innovation and change must become habituated to new ways of being and doing (**Figure 16-9**). Leaders will need to develop specific skill sets, behaviors, and competencies to work effectively within the innovation–evidence–leadership framework. Understanding and leveraging the drivers that enable this framework will be integral to moving healthcare from its siloed and mechanistic structures to more dynamic, integrated, relational and value-driven structures that can meet the needs of patients and providers today and into the future.

Figure 16-9   Leadership competencies that enable healthcare transformation

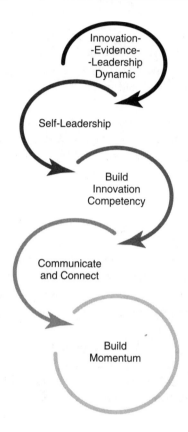

REFERENCES

Berwick, D. M., & Hackbarth, A. D. (2012). Eliminating waste in US health care. *JAMA, 307*(14), 1513–1516. doi:10.1001/jama.2012.362

Gandhi, M., & Wang, T. (2015). Digital health funding: 2014 year in review. Retrieved from http://rockhealth.com/2015/01/digital-health-funding-tops-4-1b-2014-year-review/

Malloch, K., & Porter-O'Grady, T. (2010). *Introduction to evidence-based practice in nursing and health care.* Sudbury, MA: Jones & Bartlett Learning.

Melnyk, B. M., & Fineout-Overholt, E. (Eds.). (2011). *Evidence-based practice in nursing & healthcare: A guide to best practice.* Philadelphia, PA: Lippincott Williams & Wilkins.

Porter-O'Grady, T., & Malloch, K. (Eds.). (2014). *Creating and sustaining a culture and an environment for evidence-based practice* (3rd ed., Vol. 3). New York, NY: Wolters Kluwer.

Porter-O'Grady, T., & Malloch, K. (2016). *Quantum leadership: Building better partnerships for sustainable health* (3rd ed.). Burlington, MA: Jones & Bartlett Learning.

Scharmer, C. O. (2007). *Theory U: Leading from the future as it emerges.* Cambridge, MA: Society for Organizational Learning.

Schein, E. H. (2004). *Organizational culture and leadership.* San Francisco, CA: Wiley & Sons.

Suchman, T. (2011). How we think about organizations: A complexity perspective. In A. L. Suchman, D. J. Sluyter & P. R. Williamson (Eds.), *Leading change in healthcare: Transforming organizations using complexity, positive psychology and relationship-centered care.* London, UK: Radcliffe.

Uhl-Bien, M., & Marion, R. (2008). *Complexity leadership part 1: Conceptual foundations.* Charlotte, NC: Information Age.

Weberg, D. R. (2013). *Complexity leadership theory and innovation: A new framework for innovation leadership* (Doctoral dissertation). Arizona State University.

Index

Page numbers followed by *b*, *f*, or *t* indicate boxes, figures, or tables, respectively.